Lauren

1000 QUESTIONS
ABOUT YOUR PREGNANCY

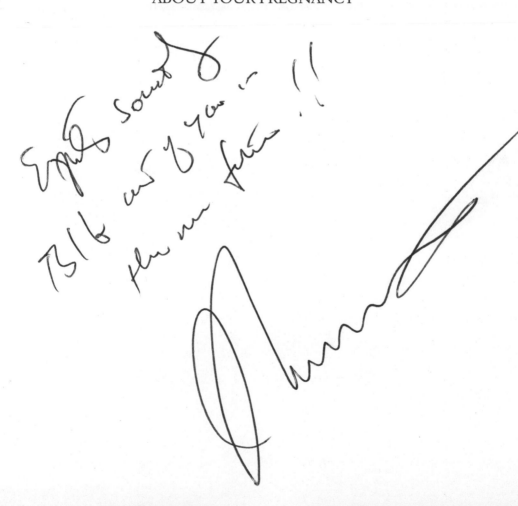

1000 Questions

About

Your Pregnancy

Fourth Edition

Jeffrey M. Thurston, M.D., F.A.C.O.G.

JT² BOOKS, INC.
DALLAS, TX

JT² Books, Inc.
P.O. Box 570614
Dallas, TX 75357

Printed in the United States of America.
11 10 09 08 07   9 8 7

Library of Congress Cataloging-in-Publication Data
Thurston, Jeffrey, 1956-
    1000 questions about your pregnancy / Jeffrey M. Thurston. -- 4th ed.
        p. cm.
    Includes bibliographical references and index.
    978-0-615-49159-2 (trade paper : alk. paper)
    1. Pregnancy--Miscellanea. 2. Childbirth--Miscellanea. I. Title. II. Title: One thousand questions about your pregnancy.

RG525.T55 2007
618.2--dc22

                    2006031891

Cover design by David Sims
Illustrations by Jamin Cunning
Book design and layout by D. & F. Scott Publishing, Inc.
Index by Michael Rossa

This book is dedicated to Evelyn Scott, RN

Her unfailing dedication and loyalty has allowed me to continue caring for my patients despite the time I have devoted to other pursuits, such as that which you hold in your hands.

CONTENTS

FOREWORD TO FIRST EDITION

I will never forget the joy I felt as I learned I was pregnant with my first child. My first response was to run to my husband's office to tell him the news. My next impulse was to contact my doctor, Dr Thurston. I had so many questions! Dr. Thurston subsequently sat down with my husband and me and answered all our questions, relieving many of our anxieties, and giving us peace of mind that carried us through all four of our pregnancies and deliveries.

I am delighted that Dr. Thurston has written *1,000 Questions About Your Pregnancy*. I know I asked him at least 900 of them during my four pregnancies! Whenever I would go for my checkups with a list of questions, I could always depend on him to answer them with straightforward, fact-filled answers and just enough humor to put me at ease. Indeed, his command of the facts combined with his sense of humor, has become his trademark.

Now he has distilled that knowledge into *1,000 Questions About Your Pregnancy*. The beauty of this book lies not only in its comprehensive nature; not only in the conversational way in which most answers are phrased; not only in its not-so-subtle good humor; but in the references it provides.

Dr. Thurston provides references to articles and texts within each section so that any question a mother-or father-to-be might have, may be thoroughly researched. Relevant Web site listings and phone numbers for useful organizations are also included throughout the book.

So pick up this volume, use the comprehensive index at the end, and find either the answers to your questions or multiple different sources wherein you might find the answers you seek. Or if you prefer, read the book straight through, laugh a little, and learn a lot, about every aspect of pregnancy that might concern you or a loved one.

But whatever you do, remember that I have two sons and two daughters, who are healthy, bright, happy, wonderful kids in some small part because of the author and his answers. Have a great pregnancy!

Maggie Murchison
October 1997
Dallas, Texas

NOTE FROM THE PUBLISHER

Not only are there references and Web sites at the end of each section, but for more general use we have included the following Medical Search Engines to help you answer any questions you may have about your pregnancy:

Search Engines
> http://www.medlineplus.com
> http://www.hon.ch
> http://www.webmd.com
> http://www.google.com
> http://www.yahoo.com
> http://www.hotbot.com

Directories and Engines
> http://www.medlineplus.com
> http://www.vh.org
> http://www.acog.org
> http://www.webmd.com

Federal Government (USA)
> http://www.fedworld.gov   *Index to all Federal Agencies*
> http://www. cdc.gov   *Center for Disease Control*
> http://www.nih.gov   *National Institutes of Health*
> http//www.fda.gov   *Food and Drug Administration*

NIH and US Department of Health and Human Services Sites
> http://sis.nlm.nih.gov/dirline/

PREFACE

We live in a world of rapidly changing technologies that has led to an explosion of both information acquisition and transference. Globalization has replaced the old world order of geographically separate nation states. The Internet has effectively miniaturized our world. Medicine is no more immune to these forces, which are rapidly altering civilization, than any other industry. There are new drugs, new pieces of information, and new uses of old drugs. There are new techniques and new attitudes, all of which are transforming obstetrics right along with every other branch of medicine.

It is in this rapidly changing environment that we address the innovations and revelations that have altered our approach in recent years to the age-old process of human reproduction. There are changing attitudes about some over-the-counter medicines, about common food additives and components, and about various prescription medicines. There are innovative new instruments to aid delivery, new drugs, and new indications for existing drugs. There are completely different perceptions of the risk/benefit ratios of everything from vaginal birth after cesarean (VBAC) to regional anesthesia to exercise and diet recommendations.

Not all of the changes can be, or even need to be, addressed. But *1,000 Questions About Your Pregnancy* has always sought to provide insights into the more common issues that arise as you prepare for and then progress through gestation, labor, delivery, and the post-partum period. As a consequence, many of the questions in this later edition have been replaced, altered, or at least had their answers updated.

The events of September 11, 2001 have forever altered the world in which we live. While the first round of terrorist attacks were horrific in and of themselves, they surely served to awaken those of us who treasure our freedoms to a new and pervasive threat. But they also focused all Americans on the very value of life itself. Now, after the horrors of the tsunamis, earthquakes and hurricanes of the last decade, it seems the whole world has a new focus on the fragility of life. We are here on the planet for only an instant, and all of us have drawn a little closer to our friends, to our families, and to our God, as we saw clearly the face of death. All of us became a little more cognizant of what a wonderful life we have been given and what a wonderful home is our planet earth. Who, now, does not see the sky a little bluer, the stars a little brighter, the ocean a little more awesome, and the mountains a bit more majestic?

So this new edition is a celebration of life from its very start! We hope that it helps to ease some of your anxieties, and in at least a small way, intensifies the joy that surrounds bringing a new life into a troubled, but still beautiful world.

ACKNOWLEDGMENTS

Even more so than with my previous efforts, I wish to thank my children, Kelly and Andy, for their patience and understanding. While I am grateful to their mother as well, my children were offered no choice about their father's occupation nor his penchant for writing! Thanks also to Ashley and Allison, their devotion to their step-father over the last decade has helped me to keep working and giving! I love you guys more than ever and I will treasure my time with each of you like never before!

Thanks to Len Oszustowicz for both the vision which led initially to this project and the first printing back in 1997. His faith in my abilities kept me going on that hectic first race to deadline.

My former publisher, Tapestry Press, and especially Jill Bertolet, deserve my unfailing devotion for their perseverance and dedication to keeping this project alive. This book could have simply died a slow death of attrition with the failure of my previous publisher, but Jill had the vision to see that the sheer usefulness of this text merited continued attempts at making the reading (and reproducing) public aware of its availability.

Thanks once more to my partners: Dr. John Bertrand, Dr. Jim Richards, Dr. Jane Nokelberg, Dr. David Bookout, Dr. Julie Hagood, and now Dr. Hampton Richards. Answering a patient's questions can be difficult enough without constantly hearing "Well, that's not exactly what Dr. Thurston says in his book." Their patience has allowed me to continue writing, as well as to continue in a group rather than a solo practice!

Thanks to J.T. Walker, my friend and mentor, who took on the task of producing the book after Tapestry. His advice, diligence and experience are all greatly appreciated. My gratitude to the tireless efforts of Erica Jennings whose expertise facilitated the production of both the fourth edition and the e-book version of he text.

Finally, my thanks always, to the God who made the miracle of reproduction an everyday reality, and whose own little boy grew up to save an entire world.

INTRODUCTION

So you're pregnant! Maybe it's the first time. Maybe it's a repeat engagement. Maybe you're not pregnant all, but you'd like to be. Maybe you are not pregnant, but the husband or partner of someone who is. In any event, just the thought of pregnancy brings a host of questions to mind almost immediately.

Finding out that you are about to be a parent, or even contemplating the process of becoming one, often elicits a common emotion. It's called fear. How can I possibly do this right? I don't know the first thing about being pregnant, delivering a baby, or taking care of a newborn, no less about being a parent for the rest of my life. Is this really the right time for this? How will this change things with my partner, my job, my friends? What will this do to my body? How can I possibly get something the size of a baby from the inside to the outside? What on earth have I done? Will I ever go to a movie on the spur of the moment again?

"Sure," you say, "I know people are busy reproducing all around me all the time, day in and day out." But that's different from me doing it person-ally, myself, right here and right now!"

Okay. Hold on there. Slow down for a second. There are at least 7 billion examples of successful reproduction in the world at this moment to which I could point by way of reassurance. People have been coming together and making little people since the dawn of man (and woman), and I might add, doing so with very little direction until recently.

So first of all, no need to panic. I guarantee there are at least three women you could name right now that fit the category of, "Well, if she can do it, I most certainly can!" While we have been having babies for some 80,000 years or so, depending on whom you believe, we have made some remarkable steps in the last century alone. True, while the process itself is by definition "natural," there are certain advances in our under-standing of that process that have led us to where we are today, in a time when we are better able to help you have a safer and thus more joyful experience than ever before.

In the course of clinical practice over the last 26 years, I have come to realize that there are many common denominators in the birth experience of all couples. While there are as many choices about how to have a baby as there are people having them, there remain 1,000 questions that everyone seems to voice consistently. I am aware that in this age of instant communication, there are a myriad of sources to which you could turn for information about pregnancy and childbirth. Although you can get the answer to virtually any question using the Internet, for example, I wanted to provide an easy to read, easy to use reference that would prove an effective means of giving you the facts you need, the reassurances you want, and maybe even a little humor that will add to the fun you have ahead of you!

These 1,000 questions and answers do appear sequentially, but as you can see, they are divided into multiple subject areas. These subject areas cover broad topic areas, each of which will become relevant at different times throughout your pregnancy. Subject areas and their subdivisions are outlined in the Table of Contents.

An extensive index is provided at the end of the book to further ease your ability to find the answers to specific questions. We also recognize that many more questions could be generated despite the answers that you find within this text, and where-ever appropriate further suggested readings are given at the end of the relevant section. Many of these suggested readings are useful, but unfortunately contain some serious errors both with respect to medical fact and with respect to emphasis. *1000 Questions About Your Pregnancy* strives to make it clear, where appropriate, which information is factual and undisputed, and which information is opinion. References are provided throughout. In every instance possible, the recommendations provided are consistent with guidelines of the American College of Ob/Gyn.

Over the years, many of my patients have become terrified by something they have read. Too many lay authors have misinterpreted and misapplied animal research in a fashion that tends to obscure the fact that God designed the system to work the vast majority of the time without our intervention at all. A pregnancy reference should provide answers to questions about common activities and occurrences.

In my practice, I have dealt with more than 50,000 pregnancies, and delivered more than 7,000 babies. While that gives me tremendous experience as a physician and childbirth educator, it remains no substitute for the relationship you establish with your care giver. Whenever possible, seek the opinion of those who have devoted their lives to helping you. Many of the issues that come up are far from black and white. The answers you find in *1000 Questions About Your Pregnancy* may occasionally conflict with the opinion of the person who is caring for you. Once you have established a trusting relationship, defer to the judgment of this individual. He or she knows your particular set of circumstances; I don't. (In fact, I tell my own patients at their first visit to remember that, no matter what they read or hear that turns out to be in conflict with what I've told them, I'm the one who's right! It keeps their lives, and mine, much less stressful.) So much of medicine is gray, not black and white, that your best option will almost always be to trust the person taking care of you. So, dive in! I hope that you'll run into many of the questions that you forgot to ask at your last visit.

It is indeed a miracle that a woman can build another human being inside of herself. The goal of this book is a simple one. It embodies a wish to be a part of this miraculous process, helping in any small way possible to lead you as a couple through the transition from uncertainty, and even abject terror, to the joyous realization of a new life created with unlimited potential.

Jeffrey M. Thurston, M.D.
F.A.C.O.G
Dallas, Texas
February, 2011

Section One

Before Pregnancy

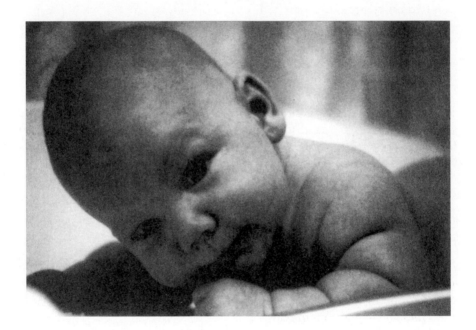

GETTING READY

1

Q *How should I take care of myself in preparation for getting pregnant?*

A There are certainly things you can do to optimize your chances of a normal, healthy pregnancy. Try to eat moderately, avoid excess fat or sugar, and increase the amount of dietary fiber you consume. Take an over-the-counter prenatal vitamin or at least a daily vitamin with a minimum of five hundred micrograms of folate (folic acid). The extra folate, added to a healthy diet, should give you the one milligram of folate recommended to help decrease the chances of certain birth defects, such as spina bifida. Do some form of aerobic exercise at least four times per week for twenty minutes.

If you still smoke cigarettes, quit! Drink alcohol sparingly if at all. Discontinue any recreational drugs such as marijuana, cocaine, amphetamines, or narcotics. Avoid diagnostic X-rays if possible, especially if you think you might already be pregnant. Consider avoiding activities in which there is a high likelihood of injury, such as snow-skiing, in-line skating, and ice-skating. There is no more miserable creature than a pregnant woman in a cast!.

2

Q *I'm on the birth-control pill. When do I need to stop taking it in order to get pregnant?*

A Doctors usually recommend three months, but not for the reason you think. Birth-control pills are out of your system in only a few days. Even if you got pregnant while on the pill and didn't find out until several weeks after your missed period, the dosage is too low with current formulations to have put your fetus at any significant risk of birth defect.

Stopping three months ahead is simply for timing. After discontinuing the pill, a substantial number of women may take three to six months to start ovulating regularly. Therefore, if you want to get pregnant in September, stop taking the pill in June, not in August. You may choose to use an alternate form of birth control during that time only if you really don't want to become pregnant before September.

Discontinuing several months ahead is also useful in that it allows an accurate date for your last menstrual period, rather than an artificial period following a pill withdrawal. This provides useful information about presumed gestational age. Knowing this can be critical at later stages in your pregnancy. (See Section 5: Drugs in Pregnancy)

3

3

Q *Are there any medicines or chemicals I should absolutely avoid when I begin trying to conceive?*

A (See also Section 5: Drugs in Pregnancy)
About 3 to 5 percent of all babies have a birth defect. Only 1 percent or so of these defects are thought to be related to drugs or chemicals. Another 10 percent are related to maternal infection and other diseases. Despite widespread public concern, only a very few common medicines are known to cause birth defects. The following *may* cause harm to the fetus. Either avoid them altogether, or at least discuss using them with your doctor.

ACE inhibitors (Captopril; Enalapril): Used to treat hypertension. Associated with fetal kidney failure, growth retardation, and underdevelopment of the bone in the skull.

Anticonvulsants: Dilantin (phenytoin) and Tridione (trimethadione). Associated with growth and mental retardation, neural tube defects such as spina bifida, and developmental abnormalities.

Benzodiazepines (Valium; Librium; Ambien): Sedatives. Associated with inguinal hernia and with midline defects such as cleft lip.

Cancer chemotherapy: Methotrexate and aminopterin. Used to treat cancer, as well as skin diseases such as psoriasis. Associated with miscarriage and multiple birth defects.

Isotretinoin (Accutane): Used to treat severe cystic acne. Associated with increased miscarriage and multiple birth defects.

Lead: Used in painting, ceramics, pottery glazing, printing, and older plumbing. Associated with developmental and central nervous system problems.

Lithium: Used to treat bipolar disorder. Associated with various cardiac defects. Quinilones: (Cipro; Floxin): Antibiotics. Used for bladder and upper respiratory infections. Associated with limb reduction defects. Tetracycline: Common antibiotic. Used especially for skin problems.

Associated with graying of tooth enamel.

Many other drugs may be associated with problems, but those listed above have long been established as potential teratogens (substances or processes that prevent normal fetal development).

4

Q *Is there anything I absolutely have to do before I get pregnant?*

A Yes! You have to be absolutely sure you are committed with your heart, mind, and soul to devote the rest of your life to the nurture, protection and development of another human being. That's about as big a step as you will ever take.

You must have already made a lifelong commitment to your mate. You must be clear that no matter what hardships are encountered, you will put the needs of your spouse before your own, and those of your children before either of you.

This is not to say that single parents are unequal to the task of raising their children. They can, and sometimes life leaves a parent with no choice. But usually, a home with two loving parents provides the greatest number of resources for overcoming a wide variety of adverse circumstances and results in a well-balanced, capable human being able to become a productive, creative member of society.

GETTING PREGNANT

5

Q *When is the best time of my cycle to get pregnant?*

A Women who release an egg every month do so about fourteen days prior to their next period, not fourteen days after the beginning of their period. So, subtract fourteen days from the total number of days in your cycle (counting from the first day of bleeding to the first day of bleeding) to find the day that ovulation is most likely to occur. The egg lives for about twenty-four hours, but the sperm may survive in your genital tract for seventy-two to ninety-six hours. Therefore, if you typically ovulate on day sixteen, sex on days fourteen through seventeen may lead to a pregnancy.

There are several well-known methods for ascertaining when you're the most fertile. Your body temperature tends to rise about half a degree Fahrenheit twenty-four to forty-eight hours after ovulation. While this does not help predict the right time for conception in the first cycle during which you plot it, the knowledge gained may be used for future cycles. Pharmacies sell special easy-to-read basal body temperature (BBT) thermometers and graphs for this purpose. For about half of women, rising estrogen levels just before ovulation lead to clear, copious, more rubbery cervical mucus at the opening of the vagina. This generally disappears after ovulation and may thus provide a clue about when to make love in future cycles. Finally, commercially available urine Ovulation Predictor Kits may be purchased without prescription. In these tests, test materials change color in the presence of LH (luteinizing hormone), a substance that tells the ovary to release the egg. Have intercourse as often as you want, and certainly within thirty-six to forty-eight hours after a positive test.

6

Q *When should I worry if I've been trying to get pregnant, but can't?*

A Infertility has been defined as the condition that results when a couple has unprotected sex at or around midcycle for the period of a year without conception. Many people find this to be a very long time when their best friends got pregnant on the first try. But remember that each ejaculate has an average of at least twenty million sperm per cubic centimeter headed for only one egg. This ratio occurs because most of the sperm don't get near the target. They are either lost in the abdomen or genital tract, trapped cervical mucus, destroyed by vaginal fluids, or end up as a wet spot on the sheets!

If, however, your periods are irregular (varying by more than forty-eight hours each month) or you're not having periods at all, you may not be ovulating and should consult your physician either when planning to conceive or after six months of trying. In about 40 to 50 percent of infertile couples, the inability to conceive may also result from lack of sperm or poor sperm motility. A semenalysis is inexpensive, easy, and can be arranged by your physician at any time.

TESTS BEFORE PREGNANCY

Infections and Immunizations

7

Q *Are there any tests I must take before I try to get pregnant?*

A (See also Section 5: Questions 399–402)
If you have engaged in unsafe sex or used illicit drugs where needles were shared, an HIV test is advisable. Roughly 25 percent of untreated HIV-positive mothers will pass the disease on to their newborns. Other sexually transmitted diseases (STDs), such as chlamydia, gonorrhea, syphilis, and herpes, can have devastating consequences in pregnancy. If you suspect that you have any STD, you should see your doctor, and be tested and treated if necessary.

All women of childbearing age should be up-to-date on immunizations for tetanus, diphtheria (booster shot every ten years), measles, mumps, and rubella (DPT-MMR).

If you do not know or cannot confirm whether you ever had varicella (chicken pox), rubella (German measles) or the vaccine for it, or Fifth's Disease (Parvovirus 19), or if you are in frequent contact with children of elementary school age, your immunity can be determined with a blood antibody titer. Titers to determine immunity to the cat disease Toxoplasmosis are also available. These diseases are *very rarely* a cause of problems in pregnancy, but women who are not immune can take certain precautions, and vaccines for chicken pox and German measles may be safely taken three months before conception.

You may have some inherited, or genetic, diseases in your family. Some of these diseases have "carrier" states for which you, and sometimes your family members, can be tested. These diseases are also referred to as "monogenic" because they only involve one gene pair. (See Inherited Diseases below)

Inherited Diseases: Genetic Testing Before Pregnancy

8

Q For which genetic diseases can I be tested to see if I am a carrier before I get pregnant?

A You may be tested for many of the diseases inherited in what is called a recessive pattern. Each of us has two copies of every gene, one from our mother and one from our father. There are twenty-three pairs of chromosomes, of which one pair are the sex chromosomes, X or Y Each chromosome has thousands of genes, or coded locations, on that strand.

Boys are genetically 46XY and girls are 46XX. With recessive diseases, you may "carry" the gene for the disease, but not have the disease yourself if your other copy of the gene is undamaged. This is because alongside the gene with the defect is a normal copy of the same gene. More common diseases in this category include Tay-Sachs disease, cystic fibrosis, sickle-cell disease, and thalassemia.

9

Q What are the chances of my baby being affected if I am a carrier of a recessive gene disorder?

A The chances are zero, unless you mate with someone else who carries the recessive gene. That's why these diseases are relatively rare. If both of you carry the gene, there is a 25 percent chance that the baby will have the disease, a 25 percent chance the baby will not even have the gene, and a 50 percent chance that the baby will be a carrier. The carrier rate is the prevalence within the affected ethnic group of the affected gene. For example, with cystic fibroses, one in twenty-two white people carries the gene; therefore, 1/22 (mother) x 1/22 (father) x 1/4 (25 percent), or one in 1,936 whites, could have the disease at birth if all fetuses survived.

10

Q *What is Tay-Sachs disease?*

A Tay-Sachs is known as a "storage disease" because cells throughout the body collect too much of a certain substance as a result of the lack of an enzyme called hexosaminidase A. Eventually, the cells can no longer function properly. Symptoms first appear at six months and eventually lead to mental retardation, blindness, seizures, and death, usually by age three. It is found most commonly in descendants of Ashkenazic Jew.

Jews of European descent should consider testing as teenagers to avoid unwittingly passing on the gene for this devastating disease.

11

Q *What is cystic fibrosis, and who should be tested?*

A Cystic fibroses (CF) is an enzyme deficiency that leads to very thick mucus in the lungs, pancreas, and bowel. It varies in severity, but usually leads to a pulmonary death during middle age (formerly in the teen years). CF patients require frequent antibiotics and supplemental pancreatic enzymes, and are often hospitalized for pneumonia.

Anyone with a significant family history of CF should consider being tested as a carrier. One in twenty-two white people carries the gene.

12

Q *What is thalassemia, and who should be tested?*

A (See also Section 9: Anemias)
The thalassemias are diseases of the hemoglobin molecule in the red blood cells and they lead to anemia. The more common Beta-thalassemia occurs in Greeks, Italians, and other people of Mediterranean descent. Alpha-thalassemia is less common and occurs in Asians. Consider being tested if you are already anemic and unresponsive to iron therapy, and of the appropriate ethnic descent.

13

Q *What is sickle-cell disease and who should be tested?*

A (See also Section 9: Anemias)
Sickle-cell disease (SCD) is also a disease of the hemoglobin molecule. In SCD, the red blood cells become deformed—into sickle shapes—so that the cells are destroyed too quickly by the spleen and liver. The end result is chronic anemia.

SCD primarily affects African Americans. The carrier rate is 1 in 12 people who have the gene; therefore, $1/12 \times 1/12 \times 1/4 = 1/576$, or one in 576 African Americans, may theoretically have the disease. There are milder forms of the disease when the sickle gene is paired with other slightly altered genes.

14

Q *What can I do if I am a carrier of one of these recessive genes?*

A If you are a carrier of a recessive gene and so is your partner, both of you can be forewarned. Plan on a chorionic villi sampling (CVS) before the eleventh week or an amniocentesis early in the second trimester, around thirteen to sixteen weeks. This can determine if your fetus is affected. If it is, you may choose to either terminate or continue the pregnancy. At least you will know the nature of your child's condition from the outset. (See Section 3: Amniocentesis/CVS)

15

Q *What other forms of inherited diseases are there?*

A There are many types of inherited diseases, but only two other major patterns of inheritance: X-linked Recessive diseases and Autosomal Dominant diseases.

X-linked Recessive diseases are similar in inheritance to the other recessive diseases mentioned above, except that they affect males almost exclusively. Women carry the abnormal gene on the X chromosome and are unaffected because they have a second X chromosome to mask the abnormal one. Men, on the other hand, have one X and one Y chromosome, so the abnormal gene on the X chromosome has an effect and causes the disease. With X-linked recessive disorders, women carry the disease but only men get it. Classic examples of this type of disease are hemophilia and Duchenne muscular dystrophy. The former causes bleeding problems in males and the latter causes the muscles to become progressively weaker.

9

Autosomal Dominant disorders are very different than recessive disorders because only one copy of the abnormal gene is needed to produce the disease; thus, there is no carrier state. In essence the bad gene is "dominant" over the good gene. Examples are polydactyly, in which the child has extra fingers or toes; achondroplasia, in which the child's arms and legs are so short that he or she is in essence a dwarf; Huntington's chorea, in which loss of control over movements and mental function is progressive and usually starts in middle age. Polydactyly and achondroplasia may sometimes be diagnosed before birth with ultrasound. Huntington's chorea can be detected by amniocentesis.

Chromosomal Errors

16

Q *What is the difference between genetic and chromosomal disorders?*

A Genetic disorders can be passed on to the next generation, and the likelihood of them occurring can be calculated. Chromosomal disorders, on the other hand, are usually caused by an error in the way the sperm or egg divided when it was formed. Many chromosomal errors are possible.

17

Q *What percentage of babies are born with a birth defect?*

A The background birth defect rate is about 3 to 5 percent. Many of these defects are either readily fixed or need no correction. For example, in hypospadias, the urethra comes out on the bottom side of the penis instead of at the end; in polydactyly, there are extra fingers or toes; in ventricular septal defect (VSD), there is a small hole in the heart.

Because even 5 percent of births is such a large number, common environmental factors such as over-the-counter drugs are blamed, despite the lack of scientific proof. Only 1 percent are thought to be caused by drugs or chemical exposure. About 30 percent of defects are genetic. The rest result from either a combination of gene effects and environment, or from the environment only. The cause of most defects is unknown.

18

Q *What are the most common chromosomal disorders?*

A (See also Section 5: Questions 249–64)
The most common one seen in newborns is Down's syndrome, in which the twenty-first chromosome has three copies instead of two. Also called trisomy 21, (47, xy:21) this syndrome includes changes in facial features—for example, low-set ears, slanted eyes, and a flattened face—as well as diminished mental ability. It can be diagnosed in the first trimester with CVS, or in the second with amniocentesis.

The incidence of Down's syndrome increases with the mother's age. If she is thirty-five years old, the chances are about one in 270. Thus, women who will be thirty-five or over at their due date are encouraged to consider prenatal testing. Because this is higher than the expected miscarriage rate due to the test itself (about one in 600 to one in 900), amniocentesis is recommended by many doctors and almost all insurance plans will pay for it.

Other common chromosomal disorders include Fragile X syndrome, which may cause mental retardation, speech deficits, and autistic behavior; Klinefelter syndrome, (47, xxy) in which the presence of an extra X chromosome in a male leads to smaller testicles, sometimes to infertility, and occasionally to mental retardation; Turner syndrome, (45, xo) in which the presence of only one X chromosome in a female results in short stature, a broad chest, skin webbing at the back of the neck, and an almost certain inability to go through puberty and to have children. Turner syndrome is the most common genetic error found in miscarried fetuses.

19

Q *What are multifactorial defects?*

A These are caused by problems on many genes combined with harmful environmental exposure. The most common multifactorial defects are congenital heart defects and open neural tube defects. They recur in first-degree relatives only about 4 to 5 percent of the time.

20

Q *What types of congenital heart defects are there?*

A By far the most common congenital heart disease is simple VSD, or ventricular septal defect, in which there is a small hole in the wall between the large lower chambers of the heart. Small defects usually do not need repair, but larger ones may require surgery. ASD, or atrial septal defect, is similar to VSD but simply involves the upper chambers of the heart. Tetrology of Fallot is a less common but more serious problem in which there are four separate problems with the heart's structure. This, too, is correctable by surgery. Rarer still is transposition of the great vessels, in which the aorta comes off the right side of the heart and the pulmonary artery off the left. This prevents oxygenated blood returning from the lungs from circulating to the body and is always fatal unless corrected surgically. Hypoplastic left heart is very rare, impossible to correct, and always lethal, while endocardial cushion defect is similar, but in some cases surgically correctable.

21

Q *What are open neural tube defects (ONTD)?*

A In these conditions, the fetus's brain, spinal cord, or the covering tissues over them fail to form normally. Spina bifida, the most common problem in this category, usually involves the lower back. When the skin over the lesion is open, it can be detected at around fifteen to seventeen weeks with ultrasound or with the maternal blood test, alpha fetoprotein. Although some spina bifida patients have little or no difficulty, others may suffer leg paralysis, loss of sensation, loss of bladder and/or bowel control, scoliosis (spinal curvature), hydrocephalus (dilated chambers in brain), mental retardation, and death. Supplemental folic acid may help prevent this type of defect.

Anencephaly is a type of ONTD where the brain and head do not form normally. Babies are stillborn or die soon after birth.

22

Q *Are there any other multifactorial defects?*

A Other multifactorial defects include pyloric stenosis, in which the opening into the intestines from the stomach is blocked; clubfoot, in which the foot is twisted at the ankle; cleft lip and cleft palate, in which a gap appears in the lip or a hole occurs in the roof of the mouth; and congenital hip dislocations, often found in babies born in breech position and especially in girls, in which the ball-and-socket joint at the hip fits poorly.

23

Q *I've heard of defects called an omphalocele and a gastroschisis. What are they?*

A (See also Section 4: Question 298)
These are rare abdominal wall defects that are not clearly chromosomal, but which may occur with some other chromosomal syndromes. (See Section 4: Developmental Defects)

PLANNING YOUR CARE

Selecting Your Doctor, Midwife, and Facility

24

Q *How do I find the right obstetrician for me?*

A The right doctor is someone who is competent, open to your questions, and one whom you feel you can trust implicitly. If you're new to an area, or don't have an OB-GYN physician, rather than depending on commercial referral services, call the nearest private hospital and ask to speak to a Labor and Delivery nurse. Introduce yourself as new to the area, and request the names of three competent doctors. If they are not allowed to give referrals, then simply ask who they use personally and call back on subsequent shifts for other names. Nurses know.

You may then make a get-acquainted appointment. Find out where the doctor trained and if he or she is Board Certified or Board Eligible. Be alert to any personal information the doctor volunteers. Trust your feelings. You'll usually know if you've found the right doctor for you in the first few minutes.

25

Q *What does it mean to be Board Certified?*

A A Board Certified obstetrician has completed an accredited residency training program and has passed a rigorous set of examinations, including a comprehensive written examination at the end of postgraduate training, and, after completing two years in practice, an oral examination before three examiners.

A Board Eligible doctor has finished an accredited residency program and has passed the written examinations, but has not yet been in practice long enough to take oral examinations.

Doctors may practice medicine in any state without being Board Certified, although many insurance plans will exclude them from Preferred Provider lists if they have not passed their Boards.

26

Q *What if I want to see a midwife and not an obstetrician?*

A (See also Section 3: Prenatal Care; Section 6: Prepared Childbirth)
Nurse midwives in private practice are increasingly frequent in the

United States. Because of medical-legal concerns, few hospitals grant privileges to midwives unaffiliated with a doctor. Certified nurse midwives have met certain training criteria for state licensure whereas lay midwives have not, and are fully competent to care for an uncomplicated pregnancy and delivery. Certified midwives have the initials CNM after their names.

27

Q *How do I decide where I want to deliver?*

A (See also Section 6: Prepared Childbirth)
Where you deliver your baby will be largely influenced by where your doctor or midwife has privileges. Birthing centers that are close to hospitals with operating room facilities that have doctors on the premises can be a very real alternative to hospital birth. However, all across the nation there is a trend toward having the entire birth experience—labor, delivery, and recovery (LDR)—in a homey, well-appointed room rather than in the sterile, cold atmosphere of a Delivery Room. In most hospitals, you may breast-feed immediately and keep the baby in the room with you.

Where you deliver may be affected by which facilities are covered by your insurance. Both preferred provider organizations (PPOs) and health maintenance organizations (HMOs) restrict your choice of hospital or birthing center to some extent.

If you have insurance, but no maternity coverage, most hospitals will work out a cash payment at a discount, as will most doctors if you ask.

We cannot recommend home delivery under any circumstances. While most births go smoothly and safely, and sometimes without medication, when things go south, they go south in a hurry! In the United States about one hundred years ago, when all births occurred at home, the maternal death rate was fifty times greater than it is today due largely to the current availability of intravenous fluids and quick access to an operating room.

Weight Before Pregnancy

28

Q *What should I weigh before I conceive?*

A Safe pregnancies occur at a wide range of weights. At the extremes, very thin people may not have a high enough ratio of fat to muscle to allow regular periods and ovulation, while morbidly obese people may have similar problems caused by an excess of a fat-generated form of estrogen called estrone. Obesity is associated with higher rates of cesarean delivery, postterm pregnancy, gestational diabetes, very large babies, and hypertension. Very underweight patients are more likely to have malnourished fetuses, especially if little weight gain occurs in pregnancy. Body Mass Index (see Appendix B), the ratio of weight in kilograms to height in meters squared, should range from about twenty to twenty-nine for minimal risk.

Food, Drink, and Drugs

29

Q *Should I be concerned about anything I ate or drank, or medicines I took before I knew I was pregnant?*

A (See also Section 2: Dietary Guidelines; Section 5: Drugs in Pregnancy)
A good general rule upon discovering that you are pregnant is to stop drinking and smoking, and to discontinue all over-the-counter medicines except for those such as Tylenol and Sudafed until you can talk to your doctor. Prescription medicines for chronic conditions should generally be continued and may be safely changed if necessary after your pregnancy is confirmed.

While there are a few prescription medicines which have definitely been associated with birth defects, the risks are clustered approximately between days twenty-one and fifty-six of fetal life—about five to ten weeks from your last period. The "All or None Effect" means that drugs taken before five weeks from your last period almost never cause birth defects. Miscarriage due to exposure is possible if the substance in question destroys the embryonic disc. However, no organs have yet been formed, so individual systems are almost never affected. This means that anything you did before you suspected you were pregnant is extremely unlikely to cause a problem because the fetus is so undeveloped.

Most medicines for chronic conditions such as asthma, depression, seizure disorders, lupus, cystic fibrosis, Crohn's disease, ulcerative colitis, hypothyroidism, chronic hypertension, and diabetes can and should be continued until pregnancy is confirmed. There are several exceptions to this rule detailed in the Section 5: Drugs in Pregnancy.

SUGGESTED READING

American College of Obstetricians and Gynecologists. 1995. ACOG *Guide to Planning for Pregnancy, Birth and Beyond.*
ACOG Website: http://www.acog.com
Order Desk: 800-762-2264

Amis, Debby and Jeanne Green. 1993. *Prepared Childbirth the Family Way*, 5th
Ed. Plano, TX: The Family Way Publications, Inc.
To order: (972) 403-0297

WEBSITES

Calculating Due Date
www.americanpregnancy.org/duringpregnancy/pregcalc.html

Diet Before Pregnancy
www.kidshealth.org/parent/nutrition_fit/nutrition/eating_ pregnancy.html

Fetal Development
www.pregnancycenter.com and/or GET APP: "Hello Baby"

Genetics
www.marchofdimes.com/pnhec/4439_1126.asp

Infertility
www.resolve.org

Obstetrics and General Info
www.acog.com
http://www.obgyn.net/

Pregnancy Planning
www.marchofdimes.com/professionals/681_1156.asp

Teens and Pregnancy
www.webmd.com and enter teen pregnancy in search engine

Midwifery
www.moonlily.com/obc/midwife.html

Section Two

Beginnings/Physical Changes/Complaints

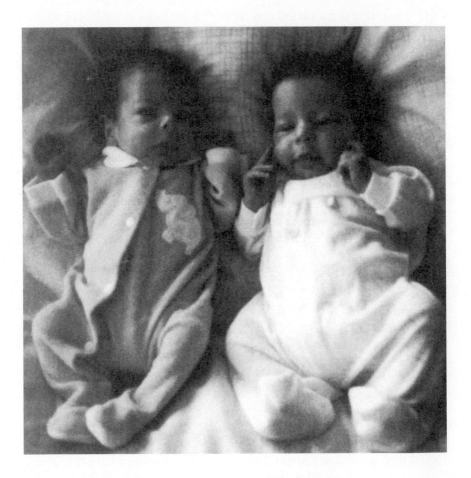

30

Q *How do I know when I'm really pregnant?*

A While missing a period can be due to stress-induced failure to ovulate, it may also indicate a pregnancy. You can easily check with a home pregnancy test, which detects minute amounts of the pregnancy hormone, human chorionic gonadotropin (HCG), in your urine. It may now detect pregnancy as early as twelve days after conception, and it is as sensitive as a blood test.

Most home tests available will definitely be positive within a week of your missed period. Buy the simplest one-step test and follow directions carefully. There are very few false negatives. Occasionally the result may be positive due to patient error in reading it or in waiting too many minutes before reading it. It's easy to make a mistake when you're nervous, whether or not you want the test to be positive. If you strongly suspect pregnancy, you should confirm the result with your doctor.

Your intuition may be accurate—or it may not. Individual women have different symptoms at different times. Signs such as breast tenderness, nausea, and fatigue usually begin at least one week after you miss your period. The embryo takes about seven days to migrate down your tube and implant on the wall of the uterus, thus establishing contact with your bloodstream. Theoretically, signs or symptoms prior to that should be impossible, so if your hairdresser tells you a week before your missed period, he was guessing! For every woman who knows she conceived ten minutes after making love, there are many others equally convinced who were wrong.

31

Q *Once I feel sure that I am pregnant, what do I need to do first?*

A Once again, don't panic! This sort of thing has been happening for some time now! Share the news with your husband and confirm any positive home pregnancy test at your doctor's office. Most of the time your pregnancy will be in your uterus where it belongs, but a little more than 1 percent of the time it could be an ectopic pregnancy either in your fallopian tube, or elsewhere in your abdomen. Notify your doctor if you have any spotting, which could be an early warning of threatened miscarriage or an ectopic pregnancy.

Unfortunately, about 15 to 20 percent of pregnancies end in miscarriage, 95 percent of these in the first twelve weeks. Wait to share your news with the world at least until you are over ten weeks and you have either seen the heartbeat on vaginal ultrasound or heard it with a Doppler device.

If you are not already taking a prenatal vitamin, start taking one—any of the over-the-counter prenatal vitamins are fine. They differ from prescription vitamins only in having slightly less folate. If you're on Medicaid, ask your doctor for a prescription even before you're seen for a first visit. Prescription prenatal vitamins are covered by Medicaid.

Otherwise, stop smoking, drinking alcohol, or taking any over-the-counter medicines other than Tylenol and Sudafed. Prescription medicines for chronic conditions should not be discontinued until you talk to your doctor.

32

Q *How do I know my due date?*

A If your menstrual periods were regular right up until you got pregnant, subtract three months from the month of your last menstrual period and add seven days. For example, if the first day of your period was January 7, 1998, then count backward (December-November-October) and add seven days: October 14, 1998, is your due date. Your doctor may make this more accurate with a vaginal ultrasound in the first twelve weeks of pregnancy.

33

Q *How long is each trimester?*

A The confusion surrounding gestational age continues with this terminology. We usually consider twelve weeks, twenty-four weeks, and thirty-six weeks the end of the first, second, and third trimesters, respectively, despite the fact that your due date isn't until forty weeks. The mean gestational age is 280 days from your last menstrual period (LMP), or about 266 days from conception. The "nine months" reflects the time to delivery from your missed menstrual period. Now, clear as mud?

34

Q *How do I know how far along I am if I don't know or didn't have a last period?*

A This circumstance is common with silent periods on the pill, if conception occurred while breast-feeding, or if your periods were irregular. Most obstetricians will perform a vaginal ultrasound in the office during the first trimester. Measurements of the baby's head to bottom (crown-rump length) can estimate gestation to within a little more or less than ninety-six hours. As pregnancy progresses, ultrasound estimates get less accurate. By sixteen weeks, ultrasound measurements give data that is accurate to plus or minus ten days; by thirty-five weeks estimates are accurate plus or minus three weeks.

35

Q *Is there anything in particular I can do to safeguard the health of my baby in the first trimester?*

A It's the same thing you can do to protect your baby in each trimester: Wear your seat belt! More fetuses are killed each year in car wrecks than are killed by poison, malnutrition, drugs, or other traumas combined. Your seat belt should be worn over your upper thighs and hips. The shoulder harness should go over (not under) the shoulder and between the breasts. It's okay for the harness to cross your belly.

MISCARRIAGE

36

Q *What is a miscarriage?*

A Miscarriage is another term for a spontaneous abortion (SAB). It implies the loss of any pregnancy from conception until twenty weeks of gestation in most states. Although viability outside the womb does not occur until after twenty-four weeks gestation, most states consider a loss before twenty weeks to be a miscarriage and after twenty weeks to be a stillbirth.

Miscarriage, meaning a loss after the patient knows that she is pregnant, occurs in about 10 to 20 percent of all pregnancies, depending on the source of the data. Most physicians accept 15 percent as the number. (The true spontaneous abortion rate may be as high as 62 percent of all conceptions, if those losses that occur prior to the patient's knowledge of them are included, i.e., SAB at about the time of your expected menses.)

37

Q *How do I avoid having a miscarriage?*

A There is essentially no way that you can either avoid or cause a miscarriage with normal activity. The fetus is incredibly well protected. The 15 percent of pregnancies that miscarry in the first twelve weeks are, more often than not, either chromosomally abnormal and/or consist of a sac and membranes with no developed fetus (blighted ovum). Rarely, abnormalities such as a uterine septum (divisions) with an abnormal placental implantation could lead to miscarriage.

Everything from a slip and a fall to nervous tension, sexual intercourse, and lifting heavy groceries has been blamed for pregnancy loss. No evidence exists to support any common activity as a cause for miscarriage in the first trimester.

38

Q *If I've had a miscarriage before, do I have an increased risk of another miscarriage?*

A The vast majority of the time the answer is "no." The chance of miscarriage is about 15 to 20 percent with each new conception. Three or more consecutive spontaneous abortions (SAB) is called "habitual abortion:' In this special circumstance, your doctor may recommend blood studies to look for antibodies like lupus anticoagulant (LAC), anticardiolipin (ACL), Leiden Factor V, protein S deficiency, as well as an enzyme deficiency called MTHFR, that may cause problems where the placenta implants and lead to repeated pregnancy loss. Depending on the findings, your chances of carrying another pregnancy to term may be greatly improved by taking one baby aspirin (82 milligrams) per day and/or being injected twice a day with a blood thinner called heparin or at some point once a day with Lovenox which requires less monitoring. MTHFR can be treated with high dose folate early in pregnancy or prenatals like Neevo which contain the active metabolite required.

39

Q *What if I've had multiple miscarriages but my antibody studies are normal?*

A Your doctor may recommend drawing blood from you and your husband to study your chromosome makeup. This is called karyotyping. He or she may also recommend office hysteroscopy, a procedure in which a fiber optic tube is placed through the vagina and cervix so that abnormalities on the inside of the uterus can be seen on a video-monitor. Some of the abnormal findings in a uterus that lead to miscarriages may then be treated surgically. These embryological abnormalities are called Müllerian Anomalies. They include heart-shaped uteri, septate uteri, bicornuate uteri (two uterine horns with one shared cervix), and uterus didelphus (two uteri, two cervices).

40

Q *My friend is taking progesterone vaginal suppositories to avoid miscarriage. Does that work?*

A This is one of those gray areas in medicine. Natural progesterone, either as suppositories or in the oral micronized form (Prometrium), has not been shown to be harmful. The rationale for their use comes from the fact that if the progesterone-producing corpus luteum cyst is removed from the ovary in lower primates before ten weeks, miscarriage will result. However, the opposite has been shown when the corpus luteum cyst has been removed in humans early in pregnancy. Even if the cyst is removed as early as six days after conception, the SAB rate is only 15 percent, or about normal. In fact, the placenta probably takes over making at least some of the essential progesterone soon after implantation of the embryo in the uterine wall.

Now that we can test blood levels of progesterone, we know there is a wide range of levels that are considered normal, but that grossly low levels imply an impending miscarriage (or even an ectopic pregnancy) because of something fundamentally wrong with the placenta and pregnancy. It's the chicken or the egg dilemma. Replacing progesterone levels probably won't prevent miscarriage since it's not the absence of progesterone causing the miscarriage, but vice versa.

However, because of the theoretical advantage and the desperation of patients with a history of multiple miscarriages, progesterone is often prescribed in the belief that it can do no harm.

41

Q *I'm about six weeks pregnant and I've started spotting. What should I do?*

A Unfortunately, there is nothing you can do to avoid a miscarriage at this point if you are destined to have one. Health professionals often advise that you "get off your feet" This advice is given out of empathy, but also impotence. They would like very much to keep you from miscarrying, but there is nothing they can do either. Sometimes they tell you to get off your feet because there's nothing else they can say. There is no evidence that bed rest, or even decreased activity, helps avert early miscarriage. The only exception would be after ten weeks, when a heartbeat is visible and actual separation of the placenta can be seen on ultrasound. In this circumstance, avoiding intercourse is good advice. Avoiding other activity may or may not be helpful.

Your doctor will be able to confirm that your pregnancy is in the uterus, rather than in your tube, with a vaginal ultrasound after five and a half to six weeks of gestation. If you are bleeding at or after this gestational age, your doctor may wish to perform an ultrasound then, rather than waiting for your first scheduled visit.

Spotting may be normal, may be a threatened miscarriage, or could be a warning sign of an ectopic pregnancy; it does *not* mean that the pregnancy might continue but with an increased chance of birth defects. Early threatened SABs are an all-or-nothing phenomenon. Either you will miscarry or you won't. If you don't, your pregnancy will continue with the same risk of birth defects as any other pregnancy—roughly 3 to 5 percent.

42

Q *My friend miscarried a few months ago. She was told that it might have been from lifting things when she moved to a new home. Could that be right?*

A No, it isn't right. This is the danger of advice like "get off your feet" when you're spotting. Vaginal spotting is a "threatened" miscarriage, but 70 percent of pregnancies with spotting and no pain before seven weeks continue normally, whether you get off your feet or not. To advise rest only plants the seeds of guilt. If you do miscarry, you will find some way to blame yourself if you were led to believe you could avoid losing the pregnancy by resting.

43

Q *How do I know if I'm miscarrying?*

A Nowadays, with early vaginal ultrasound available, many inevitable miscarriages are diagnosed at your first pregnancy visit between seven and ten weeks. First, impending miscarriage is suspected when the fetal heart rate is slower than normal (lower than 90 beats per minute) at six to eight weeks. (Normal fetal heart rate is 120 to 160 beats per minute.) If you are secure in your dates and you know when you got pregnant, then an "empty sac" after six and a half weeks, also called a blighted ovum, means miscarriage is inevitable, even if you have no signs yet. Depending on the amount of tissue present, your doctor may recommend an outpatient D & C (dilatation and curettage), in which a suction catheter is used to empty the uterus.

You may also have symptoms in which you first begin spotting, but then bleed as you would during a heavy period, with clotting and cramping. If you complete a miscarriage, the heavy bleeding and cramping usually stop suddenly when the gestational sac is passed. After about five weeks, the tissue passed in a miscarriage will look like a sphere that is slightly smaller than a golf ball. It may have tiny fronds on the surface and may be collapsed. It will not usually look like a blood clot.

If you pass what you think is tissue, try to save it in a Ziploc bag and bring it when you go to the doctor, as upsetting as that may seem. Sending the tissue to pathology may save you many blood tests that would otherwise have to be done to make sure your HCG levels return to zero.

44

Q *What will the doctor do if I'm miscarrying?*

A You might have to do nothing at all if you are at less than six and a half weeks gestation. Your doctor will advise you about what might happen if you let the miscarriage happen on its own. After about seven weeks, if you are bleeding heavily and do not pass all the tissue, or if you are discovered to have a "blighted ovum" on ultrasound in the office, your doctor may recommend a D & C.

D & C stands for "dilatation and curettage Curettage literally means scraping. In early pregnancy, however, a "suction D & C" is performed; in this procedure a small plastic cannula is inserted through the cervix and the contents of the uterus are removed. This may be done under local anesthesia with intravenous sedation in some offices, or in an outpatient operating room, depending on the facilities available. Technically, the procedure is the same as a voluntary abortion.

45

Q *I've heard that a D and C can scar my uterus and make it difficult to get pregnant in the future. Is that so?*

A This is a common misconception. Suction D & Cs in the first trimester are not associated with scarring and infertility. D & Cs performed for removal of the placenta between about twenty weeks and immediately after term delivery may, rarely, be associated with scarring. This scarring is called Aschermann's Syndrome and may be associated with infertility. It is usually treatable with operative hysteroscopy, in which a hysteroscope with attached camera is inserted through the cervix to allow visualization of procedures within the uterus. The primary symptom of Aschermann's is no return of menstruation at all after term pregnancy.

46

Q *What is a blighted ovum or empty sac?*

A A blighted ovum is the term used for an inevitable miscarriage, in which either the fetus never formed at all or it stopped growing before it became visible on ultrasound. Ovum is the Latin word for egg, and blighted ovum implies a bad egg. A blighted ovum has no implication for future pregnancies, and your miscarriage rate remains unchanged at about 15 percent. *(After our miscarriages, my wife pointed out, quite correctly, that with 150 million sperm and only one egg, a "blighted sperm" was a little more likely!)*

47

Q *I've read that eleven to twelve weeks is the most common time for miscarriage. I thought you said you were essentially out of the woods after ten weeks.*

A The statement that most miscarriages occur at eleven weeks is misleading. Modern ultrasound has allowed us to recognize missed abortions or inevitable abortions at an early stage. While most bleeding and cramping may occur at eleven to twelve weeks, the vast majority of these fetuses have been dead for many weeks, or never developed at all.

In other words, if you hear or see the fetal heart rate after ten weeks, you should feel extremely reassured. Fewer than 5 percent of miscarriages are to women whose fetal heart beat has already been heard with a Doppler device or seen on ultrasound after ten completed weeks.

Some second trimester losses are fetal demises (deaths) without any known cause. They may be due to the same type of antibodies that cause habitual abortion, to structural changes like those that can occur with DES exposure in the mother of the pregnant woman, or, rarely, to problems with implantation either over a fibroid tumor in the wall of the uterus or on a septum partially dividing the uterine cavity.

48

Q *What is a uterine septum?*

A The uterine cavity is developed embryologically from two narrow tubes that partially fuse. The unfused portion becomes the fallopian tubes; the fused portion becomes the uterus. The common wall of the fused portion is supposed to disappear. When it disappears only partially, it leaves a septum, or division, in the uterine cavity. This is one of the types of Müllerian Anomaly mentioned earlier. This wall down the middle of the cavity is mostly connective tissue with little blood supply. A fetus that implants on the septum may grow for a while and then die. Septa may be fixed surgically in the nonpregnant woman with operative hysteroscopy.

49

Q *How can DES exposure in my mother cause me to have a miscarriage?*

A DES (Diethylstilbestrol) exposure led to an increased risk of structural abnormalities in the internal genitalia of the female offspring of women exposed during their pregnancy. Ironically, from 1940 to 1971 DES was prescribed to pregnant women to help avoid miscarriage. Roughly six million women were exposed. (As of this writing women younger than twenty-seven could not have been exposed in utero.) If your mother was exposed to DES when she was pregnant with you, you have an increased risk of both a T-shaped uterus, and an incompetent cervix.

A T-shaped uterus is more often associated with infertility than spontaneous abortion. An incompetent cervix, on the other hand, is associated with repeated miscarriage during the second trimester. In this condition, the elastic tissue of the cervix is faulty and the cervix may dilate without warning or pain, leading to the loss of the fetus at around fifteen to twenty-four weeks. Unfortunately, the condition is usually diagnosed only after the first loss. In a subsequent pregnancy, it is treated at around twelve to fourteen weeks, when a suture is placed around the cervix (cerclage). This procedure can be done in an outpatient surgical setting.

50

Q *Are there causes of incompetent cervix other than DES exposure?*

A An incompetent cervix has been associated not only with DES, but also with mechanical damage from cone biopsies previously performed for cervical dysplasia (precancerous changes). Older types of cone biopsies involved the excision of a significant portion of the cervix and canal with a knife, suturing the incision afterward. Cone biopsies done in the operating room have largely been replaced with procedures performed in the office—CO_2 laser or, more recently, Large Loop Electrical Excision (LEEP). Having had a LEEP procedure in the past is rarely, if ever, associated with cervical incompetence and is not a reason in and of itself for a cerclage procedure. LEEP of the cervix is sometimes called LLETZ for "Large Loop Excision of the Transformation Zone."

51

Q *When can I try to get pregnant again after a miscarriage?*

A Everyone agrees that you should wait at least until the cycle after your next normal menstrual period. Some doctors advise waiting three months, since some feel that a slightly higher miscarriage rate exists if conception happens right away. However, very little credible evidence exists to support this precaution.

ECTOPIC PREGNANCY

52

Q *What is an ectopic pregnancy?*

A Ectopic means misplaced. Any pregnancy that implants someplace other than in the uterus is ectopic. Ectopic pregnancies occur in about 1 to 2 percent of conceptions in the normal population. People think of the word ectopic as synonymous with tubal pregnancy, but actually 10 percent of ectopic pregnancies occur elsewhere in the body, in places such as the peritoneal cavity and the ovary; they may even attach to the intestines, gallbladder, omentum, or liver.

Ectopic pregnancies are potentially lethal because once the placenta outgrows its adopted blood supply it starts to die, separating from its attachment and bleeding into the abdomen, either directly or via the fallopian tube. Tubal pregnancies, the most common type of ectopic pregnancy, may bleed out of the end of the fallopian tube or actually rupture the tube with a rapid hemorrhage, and ensuing death.

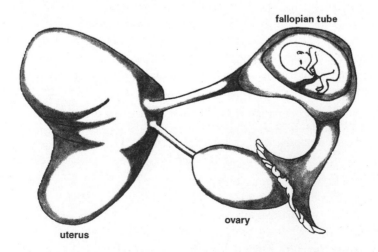

fallopian tube

ovary

uterus

53

Q *How do I know if I'm at risk for an ectopic pregnancy?*

A Anyone who has unprotected sex is at risk. About 50 percent of tubal ectopic pregnancies appear to occur with no predisposing cause, just bad luck with respect to where the embryo implants six to seven days after conception. The other 50 percent have a history of Pelvic Inflammatory Disease (PID) involving gonorrhea or chlamydia, they have previously or are currently using an IUD, or they have had a previous ectopic pregnancy.

54

Q *If I've had one ectopic pregnancy, what are my risks of recurrence?*

A That depends to some extent on your original therapy and whether or not your fallopian tube was removed at that time. If you have both tubes in place, and subsequent studies have shown them to be open, your risk is about 10 percent, or ten times higher than normal. If your next pregnancy is ectopic, it may occur in either fallopian tube, since often the predisposing factor that damaged the lining of one tube will have affected the other tube as well.

If you've already had an ectopic pregnancy, be sure to tell your doctor. You will be followed more closely than if you had never had one before.

55

Q *How do I know if I might have an ectopic pregnancy?*

A Almost all ectopic pregnancies are accompanied by abnormal vaginal bleeding. One of the insidious dangers is that this bleeding may even mimic a regular light period and lead to confusion about whether you are even pregnant.

Once a positive pregnancy is established, if you are spotting and or have pelvic pain at less than five weeks from your last menstrual period, serial blood pregnancy tests can identify an abnormally slow rise in HCG levels and alert your doctor to potential difficulty. If your home pregnancy test is positive but you are spotting, you must notify your doctor at once. If you have a slow rise or even a fall of HCG levels, that will confirm that the fetus is abnormal and will not continue to develop. You may be having either an early threatened miscarriage or an ectopic pregnancy, but at less than five weeks, even a vaginal ultrasound will show only an empty uterus and therefore cannot distinguish between the two.

After about five weeks, a vaginal ultrasound in the doctor's office can at least confirm the presence of a gestational sac and rule out an ectopic pregnancy. (See Blighted Ovum.) It is the empty uterus combined with a positive pregnancy test and a history of bleeding and/or pain that leads the doctor to suspect an ectopic pregnancy. The vaginal ultrasound usually cannot identify the tubal pregnancy; it can only confirm the absence of a pregnancy in the uterus.

56

Q *Is there a medicine I might be able to take in order to avoid surgery?*

A There are several options. If you are at less than five weeks and in no pain, your doctor may simply warn you to call if you experience increased pain or bleeding, and continue to follow blood HCG levels. (See Question 55 in this section) Many early ectopic pregnancies are thought to reabsorb on their own long before risk of rupture.

Recently, presumed ectopic pregnancies have been treated successfully with small doses of the chemotherapy agent Methotrexate. If your titers are failing to rise and meet certain criteria, your doctor knows your pregnancy has no chance of a normal outcome and he may then proceed to hasten reabsorption of the fetus with methotrexate.

If in the doctor's judgment a patient is not a candidate for medical therapy, surgery may be necessary. A frozen section may be performed on a D & C specimen in the operating room. (See D & C) If there is evidence of a blighted ovum in the uterus, the procedure is over. If the pathology shows no evidence of an intrauterine pregnancy, then a laparoscopy will be performed.

Laparoscopy involves general anesthesia. A telescope-like instrument connected to a camera is placed into your navel, after which two or more small additional punctures are made in the abdominal wall. Using a video camera and robotic instruments, the ectopic pregnancy can be removed without having to remove the fallopian tube (salpingostomy). Sometimes, however, too much of the tube is damaged, and the bleeding is too severe to be stopped without removing part or all of the tube. In this case a partial or complete salpingectomy is performed. This outpatient procedure is usually done through the laparoscope. Rarely, the situation is so urgent that an open laparotomy is performed, with a larger abdominal incision made in order to operate directly, in the more traditional fashion.

MORNING SICKNESS

57

Q *Ever since I was six to seven weeks, I've been nauseated almost all the time. What can I do to feel better?*

A Combating morning sickness varies with the individual woman. Try to avoid letting your stomach be completely empty. You can accomplish this by eating many small meals a day and constantly having crackers to munch on. It is especially helpful to keep some dry crackers on a night table and eat a few before you get up in the morning. Avoid spicy, rich, or fried foods. Try to stay hydrated. Saline solutions such as Gatorade are fine, as are soft drinks or iced tea. Iced tea settles many stomachs. The amount of caffeine in any of these drinks poses no risk whatsoever to the first-trimester fetus, and the sugar calories of the sodas, which should be avoided later on, may help relieve constant nausea.

Both vitamins and iron can contribute to nausea. If you have already begun to take a prenatal vitamin and oral iron, stop for a while. Humans have been having babies for 80,000 years without taking prenatal vitamins during pregnancy, and you can miss a few weeks in the first trimester without ill effect. The benefit of taking folate in order to avoid spina bifida occurs before the onset of nausea at about three to six weeks of gestation. After six weeks, stopping folate and other vitamins briefly is a better idea than throwing up all the time.

Despite the fact that Americans eat too much fat in burgers and fries, they are still by and large the best nourished society in human history. You may resume your prenatal vitamins as soon as you can tolerate them, which will usually be at about twelve to fifteen weeks.

Try Seabands or any form of acupressure on the inner wrist. Eat whatever you crave right away, or it may not help. If food preparation makes you sick, get someone else to do it, or eat out as often as possible. Believe it or not, try dill pickles. Dill seems to soothe some stomachs, as do Granny Smith apples, lemonade, and potato chips. Try sucking on hot candies such as Atomic Fireballs.

58

Q *What things should I avoid?*

A Motion sickness can make travel, especially air travel, tough. Traveling also traps you inside a vehicle with other people's colognes and food smells. Carry a lemon in a plastic bag so you can smell it when you feel as if you're about to throw up, or try putting lemon-smelling skin conditioner on your wrists. Avoid potent odors such as those of gas stations, coffeepots, diapers, smelly cat litter, and pet food.

Don't even open those magazines that you know are going to have cologne samples in them. Avoid watching out-of-focus video or computer screens.[1]

59

Q *I get sick before I go to bed, not in the morning, and nothing I try makes it better, Is there a medicine I can use?*

A (See also Section 5: Antinausea medicines)
Nobody knows for sure where the term "morning sickness" originated, but pregnancy can make you feel nauseous or actually vomit at any time of the day or night. A lucky 20 percent of women don't have this problem, but the other 80 percent have it to some degree. The makers of Bendectin, the most effective medicine ever formulated for morning sickness, were sued into oblivion in the late 1970s. Neither the Food and Drug administration (FDA) nor the American College of Obstetricians and Gynecologists (ACOG) ever condemned this medicine, and no definitive evidence was found to support contentions that it was the actual cause of any birth defects. Its active components were pyridoxine (vitamin B6) and the antihistamine doxylamine.

The glucose and B6 components alone sometimes help and are commercially available as Nestrex (Category A) over the counter. Nestrex, combined with the over-the-counter sleep aid doxylamine (Unisom), is safe and extremely effective, although it does have a sedative effect. Other antihistamines such as diphenhydramine (Benadryl) and dymenhydrinate (Dramamine) may be tried but seem less effective than doxylamine (Unisom). These are all Category B drugs and are considered safe in pregnancy.[2] Your doctor can also prescribe medicine after seeing you. (See Section 5 for FDA categories.)

60

Q *My morning sickness makes me feel so bad that I either can't eat, or have to eat small amounts of junk food all day long just to keep from vomiting. Isn't this poor nutrition dangerous for my baby?*

A Absolutely not. At eight weeks, your fetus is roughly 20 millimeters (3/4 inch) long. It could survive off of one tortilla chip for a month. In the first trimester once morning sickness has begun, only hydration is important. However, if you go for twenty-four hours without keeping any liquids down you should call your doctor. Dehydration can be associated with a lowered pH in your blood, reflecting more acidity, and this is potentially harmful to the fetus. Sometimes all you need is a few liters of intravenous fluids to make you feel better.

61

Q *In my last pregnancy I was hospitalized for three weeks with hyperemesis gravidarum. What can I do to avoid this problem now?*

A Morning sickness becomes the more severe hyperemesis gravidarum (nonstop vomiting in pregnancy) when the vomiting leads to dehydration. Dehydration and starvation can indeed make your blood more acidotic, but it can also be more basic or alkalotic from vomiting lots of your stomach's hydrochloric acid. This can also lead to dangerously low potassium levels, called hypokalemla.

Some newer medicines, such as ondansetron (Zofran), are available. Zofran can be very effective intravenously, but very expensive orally. Also, in many circumstances your insurance company and doctor can help arrange home intravenous fluids. Another medicine, metoclopramide (Reglan) (Category B), can also be administered intravenously to stimulate upper intestinal motility, and is sometimes helpful.

Other prescription medicines classed as Category B that are considered safe but not especially effective include meclizine (Antivert), prochlorperazine (Compazine), and ranitidine (Zantac). Just as common, however, are Category C medicines such as hydroxyzine (Vistaril), promethazine (Phenergan), Trimethobenzamides (Tigan), and droperidol (Inapsine). For the most part, they are considered safe, certainly after ten full weeks of gestation, but they also are not terribly effective. The mainstay of treatment is intravenous hydration with a balanced solution of electrolytes needed by your body. (See Section 5: Antinausea)

62

Q *Why do some women get hyperemesis and not others?*

A No one is certain. About half of all pregnant women vomit in the first trimester, and a much smaller percentage develop intractable vomiting, or hyperemesis. It used to be thought that high HCG (pregnancy hormone) levels were responsible, since women who were pregnant with twins and women with the rare molar pregnancy (a chromosomal error in which no fetus exists and only an abnormal placenta is present) developed hyperemesis at a higher rate than other women. Data from the Collaborative Perinatal Project, however, disputes this, and associates very high estrogen levels, not HCG levels, with the intractable vomiting.[3]

DIETARY GUIDELINES AND WEIGHT GAIN

Introduction

Almost every reference you read about pregnancy will stress the importance of good nutrition. The concept that during pregnancy you are "eating for two" is true in many senses, but definitely not in all. Most drugs and many nutrients do pass through the placenta with ease. The older belief that the placenta protects the fetus from harm by blocking passage of harmful chemicals is now clearly shown to be naive.

But so too is the perception that the fetus suffers unless every building block it needs is ingested by mom. Human gestation is elegantly designed to preserve the fetus's oxygenation and nutrition even in the face of phenomenal adversity. To suggest otherwise is to unnecessarily terrify pregnant women about the health of their baby if their nutritional status varies even slightly from recommended optimums.

That being the case, the answers to the following questions stick to the facts and avoid suggesting that a certain number of servings per day from this food group or that one absolutely has to be consumed.

A balanced healthy diet, avoiding excessive fat and simple sugars, increasing sources of roughage and protein such as green vegetables, chicken, fish, lean beef, and dairy products, and adding adequate daily carbohydrates in the form of grains and fruits, will support the best possible outcome of your pregnancy. Failure to eat from any particular source of nutrition even for several days at a time will not prove to be catastrophic or even dangerous to your fetus.

Dietary Guidelines

63

Q *Once I am able to eat solids regularly, aren't there certain critical foods, such as milk and cheese, that I must eat?*

A A common misperception is that it is critical to the fetus that you increase your calcium intake to build healthy bones, eat more protein to build strong muscles and grow a healthy nervous system, and stay away from salt. Tomorrow babies will be born in Dallas, Mogadishu, Bangladesh, Shanghai, and Buenos Aires whose mothers will have eaten very different foods. God designed the fetal system to be incredibly resistant and the maternal system to supply needs even in the face of near starvation. (See Question 65 in this section)

For example, if you consumed *no* calcium during your entire pregnancy it would make no difference to the fetus. If your blood calcium dropped by

34

as little as 20 percent, your bronchi would close down, your muscles would go into spasm, and you would develop heart block, heart failure, and grand mal seizures. So your body uses parathyroid hormone and leeches calcium from your bones to keep your blood level within the same narrow range. (See Hormones)

If you ate no animal protein in the form of chicken, fish, or red meat, your body would break down your muscle mass to keep the same ratios of amino acids in your bloodstream.

In short, the fetus takes its nutrients from your bloodstream. These nutrients may all come from storage forms in your body, with the notable exception of the eight "essential" amino acids, the essential fatty acids, and simple carbohydrates (sugar). The fetus depends largely on sugar for energy, and breakdown of glycogen in the liver does not provide an adequate supply. Even so, starvation diets allow fetuses to survive with little to none of these essential components for many months. (See Carbohydrates and Proteins below)

64

Q *Are there any foods I really must avoid?*

A There are certainly foods you would do better to avoid, such as extremely salty or spicy foods, those high in saturated fat, those full of "empty" calories such as simple sugars, and, of course, alcohol.

In March 2004, the FDA and EPA issued guidelines restricting intake of fish and shellfish for pregnant women and women who might become pregnant to 2 servings per week due to risk of mercury poisoning. Shark, swordfish, king mackerel, and golden or white snapper contain very high levels of mercury and should be avoided. Light tuna is preferred over Albacore (white tuna). Shrimp, salmon, pollock, and catfish are lower in mercury. Fish sticks and fast food sandwiches pose little to no risk.

Listeria is a bacteria found in soft cheeses that can lead to a flu-like syndrome in you and very rarely to death for your fetus. The USDA recommends avoiding imported soft cheeses, which tend to be unpasteurized, as well as deli meat and undercooked hot dogs. Pre-packaged vacuum sealed lunch meats from manufacturers may be substituted for fresh deli meats to avoid this tiny increased risk. Imported soft cheeses to avoid include Brie, Camembert, feta, goat, Montrachet, Neufchatel, and queso fresco. While cheeses made in the USA are made only from pasteurized milk, which kills listeria, they can be contaminated later in the process. Less risky are Roquefort, Muenster, Havarti, Gorgonzola, blue, brick, and Asiago cheeses. Cheddar, mozzarella, cream, and cottage cheeses are always fine.

You may want to avoid sushi and undercooked meats. People have cooked their food since the dawn of human history—with good reason. Toxoplasmosis, microsporidiosis, trematode infections, cysticercosis, and trichinellosis all come from undercooked meat or raw fish. Nothing in life is without risk. Ben Franklin was right about this, as in most things, when he said, "Everything in moderation." If you have eaten sushi or deli meat already in your pregnancy, don't have a hissy fit! Your risk is infinitesimal! It would be a lot safer to eat deli meat in America than to text while you're driving, and I bet you've done THAT while you were pregnant!

65

Q *What happens if I have a poor diet throughout my pregnancy?*

A After World War II, a very famous study looked at the pregnancies of thousands of starving women held under siege in the Netherlands by the Nazis. The women received, on average, less than four hundred and fifty calories a day for a period of six months, which qualifies as a starvation diet. They were in all stages of pregnancy, and many starved to death before delivery.

While birth weight in the survivors was decreased by as much as eight ounces, perinatal mortality and birth defects did not increase even under these starvation conditions. Follow-up twenty years later showed no significant difference in IQ, school performance, or job placement.[4]

66

Q *So, if my diet isn't critical, should I just ignore dietary guidelines?*

A Absolutely not! Dietary guidelines are very important for your own health. But don't worry that your baby will have an ear on his forehead if you can't look at a glass of milk at twenty weeks without throwing up. It just doesn't work that way!

67

Q *So what are the current dietary guidelines?*

A Many "experts" in the last hundred years have painted a very confusing picture about diet in pregnancy. Prior to the 1970s caloric intake was grossly restricted, and weight gain was limited to less than twenty pounds in the mistaken belief that the rapid weight gain seen with preeclampsia (PIH, or pregnancy-induced hypertension) was fat and not the excess water that we now know it actually represents.

The Food and Nutritional Board of the National Research Council makes recommendations in dietary allowances for pregnant women periodically. (See Appendix A: Dietary Allowances)

68

Q *How many calories should I eat each day?*

A An increase of three hundred calories a day is recommended for a woman of normal weight. Less than this could cause protein to be broken down for energy rather than used for growth and development. You can calculate the required caloric intake to meet energy needs and achieve appropriate weight gain by multiplying your optimum weight in kilograms (pounds/2.2) x 35 calories and adding the additional 300 calories to the total. Your optimum weight may be obtained from the Body Mass Index (BMI) table in Appendix B. If you already overeat, which is the case with many affluent Americans, don't increase your caloric intake. Remember, do the calculation with your optimum, not your actual, weight.[5]

69

Q *Since I've been pregnant, my sweet tooth has grown to the size of a walrus tusk. Is sugar bad for me?*

A Sugar in itself isn't "bad" for anyone, including diabetics. Too much sugar can be bad, because sweets may lead you to take in inadequate amounts of other nutrients that are necessary. Obviously, diabetics need to closely regulate their sugar intake whether they are insulin-dependent or not (See Section 8: Diabetes), but you can't call the primary energy source for the brain "bad." Sugar can, of course, be lifesaving for diabetics in insulin shock.

The point is that sugars are so-called "empty calories," meaning that you don't build bodies with sugars, you just burn them or convert them to fat. Therefore, you should significantly limit your intake of added sugar, baked goods, candy, ice cream, and other sweets. Read labels. Sugars appear as fructose, sucrose, glucose, dextrose, honey, corn syrup, maple syrup, and molasses. Many sauces and dressings have considerable amounts of sugar, as do items such as barbecue sauce, ketchup, soups, gravies, salad dressings, peanut butter, sodas, and cereals.

You can still have these foods. Just avoid having them to the exclusion of fresh vegetables, fruits, chicken, meats, fish, and dairy products. Ben Franklin said, "Everything in moderation," and he was right.

70

Q *What about artificial sweeteners? It seems like Nutrasweet is in just about every-thing nowadays.*

A Nutrasweet (Aspartame) is a naturally occurring amino acid. You're already made out of Nutrasweet from head to toe. There is no evidence that aspartame causes birth defects in humans. Millions of pregnant women have used Nutrasweet without documented risk, and I tell my patients it is safe to do so with our current knowledge. Maltodextrin and sucrolose (Splenda) do not pose any known risk.

Saccharin (Sweet 'n Low), on the other hand, has clearly been associ-ated with cancers of the urinary tract in animal studies. While it has not been proved to cause birth defects in humans, it should probably be avoided. (See Section 5: Artificial Sweeteners)

71

Q *What about carbohydrates? I thought sugars were carbohydrates.*

A They are. But sugars are simple carbohydrates; starches, are complex car-bohydrates—they have larger, more complicated molecules. These larger molecules should comprise almost half of your caloric intake. Foods that contain starches include those made from whole grains such as cereals, rice, breads, and vegetables such as potatoes, carrots, peas, corn, and beans.

72

Q *What about protein?*

A An additional thirty grams of protein per day is recommended by the Food and Nutrition Board to bring the total to about 80 grams, but this is nearly twice what the World Health Organization advocates. Most experts agree that the additional protein should come in the form of milk, eggs, cheese, poultry, fish, dried beans, nuts, and meat due to their amino acid content.

Proteins are essential to your health. The amino acids, which link together to form proteins, are the building blocks of muscle, blood, bone, hair, skin, teeth, and the cells of the central nervous system, including the brain. They also serve as enzymes, which are essential to the chemical reactions involved in both storing and breaking down compounds for energy. There are more than twenty amino acids. Eight of these are called "essential" because they need to be supplied by your diet. However, in studies of starving populations, even sparse diets allow human reproduction to occur, with remarkably little adverse consequence to the fetus.

High-protein diets do not always affect birth weight or the incidence of preeclampsia, as was once thought. Eighty grams of protein per day is more than adequate and can be met by two to three servings of dairy; two to three servings of meat, poultry, or fish; and two to three servings of vegetables and/or fruit.

73

Q *I realize milk is a good source of protein and calcium, but when I drink milk I get cramps, pass gas, and sometimes have diarrhea. What can I do?*

A Up to 80 percent of black women and about 10 percent of white women have severe lactose intolerance. Milk and dairy products will cause severe cramping, gas, and bloating for them. They can take supplementary calcium in the form of pure calcium TUMS; consuming several per day helps to avoid heartburn. They may obtain protein from nondairy sources, or use one of the newly available, over-the-counter, lactase enzyme supplements such as Lactaid when they consume dairy products.

74

Q *Am I supposed to stay away from fats, too?*

A Yes and no. Fats are essential to life, just as proteins and carbohydrates are. Fats can be broken down for energy, and they are needed to help with absorption of vitamins A, D, E, and K. Certain fats, such as linoleic acid, are called "essential" because they must be obtained in your diet.

However, only about 25 percent of your calories should come in the form of fats. Fats themselves come in several forms, including saturated, polyunsaturated, and monounsaturated fats, depending on slight variations in their chemical structures. Despite their slight chemical differences, the variation in their effect on your health is anything but slight. Too much saturated fat is associated with heart disease, hypertension, obesity, and many cancers. Most saturated fats are found in red meats, pork, and dairy products. In pregnancy, you should try to substitute leaner meats, such as chicken and fish, as sources of protein whenever possible. Consider drinking 1 percent low-fat milk instead of whole milk. Do not use real butter, and use margarine and mayonnaise only sparingly. Avoid "trans-fats" whenever possible.

75

Q *I'm particularly worried about cholesterol. We had a program at work to check cholesterol and mine was over 250. Should I try to avoid all fat?*

A It is almost impossible to avoid all fat, and your cholesterol reading may have been falsely elevated by your pregnancy. It is probable that the effects of high estrogen levels on your liver are responsible. However, if you had never before been tested for cholesterol and the reading was over 350, tell your doctor about it right away.

76

Q *I've heard that fish supplies essential fatty acids. What do they do?*

A Fish is not only a good source of protein but also of Omega-3 essential fatty acids. These are necessary for proper development of the fetal nervous system. These compounds may be found in herring, mackerel, salmon, sardines, and tuna. Cod-liver oil is also a rich source, but it should probably be avoided because it contains excessive amounts of vitamin A. (See Question 64.)

77

Q *How much water should I drink? I've heard I should increase my intake.*

A One of the single best and easiest things you can do for your pregnancy is increase your water intake. You should drink at least eight to ten ten-ounce glasses of water per day. Water will avoid dehydration and its potentially dangerous metabolic changes. It will help you avoid preterm labor, constipation, urinary tract infection, excessive edema, and water retention. Water helps to perfuse the uterus and placenta, and allows your body to build the increased blood volume it needs. (See Question 64 & 386 regarding tuna and salmon.)

78

Q *Can I drink alcohol? My friend's doctor says that a glass of wine now and then is no big deal.*

A It probably isn't a big deal. But the operative word here is probably. The official position of both the Food and Drug Administration (FDA) and the American College of Obstetricians and Gynecologists (ACOG) is that no safe level of alcohol has been established.

Alcohol has been associated with fetal alcohol syndrome (FAS), in which the baby is born with an unusual (atypical) facial appearance, and is destined

to develop mental retardation, growth deficiency, and behavioral distur-
bances. It was first described in 1973, but has subsequently been confirmed
by many other studies. Data is inconclusive about the effects of one to two
alcoholic drinks a day. Even women who drink more than six drinks of hard
liquor a day are only at a 40 percent risk of their fetus developing FAS.[6]

Many Europeans recommend a glass of wine per day throughout gestation after the first trimester. In the United States, preterm labor was once
treated with intravenous alcohol right through the late 1970s. Alcohol consumed prior to six weeks of gestation, when you might not know that you are
pregnant, is extremely unlikely to cause birth defects in the fetus.

However, the fact remains, that no safe minimal level of alcohol consumption is known. The best advice is to *avoid alcohol completely* during
your pregnancy.

79

Q *What guidelines should I follow regarding minerals and iron?*

A Despite what you hear about calcium, magnesium, phosphorous, zinc,
copper, selenium, chromium, manganese, and fluoride, evidence for taking supplements during pregnancy exists only in the case of iron.[7]

Supplemental iron is never necessary in the first twenty weeks of pregnancy unless you are already anemic, since it may increase morning sickness
symptoms and constipation. Even those who find little value to added iron
now agree that some supplemental iron beyond twenty-eight weeks is probably appropriate. As little as 30 milligrams of elemental iron per day, in the
form of ferrous fumarate (easier on the stomach than other forms of iron),
ferrous sulfate, or ferrous gluconate, may add up to 500 cubic centimeters of
blood volume by the end of pregnancy.

Ask your doctor if you need supplemental iron in addition to what is in
your diet and prenatal vitamin. The single most important factor in determining this will be your starting blood count. Women with hemoglobin
(Hgb) readings starting higher than fourteen or hematocrit (Hct) readings
starting higher than thirty-eight rarely require much additional iron. You will
usually not acquire iron-deficiency anemia, since you don't menstruate during pregnancy, and you get to keep all the dietary iron and the iron in your
prenatal vitamin.

Your doctor may wish to tailor your supplemental iron consumption to
your ability to tolerate the extra iron, your starting blood count, and your
diet. Excellent sources of dietary iron are red meats, spinach, veal, poultry,
soybeans, fish, nuts, baked beans, egg yolks, and dried fruits such as apricots,
peaches, and prunes.

80

Q *Do I need to take calcium supplements?*

A There is little or no evidence that supplementation of calcium is of any benefit in pregnancy.[8] If desired, cheap forms of supplemental calcium, such as calcium TUMS, are adequate. While these are possibly slightly less well absorbed than expensive calcium supplements, this antacid form helps treat the heartburn that is common during pregnancy. Most prenatal vitamins have calcium in them and the citrate forms are best absorbed. The 1200 mg of calcium required in pregnancy (see Appendix A) however, is largely obtained in any diet containing two servings of a dairy product. (See Question 63.)

81

Q *Is iodine safe?*

A Commercially available salt in the United States is nearly all iodized and its use is recommended for pregnant women. Severe iodine deficiency leads to cretinism, a condition with mental retardation and multiple neurological defects. With large amounts of seaweed in the diet, too much iodide may be ingested, depressing thyroid function and leading to a goiter in the fetus. Avoid any commercial iodide supplement other than that in iodized salt.

82

Q *I've heard that salt isn't good for you in pregnancy. What about sodium?*

A Sodium is salt. There is no current evidence that rigorous restriction of salt is beneficial. Some recent evidence even suggests that restriction may be harmful. Either adding no salt to food after cooking, or only salting lightly to taste is reasonable. Sodium deficiency, like potassium deficiency, is seen only when diuretics are used. The use of diuretics in pregnancy, at least in the United States, has essentially ceased and is not currently recommended. (See Section 5: Antihypertensives and Diuretics)

83

Q *I'm confused about all the vitamins people recommend. What do I actually need?*

A The routine use of prenatal vitamins is widespread in the United States, yet there is almost no evidence to support their beneficial effect.[9] (See Appendix A: Dietary Allowances)

Humans have lived about eighty thousand years without vitamin supplementation, and despite our "Quarter Pounder with cheese and fries" mentality, we are still the best-nourished society to date. Therefore, it is difficult to demonstrate the benefit of additional vitamins in a normal, non-anemic, non-malnourished individual. Folate supplementation is probably the only exception as mentioned earlier to help decrease the incidence of spin a bifida. Newer formulations of vitamins since 2009 often contain docosahexaenoic acid (DHA) derived from micro-algae, or other sources of omega-3, to aid in neural development, but evidence of clinical significance is weak. Certain vitamins may in fact be dangerous to supplement. Vitamin A, for instance, should never exceed about 5,000 IU (international units) per day. Levels of as little as 50,000 IU have been associated with birth defects similar to those of the Vitamin A derivative for acne called Accutane. Taken in as little as ten times the Recommended Daily Allowances, vitamins B6, C, and D, as well as iron, zinc, and selenium may all be toxic.

84

Q *Why is folic acid considered to be essential?*

A The addition of folate, also called folic acid, has been clearly shown to be of benefit. One milligram of folate daily will prevent a type of anemia known as megaloblastic anemia, as well as statistically reduce the chances of neural tube defects such as spina bifida, if taken from conception through six weeks.

The actual recommended daily requirements of folate increase from 0.4 milligrams to 0.8 milligrams during pregnancy. Good dietary sources of folate (from the Latin word folium, meaning "leaf") include the leafy green vegetables such as spinach, romaine lettuce, broccoli, Brussels sprouts, and asparagus. Folate is found in all prenatal vitamins, but may be supplemented with 1-milligram tablets if your doctor suggests it.

85

Q *My mother said she got vitamin B12 shots when she was pregnant. Is that still done?*

A Vitamin B12 does not need to be supplemented in anyone with an adequate intake of animal protein, except for the extremely rare patient with pernicious anemia. While vegetarians may have a slight B12 deficiency, it is significant only after birth, when infants who are breast-fed by vegetarians may develop a clinically significant deficiency of this vitamin.

86

Q *I was taking vitamin B6 for PMS before I got pregnant. Do I need to continue in pregnancy?*

A Vitamin B6 should not be supplemented. The tiny increase required (See Appendix A: Dietary Allowances) is more than adequately handled by the normal caloric intake. Overdosage of vitamin B6 can even lead to neurotoxicity. Some investigators used to think that B6 helped to correct abnormal glucose tolerance in pregnancy, but this has been disproved.

87

Q *How much vitamin C do I need?*

A Doctors recommend a total of 80 milligrams of vitamin C during pregnancy. While this is one-third more than is normally recommended, it is much less than the usual dietary amount consumed.

88

Q *If I adhere to these dietary guidelines, how much weight should I gain?*

A Recommendations on weight gain have changed dramatically over the past century. Where women were once told to keep weight gain under twenty pounds, they were also told in later years that no restrictions were necessary. Neither of these recommendations is probably correct.

If you are of normal body weight with a Body Mass Index (BMI) of 20 to 26 (see Appendix B: Body Mass Index), you should aim for a weight gain of about twenty-five to thirty-five pounds, with an average monthly increase of about four pounds. If you are markedly obese, with a BMI greater than 30, you may need to gain as little as fifteen pounds. If you are very underweight, with a BMI less than 19, you should try to gain twenty-eight to forty pounds.

89

Q *I'm carrying twins. What should my normal weight gain be if I started my pregnancy at a normal weight for my height?*

A (See Section 8: Multiple Gestations)
Most doctors would recommend that you gain a total of about thirty-five to forty-five pounds, with an average monthly increase of about six pounds, after the second month.

90

Q *How do I know when I'm gaining too much weight?*

A In the first trimester, you may gain anything from no weight to about six pounds, or you may even lose several pounds. From twelve to twenty weeks you will generally gain weight much more rapidly, often putting on about six to ten pounds as you retain water to expand your blood volume. Finally, from twenty weeks on, you should gain about three to four pounds per month until delivery, with an average increase of one pound a week. Sometimes you may experience a final period of rapid weight gain within three to four weeks of delivery as your swelling gets worse. Gaining more than three pounds in a week during this time period often means the presence of preeclampsia or toxemia. (See Section 8: Preeclampsia)

91

Q *How is my weight gain normally distributed?*

A Optimally, your weight gain will be distributed as follows: about one to two pounds in your breasts, three pounds in your blood volume, eleven to twelve pounds in amniotic fluid, placenta, and baby combined, and six to seven pounds in fat. Your uterus itself adds another two pounds and extracellular water retention adds about three to four pounds.

92

Q *If I'm being careful about what I eat, staying away from excess fat and sweets, and have increased my caloric intake by only about three hundred calories per day or less, why am I still gaining too much weight?*

A It's the same of answer whether you're pregnant or not. . . EXERCISE! In our sedentary society, many people sit at a desk or computer terminal all day. You should exercise in a vigorous aerobic fashion for at least twenty minutes at least four times a week, but work up to it gradually if you have been getting little or no exercise until now.

ACTIVITY & EXERCISE

93

Q *Are there activities I should avoid in the first trimester?*

A Very few. Scuba diving, water-skiing, and skydiving are forbidden because of the possibility of serious injury, or even death. Otherwise, essentially all exercises, including jogging, stair-climbing, swimming, NordicTrack, Power/Health Riders, and sex are permissible. None of these activities is associated with miscarriage in a normal pregnancy. Remember, God designed the pregnant women to run away from saber-toothed tigers. (Not archaeologically correct, but you get my drift!)

However, for fear of being sued, most amusement parks will post warnings forbidding pregnant women to participate in any rides in which the force of gravity is increased by dropping or rapidly turning. Avoiding these is a good idea anyway, since they may increase your propensity to vomit.

94

Q *Should I be exercising in the first trimester? I'm exhausted!*

A Most women in the first trimester want to sleep for two hours in the morning and two hours in the afternoon. They are wiped out. How could that little 20-millimeter fetus be sapping all that energy? It isn't. Your cardiovascular changes are getting you down. Your heart is the most active muscle in your body. By ten weeks of gestation, your cardiac output has increased by 15 percent. By twenty-eight weeks it has risen from five liters per minute to over seven liters per minute, an increase of 40 percent. That requires huge amounts of energy.

Somehow your body accommodates and your energy levels improve markedly by about fourteen weeks. You should then gradually return to exercise if you had stopped for reasons such as fatigue or nausea.

95

Q *Is it true that I need to limit the amount I exercise in pregnancy and avoid getting my pulse over 140?*

A In general, you do not have to exercise within a certain pulse limit as long as you avoid exhaustion (such as heat prostration), dehydration, and activities that could cause direct trauma to your abdomen.

If you accepted a pulse limit of 140, you'd never make it up a single flight of stairs at eleven weeks. It is probably reasonable, however, to not exceed a pulse of 140 for more than thirty minutes or so.[10]

96

Q *I've heard fetuses do better with less oxygen than we do. Is that true?*

A Fetuses have a special type of hemoglobin in their red blood cells, called fetal hemoglobin, that holds on to oxygen much more tightly than an adult's red blood cells. This gives the fetus tremendous tolerance for low oxygen percentages at the placental interface. (See Section 4: Blood) Even if some small degree of oxygenated blood shifted away from the uterus, there is no evidence to support brief periods of this adversely affecting fetal outcome.

If you performed regular aerobic exercise prior to pregnancy you should continue to do so when pregnant. If you were sedentary (sat around a lot), exercise in pregnancy should consist primarily of walking or swimming, with a very gradual increase in aerobic demand.[11]

97

Q *I've read that I'm not supposed to exercise lying on my back, or even sleep on my back. My Lamaze teacher agrees. Is lying on my back a poor idea?*

A Not really. Many people have misinterpreted basic science data. It is safe for most women experiencing normal pregnancies to lie on their back for exercise or for sleep.

In the late 1970s, several researchers suspended inverted pregnant ewes, among other animals, for their entire gestations. When the lambs were born, they had significant problems, and were smaller than usual. From this, the lay press concluded that lying on your back was clearly detrimental to the fetus's health.

In about 5 percent of pregnant women, blood pressure drops significantly when lying in the supine position. These patients also break into a cold sweat, get nauseous, and automatically roll onto their side. In fact, when these women experience a drop in blood pressure after rolling onto their back during sleep, they automatically roll onto their side in minutes without awakening.

Big surprise! God thought of this before the guys with the sheep! It seems unlikely that women throughout history avoided this position when it was often the most comfortable one for their aching back and hips.

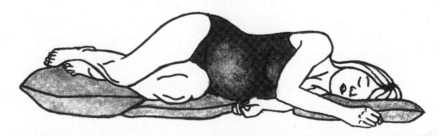

98

Q *Can I feel free to lie on my back as much as I want?*

A Not quite. It is true that the large pregnant uterus tends to compress the inferior vena cava (IVC), which returns blood to the heart from the lower body. If the supine position were chosen all the time, this could certainly contribute to sluggish blood flow in the legs, possibly worsening edema, hemorrhoids, and varicosities.

After twenty-five weeks of gestation, it is probably a good idea to purposefully avoid the supine position when you go to sleep. Use pillows behind your back and between your knees to support yourself while lying on your side. The left side is only marginally better than the right, and should be emphasized only for women whose baby is growing too slowly or who have blood pressure problems. Don't be alarmed if you wake up on your back. There is no evidence to suggest that you could have hurt your fetus. If sleeping on your back causes no symptoms, you don't have blood pressure issues or multiples, and it is the only position in which you are comfortable, sleep on your back.

99

Q *Is lying on my side sometimes necessary?*

A In conditions of poor fetal growth (intrauterine growth restriction, or IUGR) or with twins, lying on the side will increase cardiac output and thus increase the flow of nutrients to the fetus. In preeclampsia, lying on the side is a must. This position reduces blood pressure; it also increases blood and oxygen to the uterus and thus to the fetus and the kidneys. (See Section 8: Preeclampsia) If you have spinal anesthesia, the supine position also makes the drop in blood pressure greater, and care should be taken after the placement of this type of regional block. A blood pressure drop with epidurals may occur as well, but it is usually less severe and more easily treated.

100

Q *What are the generally accepted guidelines for exercise in pregnancy?*

A ACOG exercise guidelines are briefly paraphrased with additions below:[12]

1.   Regular exercise done at least three times per week is better than sporadic exercise.

2. Avoid aerobic exercise when you have a cold or the flu, and when the weather is extremely hot and humid.

3. Avoid straight leg raises, toe touching with legs straight, sit-ups without bending your knees, and deep knee bends, since all of these may injure the back in pregnancy.

4. You may exercise lying on your back if it doesn't make you nauseous or light-headed, but you should avoid the supine position for prolonged periods after twenty weeks.*

5. Use a five-minute warm-up before brisk exercise; a heavy aerobic workout should not last more than fifteen to twenty minutes.

6. Discuss peak heart rates with your doctor and follow his or her advice.

7. Always arise slowly from the floor and walk in place briefly once you are upright so that you minimize the possibility of dizziness or fainting.

8. Drink water often before and after exercise. Avoid dehydration by stopping heavy exercise when you feel thirsty.

9. If you did not exercise before pregnancy, work up to it slowly while pregnant.

10. Stop your routine if you experience vaginal bleeding, palpitations, severe back pain, extreme shortness of breath, pubic bone pain, very rapid heart beat with shortness of breath, fainting, or difficulty walking. Call and discuss what happened with your doctor.

11. Almost any form of exercise is safe if done in moderation. Some exercises are good for the heart and lungs, others for muscle tone and endurance. Pregnancy causes body changes that alter your ability to balance, which may require modification of your non-pregnant routines.

Walking is always a good choice, especially if you were not active before pregnancy.

Swimming is excellent for your body because it uses all your muscles while the water supports your weight. Do not dive in the latter months of pregnancy. Scuba diving is forbidden.*

Jogging can be done in moderation if you were used to it before pregnancy. Avoid overheating and stop before becoming overly tired. Drink a lot of water before you exercise to replace what you will lose in sweat.

Tennis is generally safe if you were used to playing before pregnancy, but be aware of your change in balance and how it affects rapid movements.

Golf and bowling are fine for fun, but do little to strengthen heart and lungs. With either of these sports, be careful to adjust your balance.

Snow skiing, water-skiing, and surfing pose some risk. You may hit the ground or water with great force and potentially hurt the fetus; you can definitely hurt yourself. Before doing these sports, speak with your doctor.*

Horseback riding is fine if you are an accomplished rider and on your own mount. There is no reason why you cannot ride through twenty-four weeks or so. As in other potentially dangerous sports, being thrown poses a risk primarily to your health, and thus to that of the fetus.* [*author additions]

101

Q *Can I continue with my weight training?*

A Weight training may certainly be continued in pregnancy if it was part of your normal exercise routine when you were not pregnant. The key concept is to avoid low back strain. Any exercises that involve bending with legs straight should be omitted. Wrist and ankle weights may be continued throughout. After twenty weeks, it is prudent to consider gradually diminishing weight routines that work the lower abdominal muscles and low back.

Exercises to strengthen the lower back, like *pelvic tilts* are described in this section: Back Pain.

102

Q *Are there certain conditions in which I have to avoid exercise?*

A High blood pressure, either chronic or as preeclampsia, may be reason for your doctor to modify or eliminate your exercise. Undiagnosed bleeding at any week of gestation, placenta previa, incompetent cervix, premature rupture of membranes, and current preterm labor are always reasons to not exercise.

103

Q *Can I exercise with twins?*

A (See also Section 8: Multiple Gestations)
Yes. Exercise guidelines are no different through 20 weeks with twins than they are for singletons. After about twenty to twenty-four weeks different doctors differ in the amount of restriction they think is appropriate. Data

has never been convincing, for instance, that preventive bed rest while carrying twins prevents preterm labor. Many women pregnant with twins may continue to walk and, particularly, swim even beyond 34 weeks. Seek your doctor's advice.

TRAVEL

104

Q *How will pregnancy affect my travel plans?*

A There is no evidence that travel itself is detrimental to the normal pregnancy.[13] Travel by car or in a pressurized aircraft poses no danger. No matter the means of travel, get up and walk briefly every hour, and remember to wear your seat belt. Avoid travel until after ten weeks, when the risk of miscarriage is significantly reduced, or at least be aware that the 15 percent miscarriage rate still applies even if you're lying on a beach in the Caribbean! You may travel anywhere you like up until the twenty-seventh or twenty-eighth week; after that we recommend only travel to cities with populations greater than 100,000. Cities of at least this size are likely to have an NICU with ventilator capacity adequate to stabilize a preemie prior to transport if necessary.

Be sure to bring a copy of your most recently updated prenatal record with you. Your doctor will be glad to provide it. In any case, you should keep one in your purse at all times.

105

Q *Do airlines have restrictions for pregnant women?*

A Most airlines will not let you fly after thirty-five weeks in the absence of an emergency and a release from your doctor. Flight attendants normally have to drop off flight status at twenty-eight weeks.

106

Q *How should I take care of myself during driving trips?*

A Whenever you drive, stop and walk around briefly every hour or so. Prolonged sitting, whether at work or in a car, decreases blood return to your heart and may decrease your blood pressure to the point of feeling faint. The enlarged uterus compresses the large central vein in your abdomen called the inferior vena cava (IVC). Sitting further decreases blood return by putting a 90-degree kink in both your femoral veins at the crease of your leg.

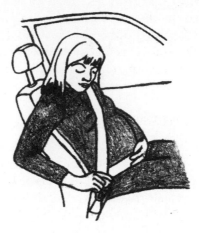

Prolonged sitting may also worsen varicosities, hemorrhoids, and swelling in your lower legs, which is why driving trips should be interrupted at least every hour for a few minutes.

107

Q *We were planning on going to the mountains for Christmas. Is altitude a problem in pregnancy?*

A High altitude doesn't have to be a problem if you plan carefully. As long as your destination is less than 8,500 to 9,000 feet, you are unlikely to encounter problems with the pregnancy or with altitude sickness. About seventy-two hours at that altitude is needed to acclimate before attempting brief trips to higher altitudes. Limiting the amount of time during which you hike above 9,000 feet to less than several hours is a prudent decision to avoid nausea, vomiting, cramping, shortness of breath, and peripheral swelling of your extremities.

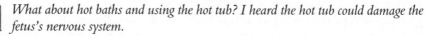

BATHING

108

Q *What about hot baths and using the hot tub? I heard the hot tub could damage the fetus's nervous system.*

Avoiding increases in core body temperature from confirmation of pregnancy until about ten weeks is a good idea. That means a drug such as Tylenol to get the fever down if you have the flu, but also avoiding hot tubs, very hot baths, and saunas. After ten weeks, a hot bath or tub is fine, but try to keep the thermostat no warmer than 102 degrees Fahrenheit. Also, be careful getting out of a warm bath, because the warm water tends to dilate peripheral veins and you could feel faint if you stand too quickly. Remember that your center of gravity may be altered as well, so hold on to something stable, like your husband, in case you slip on something wet.

It's okay, live a little! You deserve the quiet for a few moments, and the muscle-soothing qualities of a warm bath will feel wonderful. Not to mention the fact that after about thirty weeks no water from the shower is likely to see the underside of your tummy!

SEX

109

Is lovemaking safe during pregnancy?

You bet! Historically sex has continued virtually unabated despite pregnancy. Only in the presence of a threatened miscarriage, placenta previa, premature rupture of the membranes, threatened preterm labor, or pre-eclampsia can sex really be said to be contraindicated.

110

I'm more interested in sex than I've ever been, but my husband has to be threatened at gunpoint! Is there something wrong with him?

The sex drive of both partners can change in either direction and be perfectly normal. Many women find a marked increase in libido as pregnancy progresses. You may get more and more interested in lovemaking even as wearing your sexiest nightgown becomes either impossible or laughable, and your belly gets so huge that just the thought of making love is uncomfortable.

On the other hand, some women find themselves so unattractive during pregnancy that they translate this into a reticence to have sex.

But it is often the man who worries that he may injure the fetus during sex. Reassure him that even vigorous sex has never been associated with damage to the fetus.

You may be surprised to learn that your husband finds your enlarged breasts, growing tummy, and rounded posterior more alluring than ever. If he understands that he won't hurt the baby, and also respects your desires, then sex during pregnancy can be lots of fun. In the later weeks, just finding a position that's humanly possible can be worth a lot of intimate chuckles.

111

Q *My friends have told me that sex hurts when you're pregnant. Why is that?*

A Sex can hurt during pregnancy, but you can minimize or eliminate the pain with a little effort. Due to the changes imparted by huge elevations in estrogen and progesterone, the vagina does not respond to sexual excitation with elongation and lubrication as it does in the nonpregnant state. The vagina, labia, clitoris, and perineum engorge with blood rapidly after the first trimester. A lubricant such as Astroglide or Vagisil Intimate Moisturizer can be immensely helpful.

Rarely, deep pain with intercourse can occur if you've had several babies before and your uterus is prolapsing, or hanging very low in the vagina. Your husband might also have a little pain when he gets vigorous. This can be avoided by position changes; for example, he can lie behind you with both of you on your sides. With your legs together after penetration, he won't be able to go nearly as deep.

112

Q *Are there circumstances where sex is a bad idea in pregnancy?*

A It's never a bad idea, but there are times when you should keep it in the realm of the imagination only. If you have a placenta previa, sex can be dangerous. Placenta previa occurs when the placenta implants over or partially over the opening to the cervix. (See Section 8: Placenta Previa) Sex, and not just intercourse, but any activity that brings about orgasm, could lead to an uncontrolled hemorrhage. This may be due to direct contact with the cervix or due to the uterine contractions that accompany orgasm. If the condition persists to term, vaginal delivery is not possible. Most partial previas resolve by about twenty-eight weeks and can be reevaluated by another ultrasound examination at that time.

Sex may also be forbidden by your doctor after about twenty-four weeks if you are either being treated for preterm labor, or are at high risk for it. This would include women with multiple gestations, women with previous histories of premature rupture of the membranes, and/or premature delivery with an earlier pregnancy. (See Section 8: Preterm labor)

Sex is also contraindicated with rupture of the membranes, and relatively contraindicated in the presence of severe preeclampsia. In all these circumstances your husband will become familiar with the "Coyote Syndrome" where your mate learns to sit outside the cave and howl.

113

Q *Is sex ever indicated as the right thing to do?*

A Sex is actually helpful in the last couple weeks of gestation because the prostaglandin in semen helps promote uterine contractions. Orgasm will also precipitate contractions and help bring on labor. Of course, you should make sure to check with your doctor.

114

Q *Is oral sex safe during pregnancy?*

A We would say that oral sex (cunnilingus) is probably fine as long as air under pressure is not introduced into the vagina. Believe it or not, deaths have been reported due to air emboli, which can occur when air is blown into the vaginas of some pregnant women. Just as water-skiing can produce a fatal embolus with water, so can oral sex with air. This is because the placenta sits in large lakes of maternal venous blood. Air forced into these large open veins goes directly back to the heart and then into the lungs, where it blocks gas exchange, leading to death as surely as a large blood clot would.

Fellatio, on the other hand is not only safe, but may help to relieve your husband's sexual frustration if for one reason or another intercourse is contraindicated.

MATERNITY CLOTHING

115

Q *Are there any special types of maternity clothes I should consider?*

A Style is a matter of personal choice, but whatever style of maternity clothing you choose, it should be as nonconstricting and comfortable as possible.

The increasingly heavy, pendulous nature of enlarging breasts may also lead to discomfort when exercising, sleeping, hugging, or at anytime. Wear a good, well-fitting support bra of the appropriate cup size.

Avoid wearing tight calf-or thigh-length hose or socks, since these garments decrease blood return, worsen swelling and varicose veins, and increase the possibility of clotting.

Avoid wearing high heels beyond twenty weeks because the increased sway this puts in your back can lead to imbalance and falls.

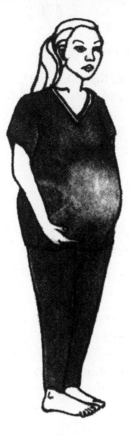

116

Q *Will I need maternity girdles and back supports?*

A Because the enlarging uterus tends to move the center of gravity forward, women compensate by altering their posture, using their large back muscles to lean the upper half of the torso rearward. (You may know this as duck-waddling.) This change in posture puts strain on the back, and wearing a support belt made of stretchy material with a Velcro closure, such as the Belly Bra, may help considerably.

Women who find a belly bra inadequate may prefer a full maternity girdle with over-the-shoulder and crotch support. The girdle supports the back, lifts the belly, takes some pressure off the pubic area, and can improve vulvar varicose veins.

117

Q *Do I have to wear those maternity panties that go up over my tummy?*

A No, you don't have to wear them, but comfort may win out over style. Most women find the loose fit and soft cotton over their enlarging abdomen preferable to bikini or thong panties. But everyone is different and some women do feel better with low-rise panties where the front edge of the panty rides below and not over their pregnant bellies.

The only important consideration is that maternity panties need to have a cotton crotch, since vaginal yeast infections may be more common in pregnancy, and their incidence can be decreased by anything that tends to keep the vulvar area cool and dry.

118

Q *I'm concerned about another aspect of my appearance. Why do friends keep telling me I look too small?*

A Looking small for your gestational age is a common occurrence, especially when your friends have already had children, and you're having your first. Assuming your uterus measures correctly in the office when lying down (fundal height), the answer is easy. You've just got better abdominal muscles than they do. The first baby stretches the rectus muscles on some women (see diastasis recti) and, because the uterus falls forward, they look huge with subsequent babies. This is somewhat dependent on the curvature of your lumbar spine as well, but it is largely good abs that hold the uterus in the body when you stand, giving you the appearance of being too small.

PHYSICAL CHANGES AND COMPLAINTS

Fatigue

119

Q *I feel so tired. How can I help myself feel better?*

A Fatigue is normal and particularly marked in the first and early second trimesters. The hormonal changes associated with pregnancy that lead to massively increased cardiac output are probably responsible. By ten to twelve weeks your heart may be pumping an extra liter of blood per minute. This, combined with the huge energy requirements of enlarging the uterine muscle, just flat out make you tired!

This fatigue seems to improve markedly by fourteen to sixteen weeks in almost everyone. If it continues or worsens after this time, discuss it with your doctor, who may test your thyroid and bone marrow function.

Get as much rest as you can. It's easy to say and hard to do. In today's society where over half the workforce is female, many of you will find yourselves working full time, at least at the beginning of your pregnancy. If you are exhausted, you need to rest. If that means a midafternoon nap, take one for thirty to forty-five minutes. If your employer objects, ask your doctor to step in on your behalf. You must listen to your body and rest when you need it.

Uterus and Ovaries

120

Q *How does my uterus change?*

A Uterine growth begins the moment the embryo implants. As the uterus is affected by HCG (the pregnancy hormone) and rising levels of estrogen and progesterone, it begins to grow and soften. There is a huge increase in blood supply to the uterus, which continues throughout pregnancy. As your uterus grows it puts pressure first on your bladder and low back, then on your lumbar spine, abdominal wall, and intestines, and finally on your stomach, gallbladder, and liver.

The normal nonpregnant uterus weighs on average about 70 grams, or one-sixth of a pound. At term the uterus weighs about 1,100 grams, or two and one-third pounds. This represents more than a tenfold increase in weight. The size of the uterus, however, grows five hundred to one thousand times its original volume.

Everyone is built slightly differently, but at fourteen to sixteen weeks, the uterus moves up out of the hollow of the sacrum deep in the pelvis, and over the small of your back into the abdomen. At this point you may start "showing," depending upon how much of your own body there is between the skin of your abdomen and the uterus, as well as how much of an inward curve you have in the small of your back. The more indented it is, the more you will show early in your pregnancy.

121

Q *I'm only twelve weeks pregnant, but I feel pressure on my right side. Sometimes it really hurts. Is this my ovary?*

A It certainly could be. If unassociated with nausea, vomiting, or light-headedness, however, it is unlikely to be dangerous. If it persists, or gets severe enough that a simple analgesic, such as Tylenol, is inadequate, call your doctor, who will do a vaginal ultrasound to see what is happening. Often the corpus luteum cyst persists a little longer than it needs to. In other words, despite the fact that the placenta has long ago taken over the task of making progesterone, the dominant cyst from which you ovulated may get a little bigger and last a little longer in some people. Simple ovarian cysts resolve without intervention during the second trimester.

A luteoma of pregnancy, on the other hand, is a rare solid ovarian growth consisting of cells that normally make progesterone after ovulation. This growth may become quite large, up to six centimeters in diameter, but always shrinks after birth. Since it also produces a male hormone, it has been known to cause masculinizing effects, such as male hair growth patterns, in the mother. The fetus, however, is not affected.

122

Q *Do I continue to ovulate in pregnancy?*

A No, you do not. The various hormonal feedback systems to the brain are altered and the luteinizing hormone surge responsible for ovulation at midcycle does not occur. While you do not ovulate in pregnancy, remember that you may ovulate while breast-feeding. There are plenty of parents with children ten months apart to testify to this reality.

Pelvic Pressure

123

Q *Is it normal to feel pressure down low?*

A Your uterus will be growing from the size of a lemon to the size of a watermelon. As this muscle enlarges deep in the pelvis, it pushes on everything it touches, especially the bladder and rectum. As the uterus fills the space deep in the pelvis behind the pubic bone and below the small of your back, you will feel like urinating frequently and may also feel pelvic pressure in the form of constipation. These are normal sensations and get better after fourteen to sixteen weeks, when the uterus moves up into the abdomen and out of the pelvis.

124

Q *The pressure I feel is more intense than it was during my first pregnancy, and I sometimes feel as if everything is going to fall out. Could there be something wrong?*

A Your first pregnancy and childbirth stretched the trampoline-like sling that supports your uterus and bladder. It will not return to its previous state because it is primarily connective tissue, which cannot be toned with exercise. The feeling of something falling out usually diminishes after twenty weeks, when the whole uterus can no longer fall into the pelvis.

This is not uterine prolapse, although it is similar. Usually, when you are no longer pregnant and the added weight of the pregnant uterus is gone, the "falling out" sensation stops. Also, the relaxing hormones from pregnancy, such as progesterone and relaxin, are gone after the baby is born. If by six months after delivery you still feel your cervix and/or bladder pushing against the inside of the labia (vaginal lips), you may have some degree of uterine prolapse or a cystocele. A cystocele occurs when the floor of the bladder, which is the roof of the vagina, expands down into the vagina behind the labia. The expansion may be minimal, or major, in which the cervix or bladder tissue actually hangs out of the vagina. This can be corrected surgically, but surgery should be delayed if at all possible until after childbearing is completed.

Back Pain

125

Q *I'm only at the end of the first trimester and my back already hurts. Is there anything I can do about it?*

A Back pain is one of the most common complaints in pregnancy. Early on, it may be due to pressure of the growing uterus against the sacrum; later, to the change in center of gravity that may cause you to waddle when you walk; still later, to the swelling around the sciatic nerve root as water retention worsens; and finally, to the pressure of the fetus's head against the low back. Low back pain is a problem throughout pregnancy, for different reasons at different times. Upper back pain may develop after twenty weeks. Your shifting center of gravity promotes the "duck waddle" that your well-intentioned husband has no doubt kidded you about. The back muscles necessary to keep you upright and prevent you from pitching forward can get sore from the tops of the hips all the way up to the middle of your back between your shoulder blades. In the late third trimester, direct pressure from the fetus's head can cause low back pain.

Exercises performed daily from the beginning of pregnancy, such as pelvic tilts, can strengthen the back. Tylenol may be used as needed. After the first trimester, a back spasm may be treated with local heat and bed rest on a firm mattress with your knees bent and supported by a pillow. (Lying on your back is usually perfectly safe. See also Question 98.) Occasionally narcotics are justified and may be prescribed for brief periods.

Supports such as maternity girdles or specific items like the Bellybra may be worn to help compensate for the muscular changes required to keep you upright when your pregnant uterus causes your center of gravity to move forward. (See this section: Maternity Clothing)

There are several preventive measures you can take:

1. Practice good body mechanics.
   Bend your knees when you bend over from the waist.
   Keep your back straight; don't lift without squatting.
   Sit upright; don't slump in your chair.
2. Do back exercises each day.

Pelvic tilt exercises: Lie on your back with your knees bent, then flatten the small of your back to the floor and hold for five counts; repeat ten times. Repeat in "all fours" position, with stomach muscles tight and low back rounded. Repeat in a standing position against a real or an imaginary wall.

Back flexion: Lie on your back with your knees bent, then bring one knee to your chest and hold. Release, then repeat with the opposite leg, and finally, repeat with both knees together.

Swelling

126

Q All of a sudden my legs have swollen like crazy! My shoes don't fit and my socks leave impressions on my skin. What's happening?

A Pregnancy leads to a tremendous increase in body fluid volume. By the end of pregnancy, your body will convert much of the water you retain into extra blood, which will be lost at delivery. If you didn't increase your blood volume, normal delivery could cause you to bleed to death.

As your kidneys retain salt and water, your blood vessels are also increasing their capacity to handle the new increase in volume. Unfortunately, the increase in fluid and increase in volume capacity of your circulatory system are not always right in step. Consequently, you may have periods of increased swelling.

Swelling is usually worse in your legs because they are dependant (low to the ground) and because the pregnant uterus falls off the spine in that direction, and so obstructs the veins and lymphatics more on that side. The obstructed blood flow may also cause swollen labia and even hemorrhoids.

To relieve the swelling, drink lots of water, at least 10 ten-ounce glasses per day. Wear support panty hose; avoid thigh-high or knee-high hose, because they constrict blood flow in the middle of your calf or thigh and can actually increase the risk of blood clots. (Properly sized Jobst stockings for severe varicosities are an exception in most cases.)

Avoid standing or sitting still for prolonged periods. Both may decrease blood return to the heart. Be sure and walk around frequently. Only by using the muscles of the calves will blood be pumped back to the heart, decreasing swelling.

Elevating your legs while sitting may be tempting. Don't do it. This worsens things by pressing on the veins in your groin. Elevating your legs while lying on your side, on the other hand, can markedly reduce your swelling.

Later in pregnancy, lying on either side increases blood supply and markedly decreases swelling. In fact, with mild to moderate preeclampsia, just strict bed rest on your side for forty-eight hours can lead to a loss of five to fifteen pounds.

Swelling accompanied by elevation of blood pressure and spilling protein in the urine are signs of preeclampsia. Swelling will usually be more marked in your hands and face in addition to your legs when preeclampsia is present. (See Section 8: Preeclampsia).

Urinary Tract (Bladder and Kidneys)

127

Q *What kind of changes happen to my urinary tract with pregnancy?*

A If you're already pregnant and reading this then you know one of them—it seems like you have to go all the time! Many structural and functional changes occur. Functionally, the kidneys receive more blood flow than normal and make more urine. The glomerular filtration reate (GFR) is a measure of flow through the "glomerulus" or first part of the kidney, and may be increased by as much as 50 percent in pregnancy. The kidneys normally retain increased amounts of salt and water in pregnancy to be converted to increased blood volume. However, with preeclampsia, this can be abnormally exaggerated.

Also, the supine position for prolonged periods late in pregnancy can lead to decreased excretion of salt and water and increased swelling.

The ureters (tubes from kidneys to bladder) both dilate and elongate after midpregnancy. This is thought to be due to compression by the enlarged uterus as well as increased progesterone levels which slow down ureteral motility. Hydroureter, or a dilatation of the ureter as seen on X-ray, is a normal finding of pregnancy.

The bladder, put quite simply, gets bludgeoned during pregnancy. First it is compressed by the uterus as it grows in the pelvis, then later squashed by the presenting part of the fetus in the final weeks. As a result, bladder capacity is diminished and the tendency toward infection is increased. The muscle of the bladder also hypertrophies (thickens) and swells with increased blood supply and partial obstruction of venous and lymphatic return caused by your enlarging uterus.

128

Q *I lose urine every time I cough, laugh, sneeze, jog, or bend over. Is something wrong?*

A The bladder undergoes many of the same physiological changes as the uterus. The muscle hypertrophies (enlarges), becomes hyperemic (engorged with blood), and swells due to blocked venous and lymphatic drainage. This is particularly marked in the last couple months when the bladder is compressed and partially obstructed by the presenting part of the fetus, whether head or breech. In short, the bladder gets squashed, just like most of your other organs. The amount of urine you can hold is lessened, and for reasons not entirely clear, small increases in abdominal pressure, as with the activities you mention above, may lead to loss of urine. This loss is called stress incontinence. The stress incontinence of pregnancy almost always resolves by six weeks after delivery unless there is significant uterine prolapse and/or a cystocele.

Kegel's Exercises in which you mimic halting your urine flow in mid-stream, may help some to prevent loss of urine in late pregnancy and post-partum. To be effective this exercise should be repeated sixty to ninety times per day!

129

Q *I feel like I have to urinate all the time. Is this normal?*

A At first urinary frequency is increased due to the pressure on your bladder caused by your growing uterus and because of your rapidly increasing circulatory volume. Toward the end of pregnancy frequent urination picks up again because of pressure on the bladder by the baby's head. You may find that you now have to get up to urinate many times during the night.

All this urination is normal, but if you develop pain or burning with urination, or blood in your urine, you should alert your doctor. Kidney infections (pyelonephritis) are more common in pregnancy because of the slowed flow of urine from the kidney through the ureter to the bladder. Both pyelonephritis and kidney stones (nephrolithiasis) may precipitate preterm labor and are particularly worrisome for that reason. (See Section 9: Kidneys)

There is a reversal of the normal diurnal (twice daily) peak of urine production by the kidneys starting early in pregnancy. This means that during the day you will tend to accumulate and retain water. Later in pregnancy the reversal will manifest itself as increased lower extremity swelling toward the end of the day. At night the kidney is better perfused, and in response to the greater blood flow, the kidney creates more urine. As a consequence, you have to urinate much more at night (nocturia). This urine will also tend to be less concentrated, looking almost like water, than it was when you were not pregnant. These changes are all normal.

130

Q *I've heard that the doctor will test my urine each visit. Why is that?*

A Urine in pregnancy has traditionally been tested with a dipstick for both proteinuria and glycosuria. Even in pregnancy the normal kidney should not allow protein to escape. Trace protein in urine is usually a simple contaminant from vaginal mucus and is not worrisome. A urine dipstick reading of 2+ protein or more may be a sign of infection or chronic renal disease in early pregnancy, or of preeclampsia (toxemia) in later pregnancy.

Sugar, on the other hand, is commonly spilled in the urine of pregnant women (glycosuria). About 15 percent of all pregnant women will spill sugar in their urine even if their blood levels are normal. In other words, the vast majority of the time, glucose in the urine of a pregnant woman is not a sign of diabetes. The kidney has increased blood flow during this time and it is so increased that the glomerular filtration rate (GFR) exceeds the ability of the tubules (last stage of the process) to reabsorb the sugar before the urine is passed from the kidney to the bladder. For this reason, urine glucose is not appropriate to follow any class of gestational diabetes. (See Section 8: Diabetes)

Abdominal Discomfort

131

Q *I feel pressure in my pelvis and I have to urinate frequently, but I also feel sharp knife-like pains down low on either side from time to time that last only a few minutes. Should I be concerned?*

In all likelihood what you're feeling are called "round ligament pains." There are extensions of the uterine muscle from the corners of the top of the uterus near where the tubes attach (cornua) which then extend out to the pelvic wall near your hips. These "ligaments," about the diameter of your little finger, then traverse under the skin back down the front of your abdomen to insert in your labia on either side of your pubic bone. (The ligaments follow the course of your extended index fingers when you place your hands on your hips.) Because they are not really ligaments, but muscles, they may intermittently contract just like a charley horse in your calf. When this happens in response to the growing uterus, you feel a severe, knife-like pain that may last several minutes, and then be sore for hours.

If pain persists, or is always on the same side, you should contact your doctor. Occasionally pain is from an ovarian cyst, which normally accompanies pregnancy, but which grows excessively large, or twists on itself. In this case, it may, rarely, require surgical treatment. If you still have your appendix and the pain is on your right side, unrelenting, and associated with anorexia, nausea, vomiting, or fever, you may have appendicitis. This does occur in pregnancy, so with the aforementioned symptoms you need to call the doctor.

132

Q *I'm about twenty-three weeks pregnant and I get occasional sharp pains right around my navel. What's going on with that?*

Navel pain is a common complaint and probably related to two things. First, there are large veins below the navel that feed back to the hemorrhoidal veins in the anus and may dilate due to the obstruction of the uterus, just like hemorrhoids. Second, the navel is attached to the bladder by a vestigial (leftover) tube called the urachus. The urachus last functioned when you were an embryo or fetus, but it still has nerves in it and the stretching of the abdominal wall may occasionally cause sharp pains to shoot from your navel down to your pubic bone. These are completely harmless.

Your navel may be starting to stick out, and you wonder if it will remain an "outie" forever. Rest assured that usually the navel returns to its original state after delivery.

133

Q How do I know if any abdominal pain might be more serious than just a usual discomfort of pregnancy?

A Abdominal pain that is persistent and is associated with other symptoms may be more serious. Any abdominal pain associated with fever, nausea, vomiting, tenderness to the touch, vaginal bleeding, or a cessation of fetal movement could be more serious than just round ligaments or navel pain.

Severe abdominal pain in the presence of preeclampsia, for instance, can be very worrisome and related to bleeding from the liver. Abdominal pain associated with vaginal bleeding late in pregnancy could represent a placental separation or abruption.

There are many medical and obstetrical complications which could lead to abdominal pain, but they rarely cause abdominal pain alone as an isolated symptom. (See Section 8: Obstetric Complications; Section 9: Medical Complications)

Constipation and Other Gastrointestinal Complaints

134

Q What is my GI tract?

A The gastrointestinal (GI) tract includes not only the small and large intestines, but also all the organs that are involved with eating and digestion. The mouth, esophagus, stomach, small bowel, gallbladder, pancreas, liver, large bowel, and rectum are all parts of the GI tract.

Quite a lot changes in your GI tract during pregnancy. Like everything else, the GI tract is also compressed by your uterus This mass effect combined with smooth muscle relaxation caused by progesterone leads to the common complaint of constipation. The relaxation of smooth muscle may also be the culprit with the increased rates of heartburn seen at all stages of pregnancy, as stomach acid gets washed up through the relaxed esophageal sphincter into the lower esophagus.

The gallbladder as well becomes less active in pregnancy. Its output is sluggish and it contracts poorly. This, combined with cholesterol saturation of the gall fluid known to occur in pregnancy, leads to a much increased incidence of gallstones (cholelithiasis).

The liver undergoes functional change as well. Most notably, the liver enzymes normally tested in the blood rise and may be confused with other hepatic (liver) disease. Alkaline phosphatase (AlkPhos) in particular rises by 100 percent, probably due to the action of enzymes made by the placenta.

Serum triglycerides are increased and cholesterol is usually doubled. Total serum albumin is decreased.

Changes occur top to bottom as demonstrated by the references to Gums and Hemorrhoids discussed elsewhere.

135

Q *What is heartburn?*

A Heartburn, or acid reflux, is a very common symptom in pregnancy. Several factors are involved, including compression of the stomach by the enlarging uterus, slowing of gastric emptying time, and relaxation of the muscular sphincter between the stomach and the esophagus. Hydrochloric acid from the stomach then washes into the lower esophagus and injures the lining there. The pain occurs in the midchest right behind the breastbone—hence the reference to the heart.

Preventive measures include eating small frequent meals, avoiding fatty foods, avoiding ice-cold, very hot, or carbonated drinks. Regular use of antacids such as Mylanta liquid or pure calcium TUMS can be helpful. However, to be effective, antacids should be used about half an hour before meals and before bedtime. The histamine blockers cimetidine (Tagamet) and ranitidine (Zantac 75) may be used in their over-the-counter doses each night after the first trimester, with excellent results in some women. Sleeping with the head of the mattress slightly elevated by placing a couch pillow between the box springs and the mattress may be helpful as well.

136

Q *I've heard my bowels may change in pregnancy. Will I get constipated?*

A Bowel movements do become more irregular in pregnancy. Pressure from the enlarging uterus combined with relaxation of the smooth muscle that controls intestinal motility may lead to intermittent hard stools or longer periods between bowel movements than you are used to. Drinking lots of fluids (for example, more than ten ten-ounce glasses of water per day), and consuming more fiber, such as wheat, barley, and oat cereal, or taking two to eight Fibercon capsules per day, will help.

Not all women have trouble with constipation, but many do. In some it could be due to higher progesterone levels and slowed bowel motility. Exercise, large amounts of fluid intake, a high-fiber diet, or supplementation with Fibercon capsules or Metamucil, and use of stool softeners such as Colace and Surfac from time to time usually proves adequate. Occasionally, iron supplements may make constipation worse. You should cut back on the iron for a period of a week or so, or switch to another kind of iron, such as ferrous gluconate to ferrous fumarate. Milk of magnesia or prune juice may be used as a laxative if necessary. Harsher laxatives (cathartics), possibly contributing to preterm labor, are discouraged.

137

Q *Can I expect to get hemorrhoids?*

A Hemorrhoids commonly accompany pregnancy even in the absence of constipation. The gravid uterus by definition increases pressure in the intra-abdominal cavity and obstructs the flow of blood through veins back to the heart. The veins in the anus are weak-walled and tend to dilate with this relative obstruction of blood flow, thus creating a hemorrhoid. Constipation and hard stools may also cause them to rupture from time to time with bright red rectal bleeding. This is not dangerous, but it is inconvenient and sometimes painful.

Use medicated wipes such as Rantex or flushable baby wipes instead of toilet paper routinely. Be sure to drink lots of water and add fiber to your diet. Other creams such as Tronolane and Anusol may be of help, so speak to your doctor.

You may develop a thrombosed hemorrhoid. "Thrombosed" refers to a blood clot. When the blood flow in a hemorrhoid becomes so slow that the blood clots, you have a thrombosed hemorrhoid, which can be very painful. Sitz baths in hot water may help these resolve, but occasionally they require the doctor to open them with a knife to remove the clot. This is done under local anesthesia and is usually more humiliating than painful.

138

Q *I have tremendous amounts of saliva, so much that I have difficulty swallowing it all. What is going on?*

A This is a relatively rare condition referred to as ptyalism. In less than 10 percent of women excessive salivation seems to be stimulated by ingestion of starches. Try to identify starches in your diet and eliminate them if possible.

139

Q *I've been craving really odd things to eat. I've even found myself actually eating potting soil, clay in the backyard, and laundry starch. Why would these appeal to me?*

A You have a rare condition called pica. Some data has suggested that your problem may be linked to severe iron deficiency, but iron replacement does not always solve the problem and some women with pica are clearly not iron-deficient. There is no specific treatment for this condition other than measures to avoid severe constipation and possible fecal impaction. Large amounts of water should be ingested and stool softeners such as Colace used if necessary. This does not appear to be a psychological disorder, but a poorly understood physical one.

Vaginal Hygiene and Discharge

140

Q *I feel "bigger" in my lower pelvis. Is that normal?*

A Absolutely. A huge increase in blood flow to the pelvic organs including the vagina and perineum (space between vagina and anus) occur with pregnancy. The lining of the vagina becomes more vascular, thicker, and the connective tissue loosens. Smooth muscle in the walls hypertrophy (enlarge) as well. Veins in the labia (inner and outer vaginal lips) may become engorged as the blood and lymphatic return to the heart is obstructed by the growing soccer ball in your pelvis.

All this combines to create a normal feeling of fullness. It's also why you should use a good sexual lubricant such as Astroglide, Vagisil Intimate Moisturizer, or liquid K-Y for intercourse during pregnancy.

141

Q *I've heard that douching is bad for you, but I seem to have much more discharge than usual. Is it safe to douche in pregnancy?*

A Increased vaginal discharge is a normal result of the physical changes of pregnancy. However, a vinegar-and-water douche can be used gently from time to time if the nozzle is not inserted more than about three inches. Avoid bulb syringes, which could introduce air under pressure.

142

Q *I know my vaginal discharge is supposed to increase in pregnancy, but now there's a foul odor and some itching. What should I do?*

A The normal physiologic increase in discharge is primarily cervical mucus and should be clear to whitish. A yellow-green vaginal discharge, especially if accompanied by vaginal odor and itching may indicate infection with Gardnerella or Trichomonas, and you should mention it to your doctor. A thick whitish discharge with little odor but intense vaginal itching may indicate a yeast infection such as Candida albicans or Torulopsis. (See Section 9: Infections)

Hair

143

Q *I have a friend who is losing her hair by the handful, and she just had her baby. Is this common?*

A During pregnancy, hormonal changes convert more hair follicles into anagen, or growing hairs, as compared to telogen, or resting hairs. As a result, hair may seem more luxuriant in pregnancy. However, one to four months after pregnancy, the anagen/telogen ratio (called telogen effluvium) is often reversed, and as a disproportionate number of hairs enter the resting phase there are fewer ones to replace the ones that fall out naturally. Some women lose virtually all their hair, but the hair loss is temporary and the hair always grows back in six to twelve months.

144

Q *I'm twenty-five weeks pregnant and have dark hair growing on my face arid abdomen. Is something wrong?*

A Mild hirsutism occurs frequently in pregnancy. It is more noticeable on darker women of Mediterranean descent and is not dangerous in any way. Moles enlarge and darken, which is also considered to be a hormonal phenomenon. Very rarely, tremendous excessive hair growth can be due to a tumor on the adrenal gland or in the ovary. Simple blood tests can rule out the more severe problems.

145

Q *Is it okay for me to color my hair or get a perm during pregnancy?*

A (See Section 5: Drugs in Pregnancy)
Hair coloring has not been associated with birth defects in any study. The chemicals contained in hair dyes have also never been studied under controlled conditions in pregnant women. Therefore, it would be wise to avoid coloring your hair in the first trimester. Vegetable products such as henna are always safe. Highlighting is probably safe in any trimester.

Permanents should probably be avoided in the first trimester. While, like hair coloring, permanents have never been associated with birth defects, it is a good idea to wait beyond the time of the fetus's internal organ formation at ten weeks.

Skin

146

Q *What cart I do to avoid stretch marks?*

A Don't get pregnant! Stretch marks (striae gravidarum) are hereditary to some extent, and if you are destined to get them, you will get them, no matter what advertising claims you may read. About 50 percent of pregnant women may get reddish, slightly depressed streaks on the sides of their breasts, lower abdomen, and, sometimes, the thighs. The best advice is to make liberal use of a moisturizer such as Lubriderm, Vaseline Intensive Care, Oil of Olay, or plain lanolin and avoid direct unprotected sun exposure. However, no preparation can either prevent or remove stretch marks. Their appearance is directly proportional to the degree of enlargement of the breasts, abdomen, and thighs.

147

Q *What are these little reddish purple spots showing up on my neck, chest, and arms?*

A They're called "spider angiomas." They are actually tiny blood vessel growths at the skin surface, which appear in about 60 percent of Caucasian women. They are common on the face, neck, chest, and arms. Spider angiomas seem to be related to the way the liver metabolizes high estrogen levels, but the important fact is that they're not dangerous in any way and do not require treatment. Often they resolve after pregnancy.

148

Q *My acne is worse than it's been since I was a teenager. What's going on?*

A Pregnancy raises progesterone levels to many times their normal values. Progesterone is chemically close to testosterone and there may be an effect on the skin glands that worsens acne, as might happen with a teenage boy. Effective treatments include oral erythromycin and topical medications such as metronidazole, clindamycin (Cleocin), and erythromycin gels, all of which are antibiotics. Drying agents such as benzoyl peroxides are also safe. Topical Retin-A is completely metabolized in the skin and may be used safely.

149

Q *My husband says that my palms seem red to him. Is this a common occurrence?*

A About two-thirds of white women notice a deeper red color to their palms from the early second trimester on, almost as though they were sunburned. This palmar erythema is quite normal and, as with the vascular "spiders," seems to be related to high estrogen levels. The condition goes away after delivery.

150

Q *I have these rough, brownish little moles popping up everywhere. What are they?*

A They're probably "seborrheic keratoses," or seb kers as they're known among dermatologists. The lesions are usually flattish, brown, and roughened, and appear to be stuck onto the skin as if they were pasted there. They are particularly common under the arms, on the neck, and over the breasts. They are not dangerous and have no malignant potential. What's more, many of them often fall off after pregnancy. They can be removed if desired, but it's usually better to wait until after delivery, since they might well come back. They are commonly confused with moles.

Moles (nevi) tend to grow and darken in pregnancy normally. Changes in color or shape should be brought to your doctor's attention.

Skin tags (acrochordons) may grow in pregnancy as well. These are elongated, nonpigmented tags of skin that occur on the neck, under the arms, and in the groin. These will not go away by themselves after pregnancy. If they become a nuisance, you may need to have them removed by cauterization after pregnancy.

151

Q *My skin is turning brown around my eyes and across my cheeks. What is going on?*

A You're one of the unlucky few who have developed the "mask of pregnancy." Its medical term is chloasma or melasma. About 50 percent of women have some darkening of facial skin. However, a few women are excessively sensitive to sunlight in pregnancy and the pigment concentrates on the sun-exposed surfaces of your cheeks, upper lip, and forehead, darkening these areas considerably. Use of a sunscreen with an SPF of 20 or greater may help prevent this. If it has already occurred, there are a few safe bleaching formulas, such as Eldoquin forte, that your doctor can prescribe.

Teeth and Nails

152

Q *Should I care for my teeth differently during pregnancy?*

A Routine dental hygiene should not be altered in pregnancy. Brushing after meals and before bed is still recommended, and all toothpastes are safe. Flossing should be discontinued only if episodes of prolonged bleeding from the gums results. Bleaching trays for whitening should probably be avoided in pregnancy, but especially in the first trimester.

153

Q *My dentist found a cavity. She wants to take X-rays and then fill the tooth. Should I wait until after I deliver?*

A There is no reason to delay dental care done under local anesthesia. Dental X-rays pose absolutely no risk to the fetus. Any concerns on the dentist's part are purely legal, so he may want your doctor's permission in writing before taking them.(See Section 5: Radiation) Fillings are safe, as is local anesthesia. After the first trimester, the dentist may administer nitrous oxide (laughing gas) if deemed necessary. (See Section 5: Anesthesia)

Incidentally, it is not true that cavities are more likely in pregnancy because of the calcium absorbed by the fetus.

154

Q *My gums seem swollen and sometimes they bleed. Should I be taking more vitamins?*

A Tissues of the gums have a much increased blood supply in pregnancy and may bleed while you are brushing your teeth or, especially, flossing. This is normal and not a cause for concern. Supplementation of vitamin C at 500 milligrams per day is considered helpful by some experts. Over-the-counter antibacterial mouthwashes such as Listerine, Scope, and Chloraseptic are safe to use during pregnancy.

155

Q *I've gotten a swollen area on the gums that looks a little like a tumor. What is this, and does it need to be removed?*

A A localized swelling of the gums made up largely of small capillary blood vessels is called an epulis. It, too, can be a normal symptom in pregnancy and almost always goes away by itself after delivery. If you have a continual bleeding problem, an oral surgeon can excise and/or cauterize the growth. This is different from the misnamed pyogenic granuloma, also known as granuloma gravidarum. These are overgrowths of granulation tissue that may result from chronic gum inflammation or gingivitis. They may require surgical excision depending on location, size, and discomfort.

156

Q *I haven't had a nosebleed since I was six years old, and I've had three in the last week. What's happening?*

A Just as bleeding gums and bleeding hemorrhoids may occur during pregnancy, so may nosebleeds. The increased vascular volume caused by fluid retention in pregnancy is manifested in some women as fragility in the tiny vessels of the nasal mucosa.

To stop a nosebleed, pinch your nostrils together while holding your head back, or while lying on your back. Cold packs may also help constrict blood vessels and decrease blood flow to the area.

Dry nasal membranes are thought to contribute to the problem, so try using saline nose drops several times per day and before bed. Humidity also improves the situation, so consider installing a humidifier in your bedroom.

Very rarely, vessels in the nose may need to be cauterized by an ENT specialist.

157

Q *My nails seem to break very frequently. Do I need more calcium?*

A Several different nail changes have been reported but none of them occurs consistently. Increased brittleness, increased softness, pitting, and transverse grooving have all been described. They are unexplained. These changes are not worrisome, and no specific treatment seems to be helpful.

Breasts

158

Q *When will my nipples stop hurting?*

A Nipple tenderness is a very common early sign of pregnancy and may occur in 80 to 90 percent of women as early as five to six weeks. Breast and nipple tenderness usually resolve by about twelve weeks, when morning sickness is abating as well.

159

Q *My breasts are already fuller and I'm only eight weeks pregnant. Will they continue to enlarge throughout the pregnancy?*

A Your breasts will enlarge and become more nodular early on as higher estrogen and progesterone levels take effect, and they will continue to enlarge throughout the gestation. This may necessitate multiple changes in bra cup size over only nine months. Veins just beneath the skin become visible as bluish, serpentine lines, signifying the engorgement of the breasts with increased blood supply. Reddish, depressed streaks may occur in the later months as the enlarging breasts stretch the skin and leave "stretch marks," or striae, in about half of women.

160

Q *My nipples stopped hurting at about twelve weeks, but now they seem bigger, too. What changes can I expect in the nipple area?*

A Not only will the nipples enlarge and become more erectile, but the brownish area around the nipple (areola) will increase in diameter and grow darker. After about twenty weeks, a sticky, yellowish fluid may be squeezed from the nipples, or sometimes may simply leak out on its own. This is colostrum, a protein-rich fluid that is the precursor of breast milk. Multiple small bumps will arise throughout the areolae. The bumps are actually enlarged sebaceous (oil) glands called Glands of Montgomery, and are completely normal.

161

Q *Will these changes in my breasts go away after I'm no longer pregnant?*

A The breasts enlarge considerably when your milk comes in and will revert to their normal dimensions several weeks after weaning is completed. Depending on the extent of enlargement and thus stretching during pregnancy, striae may remain, but fade to faint silvery streaks. Some breasts feel less firm after the first pregnancy and lactation, as the swollen milk-producing cells inside shrink back to normal. This may give the breast a slightly more pendulous appearance. Color and diameter changes in the areolae do not go away.

In fact, you can often tell when a woman has been pregnant in the past by this feature alone.

162

Q I've read that rubbing my nipples with a washcloth several times a day for several minutes, and rolling the nipples between my fingers, can toughen my nipples and make them less likely to crack when breast-feeding begins. Is this true?

A Most current lactation experts would not recommend "roughening" of the nipples. There does not appear to be any need for nipple preparation, and avoiding nipple problems with lactating seems to be much more related to breast-feeding technique than anything else. (See Section 10: Breast-Feeding)

163

Q What about nipple stimulation to initiate uterine contractions?

A Nipple stimulation in the third trimester will induce contractions just as it will with breast-feeding in the postpartum period (after-birth pains). Nipple stimulation is sometimes recommended, while monitoring the fetal heart rate electronically, to evaluate how your baby is being oxygenated by the placenta and how the fetus might tolerate labor. It should not be used to induce contractions, however, without first discussing your particular circumstance with your doctor.

164

Q I've had breast implants. Will that cause any problems in pregnancy?

A There is no evidence to suggest that breast implants (breast augmentation), whether silicone or saline, cause any problems specifically related to pregnancy. Just as in the nonpregnant state, implants may make breast self-examinations slightly more difficult. Ask your doctor how to do proper examinations in pregnancy.

165

Q I've had breast implants. Can I still breastfeed my baby?

A There are two aspects of this issue. In most cases, whether your implants are saline or silicone, or above or below the muscle, breast-feeding is not hindered. Whether breast-feeding with silicone breast implants poses a risk to the fetus is still debated. At this time, the great preponderance of belief is that the potential benefits far outweigh any theoretical risks.

166

Q *Do I need to do breast self-examination during pregnancy. It's hard enough to tell what I'm feeling when I'm not pregnant.*

A Yes, absolutely continue with self-examinations. Breast cancers are statistically more lethal in pregnant women. This is not because of high estrogen levels, not because of a more aggressive tumor type, and not because of a younger group of patients. Breast cancer is more lethal in pregnant women because they usually ignore lumps or don't look for them simply because they expect changes during gestation. Breast self-examination is critical in pregnancy. Any rock-hard lump that doesn't hurt deserves investigation. If you feel any new lumps or if you're merely unsure, ask your doctor to examine your breasts.

167

Q *Can mammograms be done in pregnancy?*

A Absolutely. The radiation exposure to your fetus from a mammogram (XMG) is approximately 1/100th of the dose known to cause birth defects or, later, increased risk of leukemia in the baby. However, a mammogram may be less accurate during pregnancy, and is in any case less accurate in women under age thirty-five. Ultrasound of the breast can also be performed with no risk throughout gestation.

168

Q *I've had a breast reduction surgery. Will I be able to breast feed?*

A This procedure is much more likely to inhibit your ability to breast-feed than is a breast augmentation. Breast reduction involves the transplantation of the nipple, and only trial and error will determine if breast-feeding will be possible. More often than not, it is.

169

Q *My nipples don't stick out, even with stimulation. Will I be able to breast-feed?*

A (See also Section 10: Breast-Feeding) Nipples that fail to become protuberant or erect are referred to as "inverted nipples." Breast-feeding involves placing as much of the areola in the infants mouth as possible, but also involves the stimulation of the soft palate on the roof of the baby's mouth with the erect portion of the nipple. Inverted nipples can be brought out to some extent by wearing a plastic breast shield designed for this purpose. Ask your doctor about these devices. You may simply have to try with your newborn and if it proves impossible or too frustrating, bottle-feed under your pediatrician's guidance. Do not be pushed into thinking that you are doing serious harm to your baby by not breast-feeding. The issue just isn't that clear-cut.

Muscles, Joints, and the Nervous System

170

Q *Is it true that my abdominal muscles may separate later in pregnancy and leave a big dent?*

A You're describing a "diastasis recti," in which the long vertical muscles of the abdominal wall pull apart in the midline over time. If they pull far enough apart, a large section of the uterus may be covered only by skin, connective tissue (fascia), and peritoneal lining. A "dent" in your abdomen after delivery is a pretty good description.

As your belly shrinks to normal size the muscles do approximate, or come together. However, their attachment to each other is often permanently disrupted. In reality this usually means that you will see the separation clearly when you do a sit-up. If the separation becomes debilitating, it can be fixed with a surgery similar to that for an abdominal hernia.

171

Q *I have pain off and on in my hip and it seems to click when I walk. What's going on?*

A The hip joint is the only one in the body that's not a "true" joint. The head of the hipbone (femur) simply rests against a shallow indentation in the pelvis (acetabulum). The "joint" is held together by the tendons of the muscles that attach across it. High progesterone levels relax the muscles and their tendons, and the joint becomes a little unstable. In fact, all of the pelvic ligaments are relaxed in pregnancy. Unfortunately, there is little that can be done about it except for getting off your feet when its particularly bad. A simple analgesic such as Tylenol may provide marginal help. The joint usually returns to normal after pregnancy.

172

Q *My right leg has already started swelling more than my left. Is that unusual?*

A (See this section: Swelling) Far from unusual, it is the most common scenario. Most of the time the growing uterus "falls off" the spine, or rotates to the right rather than the left. Think of the uterus as a basketball balanced on a fence rail. The lumbar spine is actually about three inches in diameter, and the uterus can't stay balanced on it evenly. Just as the basketball falls off the fence, so does the uterus fall off the spine. It falls to the right more often because of differences between the right and left side of your pelvic anatomy related largely to the dilated ovarian veins. When the uterus rotates to the right (dextrorotates), the veins and lymph vessels on the right side of the pelvis become relatively more obstructed, and swelling occurs more noticeably on that side.

173

Q *I've been getting calf cramps lately in the middle of the night. Even though I take extra calcium, I still get them every night. Is there any way I can make them stop?*

A Getting calf cramps, or a "charley horse" in the calves, is a common occurrence in pregnancy. They often strike between two AM and five AM, and are due to a spasm in the gastrocnemius muscle. Some experts relate an increased incidence of calf cramps to sleeping on your back, at least late in pregnancy. Again, there is no evidence that sleeping on your back in a normal pregnancy poses any actual risk to your fetus. It is theoretically possible that the slightly decreased blood flow in your legs in this position could contribute to cramps. Find the position that works best for you. Try sleeping more on your side, supported by a pillow. The actual muscle physiology is controversial and everything from calcium and magnesium supplements to various vitamins has been suggested as therapy.

Only one therapy has consistently outperformed calcium, magnesium, or a placebo, and that is a simple stretching exercise. Right before you go to bed and *every time* you get up to urinate, do this stretch and the incidence of calf cramps drops dramatically. Face the wall with your feet flat on the floor. Put your hands flat against the wall and lean forward with elbows bent. Keep your heels flat on the floor, and hold this position for fifteen to twenty seconds. Feel your calves stretch? You're cured. (See this section: Exercise)

174

Q *Why have my hands been getting numb and hurting in the morning since about thirty weeks?*

A If the numbness in your hands involves your palm, your thumb, first, second, and half of your third finger, but not your little finger, you are experiencing Carpal tunnel syndrome. CTS is common in nonpregnant people who type or work at the computer keyboard for long hours. It affects about 25 percent of pregnant women to a greater or lesser degree due to swelling in the wrist and compression of the median nerve.[14] This nerve runs along your finger tendons in the underside of your wrist. There is a band of fascia wrapped around your wrist just like a bracelet, that holds your tendons down so that when you curl your fingers the tendons don't pop up. The median nerve gets compressed between this band and the bone during the swelling in later pregnancy.

Carpal tunnel splints made of plastic with a Velcro closure are available in most pharmacies without prescription. These splints decrease swelling by holding the wrist in a neutral position while you are sleeping.[15]

Rarely, CTS may require injection of steroids into the wrist while you are still pregnant, with excellent results. Very rarely, a "release" procedure needs to be done after pregnancy by a hand surgeon.

175

Q *What is Bell's palsy?*

A Late in pregnancy, numbness of the cheek and lip accompanied by inability to completely close the eye on the same side may come on suddenly. This is called Bell's palsy. This is a weakness of the muscles served by the facial (VIIth) nerve. Its cause is unknown. It may be viral, or it may be related to swelling. Steroid injections and other traditional treatments do not seem to offer any benefit.[16]

Roughly 90 percent of women have complete recovery in the weeks to months following delivery. The only therapy required is to occasionally bathe the eye that is partially open with saline eyedrops to avoid corneal abrasions. The eye may be taped closed in sleep.

176

Q *My lower back is killing me. What can I do to help it?*

A (See this section: Back pain)
Low back pain is a common accompaniment of pregnancy at all stages. Initially the growing uterus presses on the sacrum; then postural changes to correct for the forward shift in your center of gravity (the big belly) lead to back pain; finally pressure from the baby's head on the sacrum irritates the low back as well. Pregnancy relaxes all of the pelvic ligaments and the lumbosacral joints may become tender, as may the pubic symphysis.

Low back exercises such as pelvic tilts should begin in early pregnancy before there is any pain. Belly supports that wrap around the low back and close with Velcro, such as the Bellybra, can help immensely, as can some full torso maternity girdles.

If an actual muscle spasm occurs, and you are immobilized, resting the back muscles by lying on your back with your knees bent and supported, and occasionally using prescription narcotics, will be necessary. As long as you experience no nausea, sweating, or light-headedness when supine, it is safe for you to lie on your back. (See this section: Exercises) With lower back muscle spasm, local heat may be useful as well. Hot baths are perfectly safe after the early first trimester. When your back "goes out" with these muscle spasms, it may take as long as forty-eight to seventy-two hours before you can walk.

177

Q *It's not just my lower back that hurts. I have pain down my buttocks and into the back of my leg as well. Is this just muscle strain?*

A Certainly herniated intervertebral discs can occur in pregnancy and the postpartum period just as they can at any time when not pregnant. Pain down the sciatic nerve (sciatica) could be from compression of the nerve root by a disc rupture in your lumbosacral spine. It is still more likely, however, that the pain is a combination of musculoskeletal low back pain due to the increased curvature of the spine (lordosis) and compression of the sciatic nerve root by water retention.

If sciatica occurs without back pain, try ice packs over the upper buttocks to alleviate pain.

178

Q *I have pain down my inner thigh, hut no real back pain. What's happening?*

A There is a nerve running through the inner pelvic wall that can be directly compressed by the uterus or by water retention, causing swelling in tissues around the hole where it exits the pelvis. It is called the obdurator nerve and it controls the adductor muscles of the inner thigh, which you need in order to walk. There is little you can do about it, but be reassured that it will lead to no permanent damage and will resolve after pregnancy. It may even be intermittent and thus related to degrees of water retention or possibly even a change in fetal position during the last trimester.

179

Q *I'm about twenty-eight weeks pregnant and the bottoms of my feet are really pain-ful, especially at the heel. Why am I in so much pain?*

A Foot pain is relatively common in pregnancy, especially the under-sides of the feet in later pregnancy. Probably several components are involved, including increased body weight, edema in your low back com-pressing the sacral nerve roots that give rise to the nerves supplying the bottom of the foot, and local swelling in the foot itself. The pain is always intermittent and self-limited.

Headaches

180

Q *I'm getting more frequent and severe headaches. Should I be worried? What can I do?*

A Severe headaches from about ten to twenty weeks are a frequent and normal occurrence. As your body retains more water, blood vessels must dilate to accommodate the new volume. This dilation is not always smooth and linear and thus may lead to spasm and severe headaches. Some could be due to sinusitis, but these are typically behind one eye or the other, or are accompanied by cheek tenderness. A simple analgesic such as Tylenol may be safely used in all trimesters of pregnancy. Rarely, a narcotic such as hydroxy-codone (Vicodin; Lortab) may be indicated. There have been good results with the occasional severe headache using the combination of acetamino-phen and a phenobarbital derivative (Fioricet; Flextra DS-no caffeine). These headaches almost always resolve by the beginning of the third trimester.

Occasionally abrupt elimination of caffeine can lead to severe headaches. There is little evidence that caffeine in small amounts is a problem in the first place, so caffeine may be reintroduced if it had been stopped suddenly.

Migraines which do not resolve in a day or two occasionally need to be treated with a beta-adrenergic blocker such as atenelol, 50 to 100 milligrams per day. Verapamil has been used successfully as well. (See Section 5: Antihypertensives)

A headache late in pregnancy and associated with high blood pressure is a different and potentially severe condition. (See Section 8: Preeclampsia)

Eyes

181

Q *I wear contact lenses and lately I can't see nearly as well. Do I need to have my prescription changed?*

No ophthalmologist or optometrist should agree to change your prescription during pregnancy. Just as you retain water in other parts of your body, you do so in the cornea as well. The cornea is the clear structure over the front of your eye that initially bends or refracts the light coming in. Contact lenses fit over this area and alter the angle of incident light. Glasses do the same thing, only from a slightly greater distance. As corneal edema occurs, slight changes in the clarity of your vision will occur as well. Your contacts may seem not to fit as well. These changes are transient and resolve after delivery.

182

I can see clearly, but lately I've been having episodes of being unable to see out to either side. It's as though a curtain has been pulled down to the far left and right. Do I need to be concerned?

Very infrequently pregnant women lose their peripheral (side) vision off and on. The nerves from your retina cross in an area right behind the bridge of the nose called the optic chiasm. The pituitary is right in this area. Occasionally, the normal enlargement of this gland, which directs most of your body's hormonal functions including breast-feeding, puts pressure on the nerves that supply the inner halves of your retinas. These inner halves are the ones that are directed outward, or laterally.

The condition is known as bitemporal hemianopsia. In nonpregnant women this can be very worrisome. Even in pregnancy it deserves a visit to the ophthalmologist, but you don't need to panic. The cause of your peripheral vision loss is much more likely to be because you're pregnant than because anything really dangerous is happening.

183

I see wavy lines cross my vision, and even "stars" from time to time. Should I be worried?

Minor visual changes are common in pregnancy. Not only is the eye affected by water retention in both cornea and retina, but the vascular changes and sporadic vessel spasms which accompany the normal blood volume expansion during gestation might lead to intermittent symptoms such as seeing "stars" or wavy lines. A contributing factor could also be the increased flow of vitreous fluid (fluid in the eyeball) in and out of the eye, which is known to occur with normal gestation. Unless symptoms are persistent enough to inhibit normal functioning, there is no reason to worry. However, if significant visual changes occur in the third trimester and are accompanied by high blood pressure, severe swelling, incapacitating upper abdominal pain, or the worst headache you've ever had, this could be a sign of severe toxemia or preeclampsia and you should notify your doctor. (See Section 8: Preeclampsia)

Since eye diseases that occur in nonpregnant women can occur in pregnant women as well, it is always a good idea to check with your doctor about visual changes and be referred to an ophthalmologist if necessary.

184

Q *My eyes have been red and irritated from allergies. Is it okay to use eyedrops?*

A Everyone agrees that using saline eyedrops is not a problem, likewise the occasional use of vasoconstrictive drops (Visine). Despite labeling and confusion about steroids in general, if your doctor or ophthalmologist prescribes them, ocular topical steroids (Neodecadron; Decadron Phosphate) are safe at any time in pregnancy. If your vision is altered in addition to your eyes being red, you should see an ophthalmologist.

185

Q *My son had pink eye and now I have it. Is there anything I can do?*

A Let your doctor examine you. If you have no change in your vision and your doctor diagnoses pink eye, you may safely use the common topical antibiotic ointments and drops for the eye (Cortisporin Ophthalmic; Polysporin; Neosporin; Tobradex). If your vision is altered in addition to your eyes being red, you should see an ophthalmologist.

Blood, Heart, and Vessels
(See also Section 9: Heart Disease)

186

Q *How will my heart be affected by pregnancy?*

A Your heart responds to changing hormonal signals just as do virtually all of the organs in your body. The major change is that your heart increases the amount of blood it pumps per minute (cardiac output). This increase goes from about five liters per minute in your nonpregnant state to about seven liters at thirty weeks, and to about nine liters in the second stage of labor.[17]

Your pulse will increase about ten to fifteen beats per minute. Your doctor will also be able to hear a heart murmur during systole (while the heart is ejecting blood) about 90 percent of the time.

Your blood vessels will dilate gradually and sporadically to accommodate your new increased blood volume without a significant increase in your blood pressure. In fact, because of your body's relationship to your placenta, your blood pressure actually drops in the second trimester and then gradually rises to normal or slightly higher than normal levels in the third trimester.

Preeclampsia (toxemia), or pregnancy-induced hypertension, is a medical complication of pregnancy that involves your cardiovascular and renal (kidney) systems. (See Section 8: Preeclampsia)

Experts think a good part of first trimester fatigue may be related to the tremendous cardiovascular changes going on. Why pregnant women accommodate and feel so energetic in the second trimester is the real mystery.

Dizziness may frequently occur in any trimester. Blood is returned to the right side of the heart via a large vein that passes beneath the pregnant uterus and which can be compressed, leading to near fainting spells. These occur often when standing still or even sitting without moving for prolonged periods. When you feel light headed, *you must lie down* on your side, not sit down, and the sensation will rapidly pass, usually within a moment or two. Dizziness is not worrisome unless persistent or actual loss of consciousness occurs (See 97).

187

Q *Why have my extremities, especially my legs, started to swell by the end of the day?*

A Most of the increased water retention of pregnancy goes toward expanding your blood volume so that by the end of pregnancy you will have about 45 percent more blood than in the nonpregnant state! The extra blood comes in handy at delivery, when on average you lose about 500 to 1,000 cubic centimeters of blood. Without the natural increase in blood volume, such a loss would create a serious situation.

As for swelling in your extremities, in the absence of increased blood pressure, it is perfectly normal. The kidneys retain more water in pregnancy, and you tend to make more urine at night. By the end of the day, while less urine has been made, some of the water retained is simply not contained in the vascular space and leaks out into the tissue beneath your skin.

188

Q *I've heard that if I don't take iron supplements I may need a blood transfusion. Is that really true?*

A (See section 2: Dietary Guidelines)
You could need a blood transfusion whether you take iron or not; but it's not likely. The 40 to 50 percent increase in blood volume during

gestation (1,000 to 2,000 cubic centimeters, on average) is adequate to allow you to tolerate even excessive blood loss without transfusion. (See Section 8: Obstetric Hemorrhage)

The need for iron pills in all pregnancies is somewhat controversial. Humans have gone for about 80 millennia without extra iron to supplement the diet. However, maternal deaths have been cut fifty to one hundred fold in the last hundred years, largely due to the avoidance of obstetric hemorrhage, and to prompt treatment when it occurs. The need for iron supplementation depends on your diet, your starting blood count, and the amount of iron in your brand of prenatal vitamin.

There is no controversy about the fact that the body's need to supplement iron stores increases in the latter half of pregnancy. Without additional iron in the diet or as a supplement, the blood volume will continue to rise because of water retention, but the hematocrit (blood count) will fall because of dilution. The hematocrit is really just a ratio of packed red blood cells to water in your blood, but it's the red cells that carry the oxygen. As you approach thirty weeks of gestation, your hematocrit will normally fall from around 38 to about 30 percent. Some experts feel that patients with levels below this need to take iron in a supplemental pill form (ferrous gluconate, sulfate, or fumarate). Iron supplementation of an iron-deficient diet may provide as much as the equivalent of one extra unit of blood.

189

Q *Besides having more blood at the end of pregnancy, does my blood change in any other ways?*

A Yes. The coagulability of your blood seems to increase markedly. This means that nearly all of the factors involved in the blood clotting mechanism are circulating at increased levels in pregnancy. Incidentally, this renders a common test for nonspecific inflammation, the estimated sedimentation rate (ESR) useless in pregnancy. Platelet levels, however, tend to drop slightly as pregnancy proceeds, either due to dilution or increased destruction. The increased clotting factors are probably related to the effect of high estrogen levels on the liver production of these proteins. The only real significance of the hypercoagulable state is that you are about ten to twenty times more likely to have a pulmonary embolus or a stroke when pregnant than nonpregnant. This still puts your risk at only about 40 to 80 in one hundred thousand. (See Section 9: Deep Vein Thrombosis/Pulmonary Embolus)

190

Q *Should I give my own blood toward the end of pregnancy in case I need it at delivery?*

A (See also Section 8: Obstetric Hemorrhage)

In general, the answer is no. Your body builds an extra woo to 2,000 cubic centimeters of blood normally, which is more than enough to handle even excessive blood loss. Giving your own blood too close to delivery could undermine your own body's attempt to protect itself.

Some people feel safer if they at least get designated blood donors lined up among relatives and friends. With current blood banking techniques and screens for HIV, Hepatitis B, C, D, and E, statistically you are as likely to acquire an infectious disease from designated donor blood as you are from the blood bank.

191

Q *I have a little swelling in my legs, but I also have an area in my right calf that really hurts when I touch it. Could this be a blood clot?*

A It certainly could be. During pregnancy your risk of blood clotting problems is about ten to twenty times higher than normal. Thrombophlebitis means inflammation of a vein surrounding a blood clot. If it occurs in the superficial veins near the skin surface, it may be treated with elevation, heat, and one baby aspirin per day. However, superficial thrombophlebitis may or may not be associated with deep vein thrombosis (DVT). Blood clotting in the deep veins of the calf, behind the knee, in the thigh, or deep in the pelvis can all be potentially life-threatening. Rarely, a clot can break free and become an embolus. This blood clot then flows back into the right side of the heart, out through the pulmonary artery, and into the lung, where it may then block off air exchange. This is a pulmonary embolus (PE) and is potentially lethal.

The true danger of DVT is that it may go unrecognized. Symptoms can be mild or absent. Pregnancy often causes leg swelling, and one leg usually swells more than the other. One-sided swelling, heat, and/or redness over the area, as well as tenderness to the touch, are all symptoms and signs of DVT. Treatment includes hospitalization and intravenous blood thinners such as Heparin. (See Section 9: Medical Complications)

192

Q *I've got purple-green, knotty, raised areas over my calves, thighs, and now on my vaginal lips. What's happening?*

A You have developed varicosities. Varicose, or swollen veins, are the result of a combination of factors. Blood volume steadily increases in pregnancy, thus straining the capacity of the little one-way valves in your veins that keep blood flowing back toward the heart. As your pregnancy progresses, you develop this huge basketball that compresses the larger veins as they run through the pelvis on their way back to the right side of the heart. This compression slows flow in the veins and also increases pressure in your back. Some women inherit a tendency to have weak-walled veins, and the result is varicosities.

While these are most commonly seen on the legs, large varicosities may also be found in the vulva, running through the labia majora, or larger outer vaginal lips. In general this does not become anything more than a nuisance, but occasionally it can be debilitating.

193

Q How do I get rid of varicosities?

A You don't. At least you don't in pregnancy. About six months after delivery, and if you have completed your childbearing, you may consult a vascular or plastic surgeon and be evaluated for either injection of the smaller superficial veins, or a vein stripping (removal) of the deeper ones.

Lungs

194

Q What changes in my lungs can I expect during pregnancy?

A Like everything else in your pelvis, abdomen, and chest, your lungs are about to be compressed. As the uterus grows, it gradually pushes everything out of its way. The diaphragm is pushed up about four centimeters during pregnancy. As a consequence, the base of the lungs are compressed and the functional residual capacity (FRC) of the lungs is grossly reduced. Sounds bad, doesn't it?

Luckily, God figured this out too, and the diameter of the chest increases by about two centimeters, thus increasing the circumference by about six centimeters. Because the diaphragm actually moves over a greater distance in pregnancy, the tidal volume (air moving in and out with each breath) is actually increased.

The increased tidal volume due to an increased respiratory drive is thought to be due to the very high levels of progesterone in pregnant women. Combined with the increased amount of oxygen carrying blood and the increased cardiac output mentioned above, more oxygen is actually delivered to the tissues in the pregnant woman than in the nonpregnant woman, even though the lungs feel crunched.

195

Q *If I'm actually getting more oxygen during pregnancy, why do I feel short of breath so often?*

A All women sense an increased desire to breathe while pregnant. Some may interpret this as being uncomfortably "short of breath." Because the tidal volume is actually increased in pregnancy as described above, the amount of carbon dioxide (CO_2) may drop slightly. The fall in CO_2, which results from an increase in the amount being exhaled with each breath, can be interpreted by the brain as dyspnea. Dyspnea is the subjective sensation of feeling as if you're not getting enough air.

You can help prevent the sensation of shortness of breath by maintaining good, upright posture and avoiding positions of compression for any length of time. That means standing and walking around for at least fifteen minutes every ninety minutes or so. Do not sit for more than forty-five minutes, and be aware of the need to stand and move around on long plane or car trips. Avoid bending over with your knees locked. When you rise from a sitting position, move to the edge of the chair and keep your back straight. When you rise from a lying position late in pregnancy, get up from your side by walking yourself to the upright sitting position with your hands and arms.

Standing and taking slow deep breaths, along with reassurance, is usually all that is required to regain a normal rate of breathing. At night you may need to sleep propped up on several pillows. Occasionally, more than verbal reassurance is necessary, and a monitor of blood oxygenation can be placed on the index finger in Labor and Delivery, the emergency room, or in your doctor's office, to take an instant, painless measurement (TcO$_2$, or Trans-Cutaneous Oximeter). TcO$_2$s over 90 are usually considered normal.

Hormones and Glandular Changes

196

Q *Are there many hormonal changes that come about because of my pregnancy?*

A Yes. There are many hormonal changes in pregnancy. In fact, it is fair to say that pregnancy is almost nothing but one big hormonal change. The remarkable thing is that the greatest changes in pregnancy are not brought about by your hormones, or, for that matter, by the baby's, but by the placenta's. These hormonal changes lead to almost all of the physiologic changes discussed in this section.

197

Q *Which are the most important placental hormones in terms of the changes I'm feeling?*

A Both estrogen and progesterone are made in huge multiples of the amounts which your ovaries normally make. These two hormones and their metabolites are responsible for the lion's share of the changes you feel.

198

Q *How do estrogen levels change and how does that affect me?*

A Estrogen concentrations increase astronomically by the end of pregnancy. Levels are greater than one thousand times their normal levels. Special cells in the placenta called syncytiotrophoblasts have completely taken over estrogen production from the ovaries by about twelve weeks of gestation. The placenta converts precursor hormones (DHEAS) made by both your adrenal gland and the fetus's to various forms of estrogen. By the end of pregnancy it is your fetus's adrenal gland that accounts for 90 percent of the placental estrogen production.

Rising estrogen levels are important for fetal development (See Section 4: Fetal Development), as well as many of the physical changes described previously including breast enlargement, uterine enlargement, water retention, blood volume expansion, and even mood changes.

199

Q *Is there any reason to test my estrogen levels in pregnancy?*

A Yes. Tests include the blood test (alpha fetoprotein 3, or AFP3)at fifteen weeks to check blood estriol, a way of evaluating the fetal risk of Down's syndrome among other abnormalities, and the urine test of estrogens (estriols) occasionally performed later in pregnancy as a test of fetal well-being. (See Section 3: Tests of Fetal Well-Being)

200

Q *What about the other "female" hormone, progesterone? How do its levels change and how might that affect me?*

A Progesterone levels rise throughout pregnancy, peaking at six to eight times their normal value around term. Progesterone is produced by the placenta, which replaces the ovary as the origin of this hormone early in pregnancy.

The placenta makes progesterone by converting maternal LDL cholesterol in those specialized cells, the syncytiotrophoblast. Removal of the corpus luteum or even both ovaries after the seventh week of pregnancy does not change the levels of progesterone produced.[18]

Ovarian progesterone is, of course, responsible for the preparation of the lining of the uterus, the endometrium, in order to receive the embryo for implantation. This specialized lining after implantation is then referred to as the decidua. Its role in allowing the fetus, which is essentially a foreign transplant graft, to continue to survive is one of the great unexplained mysteries of nature. Placental progesterone is subsequently largely responsible for water retention to build your blood volume, breast enlargement, and preparation for lactation, as well as for changes in your lungs, bowels, and urinary tract.

201

Q *Is there any reason to check my progesterone levels in pregnancy?*

A Because placental progesterone production depends exclusively on maternal precursors (unlike estrogen, which depends on fetal adrenal compounds), progesterone cannot be tested as an indicator of fetal well-being. For example, fetal death causes estrogen levels to plummet in the maternal blood, but has little effect on progesterone levels. It is true that a very few infertile women may have a so-called luteal phase defect, in which the amount and timing of progesterone production by the ovary after its release of the egg may be uncoordinated or inadequate. These women are best treated with the ovulatory agent clomiphene citrate (Clomid; Serophene). Some women, however, are treated with progesterone suppositories or, occasionally, injections. This supplementation is continued after the positive pregnancy test. Human evidence suggests this may be unnecessary as early as the first week after conception; other experts say as late as the fifth week. It would seem that only animal data suggests possible dependence on the corpus luteum until as late as the eighth week after conception.

In any event, some researchers now feel that early inadequate progesterone levels may signal impending miscarriage, or possible ectopic pregnancy. Levels may therefore be tested early on and if very low, your doctor may recommend progesterone supplementation; especially after an in vitro fertilization (IVF) conception or after repeated miscarriages in the past. It is quite possible, however, that the low progesterone levels indicate a problem with the early fetal placenta's ability to convert cholesterol, and thus may be a result of the problem, and not the potential cause.

Natural progesterone is not associated with danger to the fetus; therefore, trust your doctor's advice about using it.

202

Q *If estrogen and progesterone are so important, what's the "pregnancy hormone"?*

A Human chorionic gonadotropin (HCG) is the so-called pregnancy hormone, largely because it is made immediately upon implantation of the embryo, and is normally made only during pregnancy. For this reason, it is used in both urine and blood tests to identify pregnancy.

203

Q *What does HCG do?*

A HCG has many functions, the best known of which is to keep the corpus luteum cyst functioning—that is, producing progesterone. Normally, if you don't get pregnant, fourteen days after you ovulate the corpus luteum cyst collapses, progesterone levels fall, which constricts blood vessels in the uterine wall, and you have a menstrual period. HCG produced by the newly embedded embryo prevents this cycle from occurring. HCG levels peak at eight to ten weeks of pregnancy and thus perform another critical function; this is the time when increasing levels of testosterone are being produced by specialized Leydig cells in the fetal testes. HCG stimulates these specialized cells to produce testosterone, and it is the action of testosterone that drives male sex differentiation.

204

Q *Why would my friend have had serial HCGs drawn in her doctor's office?*

A HCG levels normally rise steadily and predictably, doubling about every forty-eight to seventy-two hours, through about ten weeks of pregnancy. At ten to twelve weeks, HCG levels begin to fall and do so progressively until about twenty weeks, when they reach bottom and stay there through the rest of the pregnancy.

Your doctor would draw HCG levels early in pregnancy if there were reason to believe you might be threatening to miscarry, or if you were at high risk for ectopic pregnancy. If levels have failed at least to double in seventy-two hours, you may be sure that the pregnancy is not progressing normally. These levels are usually tested very early on—less than six weeks by dates.

After that point, a vaginal ultrasound in the doctor's office should be able to document pregnancy tissue in the uterus and thus effectively rule out an ectopic pregnancy. (See Section 8: Ectopic Pregnancy and Miscarriage)

If you seem to have completed a miscarriage on your own, and there was no tissue saved for pathology, your doctor will need to follow HCGs down to zero even if it takes several weeks. This is to rule out certain forms of premalignant and malignant growths of the placenta that make HCG. (See Section 8: Molar Pregnancy and Choreocarcinoma)

205

Q *What other hormones does the placenta make?*

A Human Placental Lactogen (HPL) is one whose levels near term are among the highest of any protein hormone in your body. The hormone is thought to be important in altering maternal metabolism to make both amino acids available to the fetus to build protein, and to break down maternal fat for energy in times of maternal starvation. It is called HPL because it also stimulates changes in the breast that allow milk production.

The placenta makes many other hormones that can stimulate the adrenal glands, the thyroid, the parathyroid glands, and the hypothalamus. Inhibin is also created by the placenta and serves to shut down the maternal brain's stimulation of the ovary by follicle stimulating hormone (FSH). This is probably the reason that women fail to ovulate when they are already pregnant.

The placenta also makes an insulinase, which actually deactivates your own insulin, presumably to help keep your glucose levels high enough to make sure sugar passes across the placenta to the baby. When this and other factors stop functioning properly, you may develop gestational diabetes. (See Section 8: Diabetes)

206

Q *What does pregnancy do to my thyroid gland?*

A The thyroid gland increases slightly in size, but any nodule should still be considered abnormal. There is a modest increase in basal metabolic rate in pregnancy, partially due to thyroid changes.

Several forms of the hormone do rise moderately in normal pregnancy. Total T4 and T3 both rise. However, pregnant women do not normally become hyperthyroid. This is because a protein made by the liver, which binds to thyroid hormone, also increases significantly. Thus the amount of free, unbound (active form) thyroid remains essentially unchanged. This increase in binding hormone (thyroid binding globulin) will also alter traditional tests of thyroid function. T3 uptake falls because of this. Despite increased production of thyroid hormone, levels of the free, unbound active hormone remain within a narrow normal range throughout pregnancy, as reflected by a value that corrects for these changes called the T_7.

It is also important to note that very little if any of the thyroid hormones T_3 and T_4, or the pituitary hormone TSH (thyroid-stimulating hormone), cross the placenta. (See Section 9: Thyroid Disease)

207

Q *I've heard about changes in my pituitary as well. What are they?*

A Your pituitary is a small gland at the base of your brain behind the bridge of your nose. This gland secretes many hormones that play a role in controlling almost all aspects of your body. Despite this, the pituitary is not necessary to maintain a pregnancy if the patient receives supplemental steroids, as well as thyroid and vasopressin hormones.

208

Q *What does the pituitary make?*

A The pituitary makes protein hormones that are secreted into the bloodstream and travel to target organs that are themselves usually glands that control growth and metabolism.

Growth Hormone: Slightly increased in pregnancy. Acts together with human placental lactogen (HPL) to control breakdown of certain tissues, which will be used by mother and fetus for energy and nutrition.

Prolactin: Rises during pregnancy to ten times normal levels. Rise caused by the estrogen effect on the pituitary and also the effect of thyroid-releasing hormone. Prolactin is necessary for breast-feeding to occur.

Beta-lipotrophin: Opioid hormone that appears to rise in pregnancy and may have a role in blunting the pain of childbirth.

Thyroid-Stimulating Hormone: Controls secretion of thyroid hormone, and indirectly metabolic rate.

ACTH: Controls the stimulation of the adrenal gland and thus indirectly the production of many steroid hormones that control salt and water balance and influence the immune system.

Vasopressin (ADH): Hormone released by the posterior pituitary that affects the kidney and helps regulate body fluids by causing water to be retained. Also known as antidiuretic hormone (ADH) because it concentrates urine and decreases urine volume.

209

Q *What is my parathyroid gland?*

A Your parathyroid gland consists of four small glands that are thus named because they surround the thyroid in the middle of the front of your neck. Drops in blood levels of calcium or magnesium lead to increased secretion of parathyroid hormone, which in turn increases bone resorption, intestinal absorption, and kidney reabsorption. This is why if your diet contained no calcium, the fetus would never be shortchanged. Parathyroid keeps calcium levels constant in your plasma.

210

Q *What is calcitonin?*

A Calcitonin is a hormone made in specialized cells of the thyroid gland, whose function is essentially the opposite of parathyroid hormone—increases in blood levels of calcium lead to increased calcitonin production. Calcitonin is necessary for moving calcium into bones and decreasing the blood level when necessary. In short, parathyroid and calcitonin work in concert to keep blood calcium within a very narrow range in your bloodstream. Calcitonin levels are increased in pregnancy.

211

Q *I thought vitamin D was important for controlling calcium in the body. Is that true?*

A It is. Vitamin D is actually synthesized in the skin with exposure to sunlight. It may also be ingested. Vitamin D is converted first to another form in the liver and then to its final active form in the kidney. In pregnancy, the final conversion takes place in the decidual lining of the uterus and placenta as well. Activated vitamin D (1,25-dihydroxyvitamin D3) functions to resorb bone and increase intestinal absorption; thus, it works in concert with parathyroid hormone to raise blood calcium and works contrary to calcitonin. The enzyme that converts vitamin D to its final form is supported by parathyroid hormone. Levels of active vitamin D are grossly increased in pregnancy as well. This makes sense, since the increase works to make calcium in the maternal bloodstream available to the fetus.

212

Q *I've heard that steroid levels are affected by pregnancy. How does this affect me?*

A Your adrenal glands are perched right on top of your kidneys. These glands are physically small, but without the steroid hormones they make, life would not be possible. There are four major groups of steroids made by the adrenal glands: cortisol, aldosterone, deoxycorticosterone, and sex steroids. All four of these are considerably increased in pregnancy.

Another part of the adrenal also makes adrenaline, or epinephrine. Adrenaline is also necessary for the body's defense and leads to increased heart rate, cardiac output, and blood vessel constriction.

213

Q *Is it true that women also make male hormone?*

A Yes, it is true. Male hormones are thought to control libido, or sex drive, in women as in men. Male hormones or their precursors are made in the adrenal gland and the ovary normally.

Maternal androstenedione and testosterone levels increase in pregnancy. They serve as precursors that are converted by the placenta to estrogen in the form of estradiol. You would thus think that levels of these hormones would drop, but the opposite is true. It is thought that the ovary may be the source of these increased male hormones, and these higher levels may play a role in the acne that women experience during pregnancy.

Emotions

214

Q *I'm nine weeks pregnant and thrilled about being pregnant, but I just fly off the handle at work. Am I turning into an ogre?*

A Your progesterone levels are rising rapidly in the first trimester and probably a myriad of hormonal changes we have yet to discover are occurring as well. If PMS can lead to easy crying, irritability, headaches, and general crabbiness, early pregnancy can do it as well.

Remember also that you are experiencing a few added stresses. For instance, you may be about to throw up 80 percent of the time, but you can't concentrate on the nausea because you're too exhausted. (See this section: Fatigue) You may also be feeling the same trepidation that any human feels when faced with significant change, whether that be moving, marriage, divorce, or a new job. You can't decide whether to be elated or terrified. Mood changes are entirely expected. All of this is normal and will pass with time.

215

Q *I'm twenty weeks pregnant and feel great physically, but I just locked myself out of my car for the third time! I've lost my keys, I never remember my list of questions for the doctor, I don't think I fed the cat for three days, and I forgot a big meeting at work. Can this be normal?*

A Forgetfulness is a totally normal part of pregnancy that often begins at about the halfway point. Rest assured, the condition is temporary. The normally active woman today has a enormous amount of responsibility. Life is difficult enough without experiencing tremendous physical changes and wondering about the unknown at the end of the gestational highway. When you've reached the point at which stepping off a curb without falling on your face has become a daily challenge, how can you expect to feel in control?

Simply be reassured that you are not alone and the world is a forgiving place when it comes to pregnant women. As you become more knowledgeable about your pregnancy, more secure in your ability to handle it, and more excited rather than scared at the prospect, your daily demonstrations of "airheadedness" will diminish.

216

Q *I'm thirty-one weeks pregnant and happy about it, and my husband is the most wonderful man I've ever met. So why am I acting like a Desperate Housewife?*

A If you're normal, a little of the novelty has worn off by thirty-one weeks. Total strangers think it's okay to touch your belly. The whale, duck, and penguin jokes are wearing thin. For the last two months you've been reassured by the baby's movement, but doesn't the little tyke realize enough is enough? You don't want to hear your best friend tell you yet again how totally wonderful her pregnancy was.

Boredom with pregnancy is a normal circumstance. You are starting to feel a little of the frustrations surrounding a long wait for anything. Your husband is probably getting a little fed up with the pregnancy by now as well. In his efforts to help out, he may inadvertently run into the aura of frustration around you.

Best advice—listen to grandma. "If you can't say anything nice, don't say anything at all." Remember, your husband loves you and he is trying.

217

Q *I'm thirty-four weeks pregnant and I've never remembered a dream in my life until the last couple of weeks. Now I can't stop dreaming the weirdest stuff. What's wrong with me?*

A Dreams may become more vivid, bizarre, and memorable during pregnancy. Not only is this normal, it is probably necessary as a defense against the anxiety generated by the pregnancy process. For maybe the first time, you literally hold the future of the world inside your own body. It is natural to worry about normalcy, about labor, about delivery, and about the life changes you will shortly face. The brain handles many of these anxieties with dreaming.

Most of us who went to college have experienced the "late for the exam, can't find the exam, never went to class before the exam" genre of anxiety dream. These dreams are easily translated into the "left the baby at home alone, forgot to feed the baby, doctor didn't show up in time, locked the keys and the baby in the car" type of dream.

Many other types of dreams are encountered in which you may be helpless to change the course of events. These include being trapped inside of just about anything; being attacked by a rapist, an animal, or any stranger; or the classic—falling off or into anything. Pregnancy represents the first time in your life that your body betrays you without permission, to some extent. You lose control of physical factors as well as temporal and emotional factors. A sense of vulnerability tied to a sense of being trapped by your circumstances is very normal and very common.

Other common dreams include ones in which the baby is abnormal in some way, usually physically. This, of course, reflects your anxiety about the baby's being normal, but probably represents your own insecurities about "making" a normal baby—that is, "doing it right" and "fear of failure." These feelings are certainly normal in our competitive, results-oriented society.

While some women might view these dreams as disturbing and in need of interpretation to make them useful, that is probably not the case. Dreams are useful simply by their occurrence, probably on a biochemical level about which little is currently understood. There is something therapeutic, healing, and rejuvenating about the act of dreaming itself.

Try to view your dreams with some perspective. Be glad that you have them, and that your brain is using them automatically to reduce your anxiety.

218

Q *My husband and I have been to all six classes, I've talked to my friends, I've read the books. That doesn't change the fact that at thirty-seven weeks and counting, I'm terrified. How can I possible remember everything I have to once I go into labor?*

A Labor nurses, doulas, and doctors will be there to help. They will remember for you, because it's what they do everyday of their lives. Besides, it's like riding a bike, or getting ready for a big exam. Once the time comes for you to concentrate on what you are doing, the anxiety usually disappears.

Women have been giving birth for a long time, and you're going to do just fine. Let the people around you who have devoted their lives to human reproduction help you. As you enter this experience, reassure yourself with this thought—your mother did it.

SUGGESTED RESOURCES AND READING

American College of Obstetricians and Gynecologists. 1995. "Exercise and Pregnancy," ACOG Educational Pamphlet.
ACOG Web Site: http://www.acog.com
Main Switchboard: 800-673-8444, (206) 638-5577
Order Desk: 800-762-2264

Artal, Raul, and Genell Subak-Sharpe. 1992. *Pregnancy and Exercise.* Delacorte Press.

Regnier, Susan. 1990. *You and Me, Baby, The Official YMCA Guide.* New York, NY: Simon & Schuster.

Motherhood After Miscarriage, Diamond, Kathleen, 1991

Surviving Pregnancy Loss, Friedman, Rochelle et al, 1996

The Pregnant Woman's Comfort Guide, Jiminez, Sherry, 1992

WEBSITES

Exercise During Pregnancy
www.childbirth.org/articles/pregnancy/safeexercise.html

Headaches
www.americanpregnancy.org/pregnancyhealth/headaches.html

Miscarriage and Pregnancy Loss/Grieving
www.resolve.org/

Nutrition During Pregnancy
http://www.nal.usda.gov/fnic/pubs/bibs/topics/pregnancy/pregcon.html
http://www.kidshealth.org/parent/nutrition_fit/
nutrition/eating_ pregnancy.html

Section Three

Prenatal Care

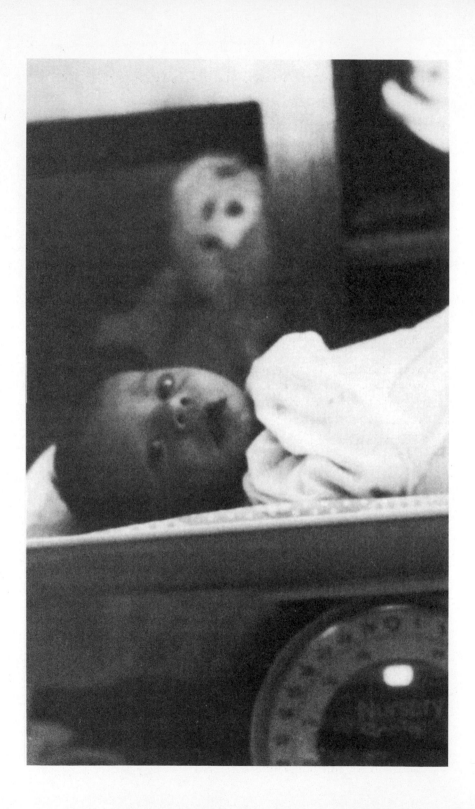

219

Q *When should I make my first obstetrical appointment?*

A Once you have a positive pregnancy test, contact your doctor's office as soon as possible. Most doctors will want to see you between about seven and eleven weeks for a first obstetrical appointment. If you are having any problems such as bleeding or severe pelvic pain your doctor will want to see you earlier to rule out threatened miscarriage or ectopic pregnancy. (See Section 8: Ectopic Pregnancy)

220

Q *Is there anything I should bring to my first visit?*

A If you are taking a large number of medicines for any chronic condition, be sure you write down their names, dosages, and who prescribed them. If you have a record of vaccinations either from childhood or as an adult, bring these as well. Much of what the doctor says will concern him directly, and together, the two of you will be able to remember more than either one of you alone.

221

Q *What will we do during the first visit?*

A Your first visit will include an interview during which the doctor will take a history that covers the following areas:

Last Menstrual Period (LMP) if known

Date of conception if known

Symptoms with pregnancy thus far

Past Medical history, including Medical: problems of heart, lungs, liver, gastrointestinal tract kidneys, bladder, extremities, and neurologic system

Surgeries

Allergies

Current Medicines

Social History: Use of alcohol and tobacco, recreational drug use, home situation, job situation, family dynamics

The second part of your first visit would normally include a complete examination unless you are transferring into the practice and have recently received care for the current pregnancy elsewhere.

You may already know the answers to these questions, but the following information should be made available to you.

1. At what institution does the doctor deliver?

2. Who does the doctor cover calls with and will that affect who might attend you in delivery? Will you get to meet his or her partners during prenatal visits?

3. Can your husband or partner be with you at all times?

4. Does the doctor's office or the hospitals he or she uses provide prepared childbirth classes? When do they start and how much time do they take?

5. Will you get an ultrasound and if so, when?

6. What can you do for the current symptoms you are experiencing, such as nausea, fatigue, and breast tenderness?

7. Save the other 993 questions until you get this book!

222

Q *What is the doctor's (or the group's) C-section rate?*

A You may certainly ask this question if you wish, but be aware that many Board Certified obstetricians may be slightly put off by it. While it is true that the C-section rate has risen nationwide in recent years from less than 10 percent in the 1960s to about 25 percent in 2005, there seems to be a public perception that this is in some part due to a cavalier approach by the obstetrician for personal reasons.

In actuality, the fifty-year-old edict that "once a C-section always a C-section," compounded by increase in the number of people having children, has caused the rise. Vaginal birth after cesarean (VBAC) is still a relatively new concept in many parts of the country, and has not had time to lower the overall rate significantly. (See Section 8: VBAC)

In addition, the specter of medical-legal ramifications has led to an increased C-section rate partly in response to continuous electronic fetal monitoring and its false positive indicators. C-sections are also safer than ever before with modern IVs, regional anesthesia, and drugs to combat infection and hemorrhage. So disincentives to cesareans have decreased at the same time as concern about fetal health has overshadowed diminishing concern about maternal well-being.

A more appropriate question might be "What is your C-section rate for first-time deliveries?"

223

Q *What will the first examination involve?*

A The first examination will involve getting completely undressed (and possibly perspiring in nervous anticipation), but essentially, it will be just like your yearly visit.

The doctor will examine your throat, neck, heart and lungs, breasts, abdomen, and then perform a pelvic examination. Normally, this will include a PAP smear as well.

224

Q *Will I be able to hear my baby's heartbeat on my first visit?*

A That depends on when you come in for the first visit. Usually, the fetal heartbeat may be heard with an ultrasound device known as a hand-held Doppler beginning at about ten weeks. Whether or not you can hear the heart, many doctors will perform a vaginal ultrasound during your first examination so that you can see the heartbeat and visualize the forming fetus. At about eight weeks you can see the brain and heart clearly. You'll be able to see the limbs forming as well. (See Section 4: Fetal Development)

225

Q *What is the normal range for the fetal heart beat?*

A You will see "120-160 bpm" printed in many places. This does not mean that a heart rate outside of this range intermittently is necessarily abnormal. Fetal heart rate in the first trimester tends to be at the higher end of the range. As pregnancy progresses it gradually falls off to the lower end of the range.

Fetal heart rate also responds to movement with acceleration in the healthy infant. (See NST)

226

Q *If we've seen the heartbeat, does that mean we're out of the woods in terms of miscarriage?*

A Not quite. Seeing a heartbeat is certainly a good thing, but at less than ten weeks, a heartbeat gives no guarantee that miscarriage will not occur. After ten weeks, however, hearing or seeing the heartbeat drops the rate of miscarriage from 15 percent to less than 5 percent.

227

Q *When can we tell people we're expecting?*

A Anytime you want. However, many doctors recommend waiting until after the completion of ten weeks. If you've seen or heard the heart and are beyond ten weeks, it is reasonable to trumpet your good news to the world. If you tell people before that, and you do have a miscarriage, you will find that "un-telling" a pregnancy is much more emotionally traumatic than never having mentioned it in the first place.

228

Q *When can we tell if it's a boy or a girl?*

A Ultrasound done abdominally after sixteen to seventeen weeks is about 95 percent reliable at determining sex, depending on the machine, the operator, and the degree of cooperation from the fetus. (See 292, 293.)

229

Q *Is it true that boys have slower heart rates than girls?*

A Despite what you may have heard, there is no relationship between fetal heart rate at any gestational age and the fetal gender. Perhaps the belief that such a relationship exists came from the fact that small animals have fast heart rates (hummingbird hearts tick at fifteen hundred beats per minute) and large animals have slow heart rates (elephant hearts thump at twenty beats per minute). Since boys are statistically slightly larger than girls at birth, one would think that perhaps their heart rates were slower, but as it turns out, no statistically significant difference exists.

230

Q *Are there biological advantages to having one sex over the other?*

A Yes. In rare instances some genetic disorders affect the sexes unequally. The primary difference though, is that boys do stupid stuff, but they CAN pee out the van door on a trip. Girls on the other hand, are easier early on, but more expensive in the long run.

Vaginal Sonogram

231

Q *What is a vaginal sonogram?*

A In about 1988, ultrasound technology advanced to the point where we could introduce a small transducer (sound emitter) into the vagina. This allowed the head of the instrument to be only centimeters away from the fetus and thus give a clearer, more detailed picture. The probe is attached with a long cable to a computer that projects an image on the monitor. The sound waves bounce off, or are absorbed to differing degrees, depending on the tissues contacted. The transducer then senses the returning sound waves and the computer interprets the signals and makes a picture.

The main thing to remember is that a vaginal sonogram (ultrasound) doesn't hurt. The probe is covered with a condom and a lubricant for reasons of hygiene, and the only discomfort you might feel is a cold clammy sensation if the lubricant is not warmed.

232

Q *Is ultrasound really safe? I've heard some people say it can be dangerous.*

A We now have over twenty years of experience with ultrasound safety in pregnancy. There is probably no other diagnostic test that has been more studied in terms of potential effect. Although in the United States insurers sometimes refuse coverage despite the more than thirty indications itemized by the American College of Obstetricians and Gynecologists, in Europe they have averaged three to five ultrasound examinations per pregnancy for many years. There is no reputable data to suggest a danger to ultrasound at any point in pregnancy.

233

Q *Is the ultrasound at the first or second visit the only one I will have during the pregnancy?*

A Ultrasound with the vaginal transducer in the first twelve weeks of pregnancy establishes only that the pregnancy is in the uterus, how many fetuses there are, if they are living, and what the gestational age is to within ninety-six hours or so. No information about normalcy is usually possible. As a consequence, we recommend another study be done at about sixteen to eighteen weeks. At this gestation, all major anomalies may be ruled out and gender may be determined if desired. Even more ultrasounds may be indicated later in pregnancy for specific problems. Even ten years ago the United States Department of Health and Human Services recognized twenty-seven indications for ultrasound during pregnancy. (See this section: Tests of Fetal Well-Being)

Laboratory Tests

234

Q *Will there be any other tests performed during the first visit?*

A Routine blood work as well as a urine specimen for culture will be collected. Blood work includes the following tests: CBC, blood type and antibody screen, RPR, HIV, TSH, HbsAg, and rubella. A urine culture and Pap smear are usually performed as well. Some states now require cultures for chlamydia and gonorrhea as well.

CBC stands for complete blood count. It is a routine test to determine if you are anemic, if you have any evidence for infections with alterations of your white blood count (WBC), and if you have the normal number of platelets to clot properly.

RPR is a nonspecific but sensitive test for the sexually transmitted disease syphilis. Syphilis is a bacterial (treponemal, actually) infection transmitted by intercourse and oral or anal sex, which, when transmitted across the placenta, can have devastating effects including stillbirth. The RPR is a good screen, but many conditions can cause false positive tests, especially autoimmune diseases like lupus (SLE). The FTA-ABS is a more specific test. If your RPR is positive to any degree, exposure to syphilis will be confirmed with the more specific FTA-ABS. (See Section 9: Infections)

TSH (thyroid stimulating hormone) has recently been recommended as a universal screen since some studies have shown small but significant IQ differences in children of women even minimally hypothyroid.[1]

Hepatitis B Surface Antigen (HbsAg) is a blood test that determines if you have been exposed to hepatitis B. This form of viral liver infection is transmitted sexually by infected body fluids, as well as by blood transfusion. It is not what is commonly referred to as "infectious hepatitis," which is hepatitis A. If a pregnant patient tests positive for hepatitis B, other more detailed studies are done to determine if she is infectious. Furthermore, when the baby is born it will be given both a specific immunoglobulin for hepatitis B as well as the recombinant hepatitis B vaccine. The vaccine is synthesized and is not live, allowing high-risk pregnant women to be vaccinated with no risk to the fetus. (See Section 9: Infections)

235

Q *What is the rubella test?*

A The blood test for rubella is an antibody titer to see if you have been previously vaccinated successfully as a child, or if you have been exposed to the disease. If your antibody titer is high enough, then you need not worry about any exposure to German Measles while you are pregnant. If your test results are too low, then you are considered nonimmune. You will need to avoid exposure to rubella during pregnancy, and should be vaccinated after delivery. The rubella vaccine is a live but weakened, or attenuated, virus. The greatest risk for congenital birth defects from rubella is infection acquired in the one week prior to and the four weeks after conception.)[2]

While no evidence of rubella-associated defects as a result of inadvertent vaccination of a pregnant woman have ever been found, vaccination should still be avoided in the three months prior to conception. (See Section 9: Infections)

236

Q *I know what "blood type" is, but what's an antibody screen?*

A The purpose of determining your blood type is, as you probably know, to determine if you are Rh-D negative or positive. Whether a blood type is O, A, B, or AB is usually not critically important to the health of the fetus. However, if you are Rh-D negative (for example, Type AB-) then there is potential danger for the fetus.

Picture red blood cells as all having a "positive" sign, or alternatively, no sign at all, which indicates "negative." Now let's suppose that your husband's blood cells are positive, and yours are not. If your fetus has a positive blood type, and there's at least a 50 percent chance that it will, and even a few of its blood cells get into your bloodstream across the placenta during pregnancy, your immune system learns to recognize those positive cells as foreign invaders. In the process of destroying them, it will make antibodies to Rh+ cells that will be able to cross the placenta in future pregnancies, attack the fetus's red cells, and cause a severe enough anemia to lead to fetal heart failure (immune fetal hydrops) and, eventually, death (Rh Disease, or Erythroblastosis fetalis).

The antibody screen tests for the presence of these antibodies in your bloodstream to see if you've already come in contact with Rh+ cells, in other words, if you have been Rh-sensitized, or isoimmunized. Usually, the only time your blood mixes with the baby's is at birth, so in a first pregnancy the risk to your baby of Rh disease is considered to be almost zero.

For that reason, if the baby's blood type is determined to be positive after birth from testing the umbilical cord blood, you will be given Rhogam to protect you for future pregnancies.

It is now known that a minuscule percentage of mothers may become sensitized during pregnancy, either when they bleed spontaneously, go through a threatened miscarriage, or by having an amniocentesis. For that reason, you will receive Rhogam at 28 weeks of gestation if you have a negative blood type. (See Section 8: Rh isoimmunization)

237

Q *Why is a urine culture performed if I have no symptoms?*

A Urinary tract infections (UTIs) of both the bladder and the kidney are more common in pregnancy, and can have severe consequences. In 1 to 3 percent of pregnant women, UTIs develop. About 8 percent of pregnant women have asymptomatic bacteriuria, or bacteria in their urine but no pain. If the colony count on a culture is greater than 100,000, this constitutes infection and your doctor will treat it. While one-day therapy for UTI works 90 percent of the time in nonpregnant women, three-day therapy is appropriate for pregnant women. Antibiotics are safe at all gestations with the following exceptions: the quinolones (Floxin; Cipro) because of effects on fetal cartilage, sulfa drugs (in the late third trimester) because of bilirubin binding in the newborn, and tetracyclines because of their effect on fetal teeth. (See Section 5: Antibiotics)

It is important to identify UTIs or asymptomatic bacteriuria as soon as possible because they can be associated with preterm labor later in gestation.

238

Q *I had a Pap smear six months ago. Why do I need another one?*

A The Pap smear is a screening test for cervical cancer. Despite all the criticism in the American national press during the 1990s, it remains the most successful, lifesaving medical screening test ever. Pregnancy is a time when the human papilloma virus (HPV) seems to like to grow. Women who have venereal warts tend to see them spread and sometimes grow extremely rapidly in pregnancy. Since we know that 95 percent of precancerous disease in the cervix is caused by the sexually transmitted HPV virus, it makes sense to get a baseline evaluation. If precancerous changes do exist on the first Pap smear, more vigilance will be required with closer follow-up than normal both in and after pregnancy. (See Section 9: Infections; Cancers)

239

Q *I'd like to know what to expect in the way of recommended tests. Is there a schedule that applies to all pregnant women?*

A Doctors recommend tests to individual patients as needed, and the testing intervals may differ from patient to patient. However, the American College of Obstetrics and Gynecologists does have some general guidelines.

RECOMMENDED INTERVALS FOR ROUTINE AND INDICATED TESTS★

Week of Gestation	TYPE OF TEST
Initial	Blood type, Rh, antibody screen, Hgb/Hct (blood count), rubella, syphilis (RPR), GC and chlamydia, hepatitis B (HbsAg), urine culture, TSH, HIV.
8-18	Ultrasound, maternal AFP3, CVS, or amniocentesis as indicated. Nuchal fold sono optional.
24-28	Diabetes screening, 3-hour glucose tolerance test if screen abnormal, repeat antibody screen if Rh negative, Rhogam administration, if indicated to Rh negative mothers.
32-36	Ultrasound if indicated; repeat RPR and GC culture (some states require), blood count, Group B strep cult. Repeat Hgb/Hct, HIV
Optional	HIV testing (some states require by law), hemoglobin electrophoresis, chlamydia culture.
Every visit	Blood pressure, weight, urine, fetal heart rate, fundal (tummy) measurement.

★American College of Pediatrics, American College of Obstetricians and Gynecologists, *Guidelines for Prenatal Care*, 4th Edition, Elk Grove Village, IL; AAP; Washington, DC: ACOG, 1992.

AFTER THE FIRST VISIT

240

Q *After my first prenatal visit, how often will I see the doctor?*

A This may vary considerably from clinic to clinic, but the usual distribution is visits at intervals of four to six weeks until twenty-eight weeks, visits every two weeks until thirty-six weeks, and weekly visits thereafter. The average total number of visits recommended if begun in the first trimester is about twelve to fourteen.

241

Q *Will I have to undress at every visit?*

A Unless you have a specific problem that requires examination of a certain area such as the breasts, cervix, or vaginal area, you will only have to undress completely at your first visit, and from the waist down for your final two or three visits. You will also have to undress from the waist down in the last trimester at some point for a Group B Strep Screen, which is a culture with a Q-tip swab from the outer third of the vagina. (See Section 9: Infections)

Ultrasound: Second Trimester

242

Q *What is a second trimester ultrasound?*

A Any ultrasound performed between twelve and twenty-four weeks would be considered a second trimester ultrasound. However, the term usually refers to an ultrasound study done between about fifteen and twenty weeks. Any time after about sixteen and a half weeks, an abdominal scan can give you a good cross-sectional view of the spine, head, and chest, as well as the heart and lungs, stomach, liver, kidneys, and bladder, and an assessment of the extremities. You can determine sex with about 95 percent accuracy simply by imaging the external genitals. While you may not want to know the sex, it is important for your doctor to know, because certain genetic disorders affect a particular sex.

Measurements are also taken of the length of the long bones, the circumference of the abdomen and head, the diameter of the head and the total length of the fetus. There are more detailed measurements done of the brain, the heart, and volume of amniotic fluid. If your doctor has experience with second trimester ultrasound and feels comfortable ruling out anomalies or birth defects, then he or she or a technician will do the scan, usually in the office. Many obstetricians have either radiologists who specialize in ultrasound do these studies, or sometimes perinatologists, who evaluate high-risk patients, perform sophisticated ultrasound examinations, and do amniocentesis and CVS.(See this section: Tests of Fetal Well-Being)

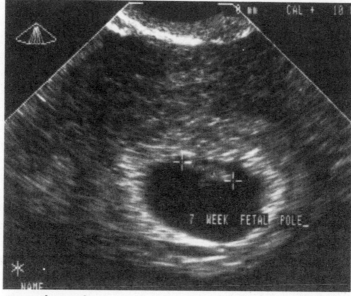

seventh week

243

Q *Is it really necessary that I have this second trimester ultrasound?*

A (See this section: Tests of Fetal Well-Being)
The American College of Radiology lists 12 indications for 1st trimester sono and 27 for 2nd trimester sono. (See Appendix C)[3] Medical necessity is a topic with hazy outlines and definitions when third-party payers get involved. Many insurers feel that unless there's a problem there is no justification for the expense. Most obstetricians feel that ultrasound has been far and away the single most important advance of the second half of the century. It is the way in which many, many problems that would otherwise have been unsuspected come to light.

This study is important for obtaining knowledge about defects. Six months of learning and psychological preparation about babies with these defects can make a major difference to your birth experience. Some defects are actually incompatible with life, or at least anything close to normal life, and termination may be an anguished choice. Some problems lend themselves to immediate surgery after birth by highly trained specialists, and knowledge ahead of time could change the desired route of delivery and even the hospital at which you deliver.

Remember that second trimester ultrasound only estimates gestational age to within ten days, more or less, while first trimester dating is more reliable at about roughly ninety-six hours. Even though the image may be better, fetuses at sixteen weeks have already started to diverge in growth , with one destined to be a ten-pounder and another destined to be a six-pounder. Naturally, relying on measurements of their body parts to determine their age becomes less and less accurate over time.

Other findings such as placenta previa, in which the afterbirth lies over the cervix, or over the opening to the uterus and birth canal, can lead to a fatal hemorrhage if not diagnosed ahead of time.

Multiple gestations are occasionally found when missed in the first trimester, or when an early study wasn't performed at all.

The length of the cervix, if shortened with "funneling" of the membranes, can be a warning sign of incompetent cervix, in which you can lose the baby with no warning whatsoever. Once diagnosed, it may sometimes be treated with a cerclage, or stitch, placed around the cervix to keep it closed until near term when the stitch is removed.

Uterine abnormalities, such as fibroids or leiomyomata (benign muscle tumors of the wall of the uterus) and septa (divisions of the cavity), may be found and lead to preventive therapy for preterm labor.

There are many, many reasons for a second trimester ultrasound. (See Appendix C: Indications for Ultrasound in Pregnancy) If your insurance plan doesn't cover it, first get your doctor to take up the issue with them. If they still refuse to cover it, find the money yourself and get it done. Consider it an extra premium if you must, but get it done.

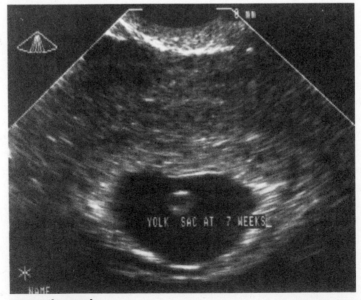

seventh week

Routine Visit Parameters

244

Q *What will be done at my prenatal visits after the initial one?*

A Each visit should give you the opportunity to ask questions about the way you feel, and any worries that you might have. Remember, no question is too stupid or too embarrassing. Ask as many questions as you like, and be sure to write them down ahead of time. You are not wasting the doctor's precious time—that's what he or she is there for!

In most offices, your visit will begin with the dreaded measurement . . . your weight! In the later months you may be tempted to take off more than your shoes and coat for the weigh-in!

Next the nurse will take your blood pressure and dipstick a sample of your urine. Your gestational age may be recalculated and recorded along with the other information in your chart.

After reviewing data on your weight, blood pressure, and urine, the doctor will examine you. Usually after the first visit this will include only a "tummy check." The size of the growing uterus is measured, the heartbeat is heard with a handheld Doppler device so that you can hear it as well, and swelling is evaluated. At this point, the doctor should be receptive to your questions.

245

Q *Why is my weight gain important, other than the fact that I don't want to have to lose it later?*

A Adequate weight gain combined with adequate fundal height measurements are a good indication that your baby is growing normally. Too little weight gain can be an indication of intrauterine growth restriction (IUGR) or a sign that the fetus is not getting enough nourishment through the placenta. A weight gain that is too rapid could be an indication of preeclampsia or toxemia later in pregnancy. It can also be associated with gestational diabetes. (See Section 9: Obesity)

246

Q *What does "dipstick" the urine mean?*

A Throughout most of your pregnancy your urine will be tested for glucose (sugar) and protein. Glycosuria, or sugar in the urine, was long thought to be a sign of diabetes. While that may still be the case, often in pregnancy sugar is spilled in the urine even though the blood glucose is normal. This is related to physiologic changes in the kidney. (See Section 2: Bladder and Kidneys) Although unreliable as an indicator of a problem, the urine dipstick might still prompt a test of blood sugar that proves revealing.

Proteinuria, or protein in the urine, can be a sign of preeclampsia. Preeclampsia is a disease in pregnancy that is associated with high blood pressure, excessive swelling, and a placenta that may not adequately supply the baby with nutrition. (See Section 8: Preeclampsia) A trace amount of protein in the urine is usually just contamination from vaginal mucus. It can also occasionally be an indication of a bladder infection.

247

Q *Why is it important to have my blood pressure taken at every visit?*

A The primary reason to record blood pressure at each visit is to identify any worrisome trend from week to week in your gestation. While preeclampsia may have its physiological cause in events that occur at the very beginning of pregnancy, symptoms usually don't occur until the mid to late third trimester. These include swelling, proteinuria, and increased blood pressure. Classical criteria for hypertension in pregnancy include an increase in the diastolic blood pressure (bottom number) of more than 15 mmHg (millimeters of mercury), or an increase in the systolic blood pressure (top number) of more than 30 mmHg. These changes, however, can easily occur and still have a resultant blood pressure in the normal range. So, for all practical purposes, anything consistently over 140/90 may be thought to constitute pregnancy-induced hypertension (PIH).

If your blood pressure was greater than 140/90 at the onset of pregnancy, and worsens toward the end of pregnancy, the condition is called pregnancy-aggravated hypertension, and can become either superimposed preeclampsia, or superimposed eclampsia. (See Section 9: Chronic Hypertension)

248

Q *What will happen if my blood pressure does stay up and I'm told I have preeclampsia?*

A The process of preeclampsia may be slowed, sometimes for weeks, by strict bed rest. The disease process is only cured however, by delivery. This is probably the case because the placenta may be the source of certain compounds that lead to the chain of events causing blood pressure to rise, and removal of the placenta halts the process.

Thus, if you develop preeclampsia, your doctor will either try to abate the process with bed rest until the fetus has reached a safe maturity, or deliver you depending on both gestational age and severity of preeclampsia. (See Section 8: Preeclampsia)

Alpha-fetoprotein 3 Test

249

Q *Are there blood tests to detect Down's Syndrome early in pregnancy?*

A It is true that certain proteins and steroid hormones made by the placentas of babies with some abnormalities tend to show a certain pattern of increase at identifiable gestational ages that varies statistically from the normal.

There are tests, such as the alpha-fetoprotein test (AFP) and the triple test, (AFP3), which will predict your fetus's risk of Down's syndrome, trisomy 18, and open neural tube defects. These tests *do not* tell you if your fetus is normal or abnormal. A new test including HCG and PAPP (pregnancy associated plasma protein A) has been combined with nuchal fold ultrasound (Ultrascreen®) to achieve 97% sensitivity for Down's and 99% for trisomy 18 before 12 weeks. The nuchal fold is the skin behind the neck area. Ask your doctor.[4]

250

Q *What is an open neural tube defect?*

A Open neural tube defects (ONTDs) are conditions in which an error occurs very early on in the embryo, before day 26 of life, or about five and a half to six weeks from your last period.

The central nervous system, including your baby's spinal cord and brain, are derived from an embryonic structure called the neural tube. If this tube fails to close completely by day 26, then a whole spectrum of abnormalities involving the brain and spinal column can result.

The most severe defect is anencephaly, in which the skull and higher brain centers never form. It is always fatal. Spina bifida, also known as a meningocele, occurs when tissues that normally surround the spinal column protrude through an opening in the lumbosacral vertebrae. If these tissues contain actual spinal cord material, the defect is called a meningomyelocele and is more severe. If skin covers the defect, it is known by the prefix "closed" instead of "open." The severity of the debility is related to how much and which portion of the nervous system is affected. Spina bifida may be severe and involve paralysis of the lower extremities with no control of bowel and bladder function, or cause no appreciable deficit at all.

All of these defects are known as "multifactorial" in origin. This means the defects don't have straightforward Mendelian inheritance patterns, but instead involve multiple genes in combination with environmental factors.

Some women are concerned that their risk of spina bifida or other open neural tube defects might go up with their age or their husband's age, but it does not. Your risk is approximately 0.7 per 1,000 births for open spina bifida and about the same for anencephaly. Therefore, your total risk is about 1.4 per 1,000 births for any ONTD.

251

Q *I've had three friends who had the AFP3 test done and they all had false positives. Amniocentesis showed that nothing was wrong. What does a false positive mean?*

A The AFP3 test includes measurements of three hormones—HCG, estriol, and AFP, or alpha-fetoprotein. The patterns of these hormones at various gestational ages can be plotted against those of a few hundred thousand other pregnant women, and predictions can then be made about your personal risk for ONTD (Open Neural Tube Defects such as spina bifida), and your personal risk for Down's syndrome (trisomy 21). Predictions can also be made about the less common but more devastating trisomy 18.

Because the test gives you a risk statistic, there can be no false positives. The test is simply a way for you to get more information. Under age thirty-five, insurers will not pay for amniocentesis without a reason. If your risk is higher than it should be at your age, the test is reported as increased risk, and then insurers will pay for the amniocentesis. AFP3 is now often replaced by a "Quad test" combined with Nuchal fold. (See 253)

252

Q *So trisomy 21, trisomy 18, and open neural tube defects are the only conditions that can make my AFP3 abnormal?*

A Hardly. These are simply the most common. Abnormal-AFP3 has been associated with many findings, including those that do not show up until much later in pregnancy or until the time of delivery. All of the following have been associated with abnormal AFP3 findings when the AFP component is elevated: congenital nephrosis, cystic hygroma, esophageal obstruction, gastroschisis, liver necrosis, low birth weight, osteogensis imperfecta, oligohydramnios, renal anomalies such as polycystic or missing structures, and sacrococcygeal teratoma. False elevations of AFP can come from low maternal weight, multiple fetuses, and underestimation of fetal age.

Abnormal AFP3 findings with decreased AFP levels include chromosomal trisomies such as Down's syndrome, gestational trophoblastic disease (molar pregnancy or choriocarcinoma), and fetal death. False decreases in AFP can come from increased maternal weight and overestimation of fetal age.

253

Q *What is Nuchal Fold Testing and what is my risk for Down's Syndrome?*

A Assuming no significant family history of Down's syndrome, your average risk may be assessed by knowing your age at the time of delivery. Nuchal Fold Testing, which is a 12 week ultrasound to measure the skin fold thickness in the back of the neck, combined with blood testing like the AFP3, can provide additional risk assessment without amnio or CVS. The following are generally accepted as indicators of risk of Down's syndrome (trisomy 21) at birth for given maternal ages.*

Age	Risk of Downs Syndrome	Risk of Any Chromosomal Abnormalities
20	1/1667	1/526
25	1/1250	1/476
30	1/952	1/385
31	1/909	1/385
32	1/769	1/322
33	1/602	1/286
34	1/485	1/238
35	1/378	1/192
36	1/289	1/156
37	1/224	1/127
38	1/173	1/102
39	1/136	1/83
40	1/106	1/66
41	1/82	1/53
42	1/63	1/42
43	1/49	1/33
44	1/38	1/26
45	1/30	1/21

These numbers are risks for liveborn infants. Relative risks for findings at amniocentesis are slightly higher due to terminations, late miscarriages, and stillbirths. For example, the risk of Down's syndrome at amniocentesis in a thirty-five-year-old is about 1/270, not 1/378.

254

Q *No one in my family has ever had Down's syndrome. Why does my risk of Down's and other chromosomal abnormalities increase with age?*

A Unfortunately, negative family history is in no way protective. Trisomies occur with increasing maternal age because women carry the egg. That egg has been stuck in meiotic prophase (mid-division) since you were in puberty and right up until it answered the call for this cycle. It has been exposed to ambient ultraviolet light, infrared waves, microwaves, X-rays, and all kinds of electromagnetic fields. Over time, your chromosomes may experience breakage or "stickiness." When your egg is formed, if the first division of chromosomes messes up at chromosome 21, your egg ends up with two sets of chromosome 21 instead of only one. Yours added to your husband's makes three sets, thus the "tri" in trisomy 21.

255

Q *My husband is 51. Does his age increase my genetic risk? Are there other risks as I get older?*

A In general, the answer to the first question is "no." Experts think this is because new sperm are made every ninety days or so, while your egg has been exposed to the environment ever since birth and has been stuck in the same division since puberty. Some recent reports suggest very slightly increased risks with paternal age, but these are minimal and controversial.

While increasing maternal age affects your risk of chromosomal errors, it also statistically increases the risk for pre-eclampsia, pregnancy induced hypertension, gestational diabetes, placental insufficiency, preterm labor and stillbirth. For a healthy patient however, the increase in these risks are small. Your doctor may, however, recommend more frequent sonos in the third trimester to evaluate placental efficiency and fetal growth.

Amniocentesis and CVS

256

Q *What is amniocentesis and isn't there a blood test you can do instead?*

Amniocentesis is the definitive test in which a small amount of amniotic fluid is removed with a needle under ultrasound guidance. (This needle does not go through the navel, contrary to popular belief, but does go through the abdominal wall.) Fluid is then sent to the genetics laboratory, where fetal cells are grown in culture, and after ten to fourteen days the number of chromosomes within each colony of cells can be counted. A preliminary result called flourescent in situ hybridization or "FISH" may be available in 3 days for limited chromosome sites, usually 13,18, 21, X and Y. The actual number of chromosomes can be reliably determined, and diseases with abnormal numbers of chromosomes, such as Down's syndrome, Edvard's syndrome, and many others can be prenatally diagnosed. In concert with a thorough genetics history, there are also over six hundred errors of metabolism that can be diagnosed.

As of spring 2011, the technology for an 8 week simple blood draw to rule out Down's had been confirmed but was not yet commercially available. When released it could well replace the need for many CVS and Amnios.

257

Q *Why should I be tested if I'm under thirty-five years of age?*

A Contrary to popular belief, considerably more children are born with Down's syndrome to women under thirty-five than over thirty-five. This is simply because although your risk is higher over thirty-five, many more women under thirty-five are having babies. Because the risk for Down's syndrome at thirty-five years old is 1/270 (at sixteen weeks), the American College of Obstetricians and Gynecologists feels that all women over 55 should be offered amniocentesis.

If you are going to be less than thirty-five when the baby is born, you may consider the AFP3 test. Remember to stay calm if your test comes back with an elevated risk. This does not mean your baby has any problem whatsoever—it merely provides your doctor with a reason to check further.

258

Q *Is if true that amniocentesis can cause you to miscarry?*

A Yes it is, but the numbers are changing. Up until about 1980, most places in the country did amniocentesis "blind." That means they stuck the needle in, and if they got blood, they simply pulled it out and kept going until they got one with amniotic fluid. The miscarriage rate with this procedure was quoted at about 1/300, roughly the same as the risk at thirty-five of Down's syndrome. That's the origin of the concern about a maternal age of thirty-five, when the risk/benefit ratio of testing or not testing crosses over.

But now, with much more sophisticated color flow Doppler ultrasound devices, the test can be done more carefully than when the doctor couldn't see inside your body. Most experts estimate the true amniocentesis-related miscarriage rate at about 1/800 to 1/900.

259

Q *I'll be thirty-eight when the baby is born. I don't want to take any risk of miscarriage to do genetic testing. Besides, we would never terminate a pregnancy, so what's the value of knowing this information?*

A You certainly don't have to get an amniocentesis, or an AFP3 test, for that matter. But recognize that reality is often different than the hypothetical. Nothing is real until it happens to you or a loved one. It's also good to remember that, in general, finding out the facts isn't dangerous in and of itself. We've had patients who would never terminate for Down's syndrome, but who discovered they had trisomy 18 and decided not to put the mother's life at risk with a term pregnancy and delivery.

By the same token, other mothers have discovered that their baby had a lethal anomaly In tin the amniocentesis data. Instead of aborting, they chose to carry to term knowing that the baby would die in the first few hours. Still, they were given the opportunity by the amniocentesis to grieve so that when the birth occurred they were prepared, a much better option than being unaware at the time of delivery.

260

Q *I'm forty rears old and already have a child with Down's syndrome. Is there a way to determine genetic abnormalities without waiting until fifteen weeks and doing an amniocentesis?*

A Chorionic villus sampling (CVS) has been around since the early 1970s and in wide use over the last fifteen years. A small portion of the placenta is removed via a catheter placed through the vagina and cervix. In recent years, this has been done with a needle transabdominally as well. The procedure is usually done at about ten to twelve weeks, with results by the end of the first trimester, thus making the potential need for a termination much easier technically, and therefore safer.

261

Q *Why doesn't everyone who wants genetic testing do CVS instead of amniocentesis?*

Initial reports of CVS tended to point to CVS miscarriage rates not in the range of 1/800, but of 1/50 to 1/150. Subsequently, miscarriage rates that high have been at least partially attributed to the inexperience of the doctors performing the technique in large residency programs. Nevertheless, it cast a pall on the procedure for a number of years. Then, when its popularity was back on the rise, reports of limb defects began coming out, and its role diminished yet occurred again, despite the fact it was later established that limb defects occurred only when sampling was done prior to nine weeks. Now, with abdominal CVS, it would seem that the infection, miscarriage, and limb defect rate are all reported to be on the way down. Certainly the abdominal route would seem to cause less bleeding and less chance of infection than the vaginal route. The miscarriage rate of CVS in experienced hands is now felt to be the same as amniocentesis. But the test has a few other shortcomings.

Any test such as the AFP concentration requires not just the cells to grow, but also the actual amniotic fluid that can be obtained only by amniocentesis. CVS, because it is done four to six weeks earlier, will pick up more chromosomal errors. Why? Remember that 20 percent of pregnancies miscarry on their own in the first trimester. Many of those with severe chromosomal defects never survive long enough to make it into the statistical pool for amniocentesis beginning at fifteen weeks or so.

262

If I decide to have amniocentesis, is fifteen weeks the earliest it can be done?

No. Amniocentesis may be performed as early as thirteen weeks in some cases, but early amniocentesis has been associated with a higher miscarriage rate. Also, valid statistics for AFP3 really start at fifteen weeks. Consequently, unless you are over thirty-five, you won't know if your risk of trisomies such as Down's syndrome is significantly increased until sometime after about fifteen and a half weeks. It should be noted that a 2005 study found a fourfold increased risk of clubfoot after very early amniocentesis, i.e., less than 15 weeks, as compared to CVS. This is still, however, a very small risk (on the order of 8/1000) when weighed against the potential benefits of the procedure.[5]

The actual procedure takes only a few moments. First, a good pocket of fluid is identified by ultrasound. Then a needle is introduced through the skin directly into this pocket of fluid. Some doctors use a local anesthetic and others do not. In any event the needle is usually in place less than thirty seconds and the discomfort is less than that of having an IV put in your arm.

263

Q *What do I have to do afterward?*

A Although there is little data to support its necessity, most doctors will have you stay off your feet and avoid travel for the next twenty-four to forty-eight hours. It's a good idea to plan on someone else driving you home in any event.

264

Q *How long will it take to get the results?*

A Usually a minimum of twelve to fourteen days is required for the results because the cells in the amniotic fluid must be grown in culture. There are a few specific tests that have faster turnaround time, and if appropriate, your doctor will discuss these with you.

265

Q *When will I be able to feel the baby move?*

A Most women who are carrying a pregnancy for the first time feel their first definitive movement around twenty weeks. The first sensation of fetal movement is called "quickening" If you're over twenty weeks and haven't felt the baby move, don't be alarmed. It's different for everyone. Often if your placenta is in front (anterior), you may not feel movement until later than your friends did.

If this is not your first pregnancy, you might well feel movement as early as sixteen weeks. Whether this is your first baby or your sixth, your placenta is in front or in back, you may well not feel consistent daily movement until after twenty-five weeks.

Glucose Screening

266

Q *My doctor said I need an Oral Glucose Screen (OGS) to lest for diabetes between twenty-four and twenty-eight weeks. What does that mean?*

A Gestational diabetes, meaning glucose intolerance that is thought to be caused by the gestation itself, occurs in 1 to 4 percent of pregnant women.[6] Some experts feel that this is actually adult onset diabetes unmasked by the physiological changes of pregnancy, but the practical result is the same.

Due to the potential obstetric complications, including huge babies (macrosomia), increased frequency of infections, increased risk of pre-eclampsia, increased risk of C-section, increased risk of polyhydramnios (too much fluid), increased risk of preterm labor, and increased risk of neonatal problems with breathing, calcium, and glucose levels, all pregnant women should be offered glucose screening. Gestational diabetes in general has no symptoms, no signs, and is only weakly related to family history. As a result, blood glucose screening tests are the only way to discover the majority of gestational diabetics.

It should be noted, however, that a considerable controversy has raged for years over whether all women should be tested or just those thought to be at high risk—that is, women who are obese, have a history of previous macrosomia, a stillbirth, or a malformed infant, have a strong family history of diabetes, or have hypertension and/or glucosuria.

267

Q *How does the screen determine if I have gestational diabetes?*

A It doesn't. The oral glucose screen (OGS) currently consists of an oral load of 50 grams of glucose, usually as a cola, orange, or lemon-lime drink. The glucose load is taken theoretically without regard to previous meal, although as a practical concern most doctors will tell you not to have any sugar in the several hours beforehand.

A value of greater than 140 milligrams per deciliter of plasma at one hour after ingestion is a positive screen. This does not mean you have gestational diabetes, but that you qualify for further testing. While 15 to 20 percent of women flunk the screen, only about 15 percent of this select group, or 4 percent of all pregnant women, actually have gestational diabetes.

If you have an abnormal OGS, you will be encouraged to undergo a three-hour glucose tolerance test. This will consist of a drink containing 100 grams of glucose and blood drawn beforehand, and at one, two, and three hours afterward. You will be instructed to fast for twelve hours beforehand. Plasma values that exceed 105 fasting, 190 at one hour, 165 at two hours, and 145 at three hours are considered abnormal. The test is considered positive if any two values are abnormal.

268

Q *Once I have the diagnosis of gestational diabetes, will I have to get insulin shots?*

A Probably not. The vast majority of gestational diabetics may be managed with diet alone. You will first receive dietary counseling and be taught how to test your own blood sugars at home. (See Section 8: Diabetes)

Rhogam

269

Q *I just had my glucose screen done and my doctor said I needed an antibody screen again because I'm Rh negative. Why do I have to do it again?*

A Some people have Rh-negative blood types. This means that their red blood cells are missing a certain glycoprotein on their surface known as the Rh-D factor. If the baby's blood Rh type is positive (from the father's type), then his or her cells could leak into your bloodstream in tiny amounts. Your immune system could then learn to recognize positive cells as foreign invaders and attack them with your next pregnancy. If this occurs the baby develops Rh disease, otherwise known as erythroblastosis fetalis. (See Section 8: Rh Isoimmunization)

The repeat antibody screen at twenty-five to twenty-eight weeks is to determine if you are one of the rare persons in which this has happened, because if you are, you will not be a candidate for Rhogam.

270

Q *I'm supposed to get a Rhogam shot at my next visit. What is it?*

A Rhogam is actually a brand name for the Anti-D Rh immunoglobulin. In other words, Rhogam is the antibody that your body should not learn how to make. If your antibody screen is negative, then the doctor knows that any fetal positive cells that might have sneaked into your bloodstream have not yet alerted your immune system to their presence. The job of Rhogam is to make a preemptive strike and kill those fetal positive cells before your immune system counterattacks.

Most of the time the fetus's blood only leaks into yours at delivery. That's why until about fifteen years ago Rhogam was only given after birth, and only if the baby had a positive blood type. Now it is known that a few percent of people get "sensitized" during the second and third trimesters. Rhogam given at twenty-eight weeks seems to eliminate this risk. Rhogam is still required at birth if the baby is Rh positive.

271

Q *When will we be able to tell what position the baby is in?*

A At about thirty weeks your doctor can usually tell what position your baby is in by feeling your tummy with his hands. There is a series of maneuvers to do this systematically called "Leopold's Maneuvers."

Even though your doctor can probably tell you your baby's position at about thirty to thirty-two weeks, it may change from hour to hour. At thirty weeks about forty percent of babies are in breech position (butt down). At thirty-seven weeks only about 5 percent are in this position. That means that in the last few weeks a considerable amount of shifting is going on.

Third Trimester Anemia

272

Q *I'm thirty weeks pregnant and the nurse pricked my finger today to test my hemoglobin and hematocrit. She said it was low and I would need to take iron. Am I anemic and is that why I'm so tired?*

A It would be reassuring to be able to say that a lack of sufficient iron is responsible for making you tired, but it's probably not the case. The odds are that you're tired because you're supposed to be superwoman and supermother in today's society. So, you work a ten-hour day and then come home to take care of the other baby, if you have one, and your husband. Add to that the fact that you're carrying at least an extra twenty pounds by now and you've got the recipe for fatigue.

Your blood count is *supposed* to drop in the third trimester. The hematocrit is just a ratio of red blood cells to serum (water), and you will remember that you are retaining massive amounts of water. Your blood count is simply diluted. You can't actually be losing blood because for once in your life, you haven't had to bleed each month.

The bone marrow really turns on at about 30 weeks and it can use the extra iron. However, if iron makes you nauseated or constipated, you can certainly use it sparingly. No matter what the preparation of the supplement is, if your hemoglobin is at least greater than 10.5 and your hematocrit is greater than 30 percent, taking iron every other day is more than adequate. (See Section 2: Dietary Guidelines)

Most of the time you're meeting or exceeding your daily iron requirement with diet and your prenatal vitamin.

Ask your doctor for advice regarding your particular circumstances.

Fetal Movement

273

Q *My baby has been moving less now that I'm over thirty weeks. Is that normal?*

A Fetal movement is always considered a sign of health. Conversely, decreased fetal movement may be a sign of an ongoing disease process or inadequate support from the placenta. As such, it should always be taken seriously and mentioned to your doctor.

That being said, decreased or at least altered fetal movement is the rule after 30 weeks. The baby may move several times from breech position to head down (vertex) and back again. The quality of movement in each position may be markedly different.

In addition, the sheer mass of the placenta and baby are now increasing substantially. In short, the ratio of baby to swimming pool is rising. Especially after thirty-four weeks you may notice that kicks have diminished and have been replaced by rolling, squirming, "let me out" type of movements.

Feeling "shudders" is also normal and does not represent a seizure, but simply incompletely developed nerves which is normal for the fetus.

274

Q *It isn't just that my baby's movement is different—it seems to always be on one side. Is there something wrong?*

A After thirty weeks, movement is often concentrated on one side of your tummy or the other. Just as the baby is getting bigger—it is about three and a third pounds by thirty-one weeks—so is your placenta. It is often located more to one side than the other, and the placenta and the baby can't occupy the same space.

275

Q *I feel the baby hiccup a lot, sometimes for twenty to thirty minutes when I lie still. Is that okay?*

A Fetal hiccups certainly do occur as the neuromuscular connections for the baby's diaphragm mature and become more coordinated. However, babies hiccup like anyone else, in an irregular pattern. Check to see if what you're feeling is in a perfectly rhythmic pattern that occurs about every second or so. If it is, you're feeling your own aortic pulse transmitted through the wave of amniotic fluid in the uterus.

Next time you think that the baby is hiccuping, check your own wrist or neck pulse to see if it matches the twitch in your tummy.

TESTS OF FETAL WELL-BEING

276

Q *A friend told me her doctor said that the baby should move ten times an hour. I never feel the baby move that much, and mostly I feel movement in the evening at home, not at work. Could something be wrong?*

A "Could something be wrong?" is never a good question to ask because the answer will always be "yes." Is it likely that something's wrong?

Certainly not. It is very normal to feel the baby move primarily in the evening when things have quieted down and you can pay attention.

Kick counts have long been suggested as a test of fetal well-being, and indeed very sick babies tend to be limp and move very little if at all. Most obstetricians would tell you that if you lie down during the time of day when the baby seems to move the most (or you attend to it the most), and count movements, you should feel ten movements within two hours. If indeed it takes longer than two hours to feel ten movements, you should contact your doctor.

When you're counting kicks, you can get the baby to move more by tickling him or her just like you will after the birth. Shove the baby around a little and see if there is a kick back. Gently moving the baby with your hands won't be harmful. Talk to your baby, who can certainly hear you in the third trimester. In fact, you can usually get the baby to respond to a loud noise if you clang a pot and pan over your tummy. Many experts have suggested that you drink something with sugar or caffeine in it to "wake up" the baby. Recent studies have concluded that these methods may not actually affect fetal movement. Most obstetricians seem to think they do, however, and it won't hurt to try.

277

Q *I told my doctor that I haven't felt the baby move more than once or twice a day and he wants me to get a non-stress test. What is that?*

A A non-stress test (NST) is a simple test of fetal well-being that is painless and usually takes less than half an hour. It is called a non-stress test to distinguish it from other tests in which the fetus is under the "stress" of uterine contractions. You will be asked to lie back in a recumbent position or on your side and wear a stretch belt around your waist. The belt holds a Doppler ultrasound transducer in place over wherever the fetal heart is heard best. Each time you feel the baby move, you will be asked to press a hand-held button that marks a paper readout of the fetal heart tracing. Many times when a healthy fetus moves, its heart rate will increase by at least ten beats per minute for at least ten seconds. Two such increases in a twenty-minute period constitutes a reactive NST.

A reactive NST suggests that the fetus is generally healthy at the moment it is being tested. However, a non-reactive NST does not necessarily indicate a sick fetus. In fact, 80 percent of fetuses with non-reactive NSTs are found to be perfectly normal.

There are other reasons that NSTs may be done. They are also useful for surveillance of any fetus at risk due to a chronic disease of mother or baby. NSTs are used in gestational diabetes, preeclampsia, chronic hypertension, systemic lupus erythematosus (SLE), premature preterm rupture of the membranes, intrauterine growth restriction (formerly called Intrauterine Growth Retardation, or IUGR), and post-term pregnancy. (See Section 8: Obstetric Complications)

The NST can be extended to ninety minutes. Vibroacoustic stimulation can be applied to the area of the head to stimulate heart rate acceleration. If these things fail, until very recently it was recommended that you either repeat the NST in twenty-four hours, or proceed to a contraction stress test (CST).

More commonly today the next move would be to perform another ultrasound and combine it with another NST. This is called a biophysical profile (BPP).

278

Q *What is a contraction stress test?*

A The contraction stress test (CST) is simply the real-time recording of the fetal heart rate changes in response not to movement as with the NST, but to repeated uterine contractions, as would be found to a greater degree in labor.

During uterine contraction, oxygenated blood from the mother no longer reaches the placental interface. The muscular contraction of the uterus squeezes the uterine vessels closed. Therefore, the fetus must survive the duration of the contraction on the oxygen already stored in the placenta.

If either the fetus is sick, or the placenta is inadequate due to disease, malformation, misshapen blood vessels, or umbilical cord constriction, the fetal heart rate will decelerate with uterine contractions. Although repeated decelerations during a CST is a cause for concern, the test would be called "Positive" in this circumstance. In other words a negative CST is a good thing, and implies fetal well-being. A positive CST is potentially worrisome, and implies fetal or placental compromise and the possible need for delivery. Even with repetitive "late" decelerations on a CST, however, over 50 percent of those fetuses go on to do normally in labor and after birth. Thus, the CST has a 50 percent false positive rate.

These problems with the CST have led to the widespread use of the BPP as a safer and more accurate test of fetal well-being. However, an attempted Pitocin induction that fails may occasionally serve as a prolonged CST and be reassuring enough to send the patient home to return another day for attempted induction.

279

Q *What is a biophysical profile?*

A A biophysical profile (BPP) is another test of fetal well-being that has gained in popularity over the last fifteen years. It combines ultrasound evaluation of amniotic fluid, fetal movement, breathing efforts, and limb position with an NST. A 10 out of 10 is a perfect score. Less than a 6 out of 10 is worrisome. It has long been known that movement is a sign of fetal health. (See this section: Non-Stress Test) It has also long been known that adequate amniotic fluid is an independent and very strong indicator of fetal health as well. Amniotic fluid in the third trimester is largely fetal urine. Therefore, adequate amniotic fluid levels imply good urine output, which in turn implies good perfusion (blood flow) to the fetal kidneys. If the kidneys have good blood flow then the fetal cardiac output is adequate. Since the fetal kidneys are functioning, the implication is that the placenta is doing its job and adequately oxygenating fetal tissues as well.

Amniotic fluid is known to decrease with many fetal and maternal conditions. Below a critical level it is referred to as oligohydramnios.

Oligohydramnios commonly accompanies IUGR, chronic hypertension, preeclampsia, some genetic disorders, and fetal kidney problems, and post-dates pregnancies. (See Section 8)

The traditional method of scoring the BPP is the most widespread. Either two points or zero points are assigned for each of five criteria, the fifth being the repeat NST. Adequacy is determined in the areas of fetal breathing, fetal body movements, fetal tone (limb position and flexion), and amniotic fluid volume. Amniotic fluid volume is quantified with a unit called the amniotic fluid index (AFI), which takes into account the number and square areas of fluid pockets found on ultrasound.

If your score for each parameter is 2/2, then your total is 8/8 and it is considered a normal reassuring study. In this case there is no need to repeat the NST. A score of six is considered equivocal and mandates retesting in less than twenty-four hours. A score of four or less indicates a severely compromised infant and essentially mandates delivery in the very near future no matter what the gestational age.

The BPP seems to have a significantly lower false positive rate than either the NST or the CST Unfortunately, its false negative rate (that is, the test is normal, but baby gets sick) has not been found to be much better than either of the other tests.

280

Q *My doctor said that my baby's umbilical resistance was good and encouraged me not to worry. What is umbilical artery resistance?*

A A special component of the ultrasound machine exists that allows the doctor to measure speed of blood flow in the umbilical blood vessels, called the umbilical artery resistance. If flow is sluggish in the umbilical artery, it implies high resistance in the placental vascular bed. This could mean that the placental vessels are "hardened" or that the placenta is "stiff". The complete absence of flow during diastole (time when the fetal heart is filling) implies potential compromise. Reversal of flow during diastole can mean impending fetal death. At the moment this technique is still considered by most to be investigational, but is widely applied.

GROUP B STREP

(See Section 9: Infections)

FETAL FIBRONECTIN AND SALIVARY ESTRIOL

281

Q *I delivered my last baby at twenty-nine weeks and now I'm having a lot of Braxton-Hicks contractions and I'm worried. My doctor mentioned two tests, Fetal Fibronectin (Ffn) and Salivary Estriol (SalEst.) What are they?*

A Fetal Fibronectin (Ffn) is a vaginal swab test introduced in 1996 and Salivary Estriol (SalEst) is a saliva introduced in 1998. Both are intended to help manage those at risk for pre-term labor. (See question #725)

PELVIC EXAMINATIONS

282

Q *I am now thirty-six weeks pregnant and my doctor says he wants to see me each week. When will I start getting pelvic examinations?*

A Most doctors recommend visits every two weeks from twenty-eight to thirty-six weeks and weekly thereafter. Visit frequency increases because the likelihood of problems such as bleeding, high blood pressure, decreased movement with decreased fluid, and malposition of the fetus increase when you are close to term.

Pelvic examinations are usually done from thirty-eight weeks on. The examinations are usually performed with one or two fingers only and with lubricant and a gentle doctor, they should be tolerable and brief. The discomfort from a pelvic examination late in pregnancy seems to vary tremendously from one patient to the next. At this point in your pregnancy, however, your curiosity usually overcomes reluctance.

283

Q *What does the doctor check with these pelvic examinations?*

A There are five parameters to these examinations, all more or less related to your cervix. They are dilation, effacement (thinning), position, consistency (firm to soft), and station (descent). A pelvic examination also allows one to assess presentation, that is, to feel which part of the baby is coming out first: vertex (head down), breech (butt down), footling breech (feet down), or other.

The results of your pelvic examination cannot help predict when you will go into labor, although it does give some information. As you get closer to labor, the baby may "drop," meaning that the head snuggles down into the pelvic inlet (engages) and you can breathe again. But it could be two days or two weeks after the baby drops before labor begins.

Furthermore, the baby may "dip," meaning that it may be engaged one day and not the next. The cervix begins to efface, or thin, move forward in the vagina, soften, and occasionally dilate one to two centimeters as you approach a first labor. With first pregnancies it is common to efface without dilating before labor. However, these things have no consistent relationship to the time that labor actually begins. With subsequent pregnancies you are less likely to do any of these things, including dropping, but you may dilate without effacing. In fact, you can easily walk around for weeks at four to five centimeters.

284

Q *Can the doctor tell how big my baby is?*

A No. Estimated fetal weights (EFW) by physical examination are extremely inaccurate. In fact, they are no better than plus or minus about 15 percent, which is very close to the accuracy of third trimester ultrasound. One study reported that the accuracy was not statistically different, whether the EFW at term was given by full professors of obstetrics, by ultrasound with the computer algorithm, or by inner-city high school students. In short, there are simply too many variables with abdominal wall thickness, uterine wall thickness, amount of amniotic fluid, position of the baby, lumbar curvature of the spine, and actual baby weight to make estimates worthwhile.

285

Q *How long should I be allowed to go past my due date?*

A Usually about ten days. One of the meanest tricks ever played on womankind was instilling in her the belief that there is such a thing as a due date. Pregnancy is two hundred eighty days or forty weeks from the last menstrual period, or two hundred sixty-six days, on average, from conception. However, "term" is considered thirty-eight to forty-two weeks. It would be kinder to tell prospective parents that the baby will arrive "sometime in the spring" instead of May 14th.

In any event, post-term is defined as past forty-two weeks of gestation, while post-date simply means "past your due date." Most doctors get almost as anxious as you do to get your baby out after forty-two weeks. In some institutions, tests for fetal well-being are begun in the normal pregnancy at 41 weeks, usually the biophysical profile described above. Adequate amniotic fluid is a very reassuring finding at BPP for post-date pregnancies. Extra instruction about attending to fetal movement is reiterated as well, and if after two hours the patient has felt less than ten movements, she is instructed to call the doctor. (See Section 8: Post-Term)

286

Q *Is it true that_____will help to get my labor started?*

A You may fill in the blank with castor oil, Mexican food, cheese pizza, washing the floors, riding over the railroad tracks during the full moon, eating prunes, or just about anything you would like. The answer would still be no. If you think about it, the further you get past your due date, the more likely it is that standing on your head eating alfalfa sprouts will work. This makes it very hard to determine what seems to work best.

Your due date is the middle of a bell-shaped curve. About 50 percent deliver before and 50 percent after, most of these between thirty-eight and forty-two weeks. Actually, the only thing which has uniformly been shown to help is making love, which allows the prostaglandins in your partner's semen to bathe your cervix, which in turn helps with thinning of the cervix.

(Some say that the baby will come out if you go to bed with an Oreo cookie between your knees. Usually, however, you wake up with your husband's feet on the pillow and the Oreo gone!)

287

Q *I'm two days past my due date, my parents are in town, my husband skipped a trip to Europe, and my doctor won't induce me! Why not?*

A Medical induction of labor, whether with Pitocin alone or with prostaglandin cervical ripening followed by Pitocin, should not be undertaken lightly. An unripe cervix, meaning one that is hardly thinned out or dilated, where the head is still out of the pelvis (not dropped), is sometimes hard to change. Inducing an unripe cervix may in fact lead to a much higher chance of C-section, particularly if you are having your first baby.

The American College of Obstetricians and Gynecologists set out strict criteria for induction, and your doctor may either wish to abide by them in your best interest and or be restricted by the hospital's protocols. Inductions may certainly be done in the face of medical indications such as post-term gestation (greater than 41 weeks) and preeclampsia. (See Section 8: Induction)

SUGGESTED RESOURCES

American College of Obstetricians and Gynecologists. 1995. *ACOG Guide to Planning for Pregnancy, Birth, and Beyond.*
ACOG Web site: http://www.acog.com
Main Switchboard: 800-673-8444, (206) 638-5577
Order Desk: 800-762-2264

Eisenberg, A., Murkoff, H., Hathaway, S. 1991. *What to Expect When You're Expecting.* New York, Workman Publishers.

MacDougall, Jane (Ed.). 1997. *Pregnancy Week By Week; Everything You Need to Know.*

Schroeterbae-Cox, Kathryn. 1989. *Pregnancy Over 35.*

Sears, William, et al. 1997. *The Pregnancy Book; A Month by Month Guide.*
To Order Call: 1-800-299-3366 ext. 287. Childbirth Graphics. Div. of WRS Group Inc. Ask for item #HX46632
Web site: http://www.childbirthgraphics.com

WEBSITES

Genetic Testing

http://ucsfhealth.org/childrens/medical_services/preg/prenatal/

http://www.npr.org/about/press/980929.palca.html

http://www.wdxcyber.com/npreg08.htm

Amniocentesis

http://www.marchofdimes.com/professionals/681_1164.asp

CVS

http://www.marchofdimes.com/pnhec/159_521.asp

Nuchal Fold Test

http://www.pregnancyweekly.com/pregnancy_information/ nuchal_translucency_screening.htm Alpha FetoProtein/Triple Test

http://www.webmd.com/hw/being_pregnant/hw1663.asp

http://www.americanpregnancy.org/prenataltesting/tripletest.html

Ultrasound in Pregnancy

http://www.americanpregnancy.org/prenataltesting/ultrasound.html

Section Four

Fetal Development

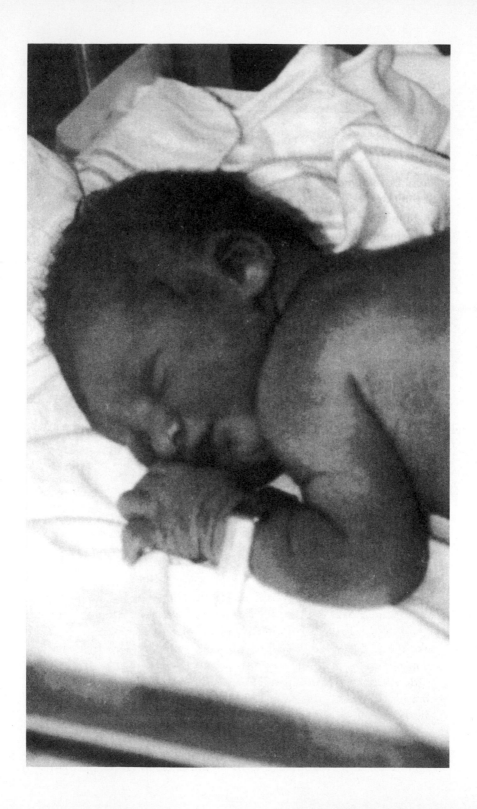

First Trimester

288

Q *When and where does conception take place?*

A It is thought that conception takes place within twenty-four hours after the release of the egg by your ovary, and most frequently in the fallopian tube. Recall that sperm can live in your genital tract for about seventy-two hours, so that sex even three days before ovulation can lead to pregnancy, but sex only thirty hours after ovulation probably will not.

Unlike bunny rabbits, the human fallopian tube isn't attached to the ovary. In other words, the egg doesn't come out of the ovary and go right into the tube. It is instead released into the pelvic cavity. The fimbria (structures on the ends of the tube that look like the strings on a mop head) pick up the egg out of the pelvic fluid. Sometimes when the sperm pass all the way through the tube and find no egg until they get to the pelvis, they form an embryo there. Six days later it implants where ever it is, and you've got an ectopic pregnancy. (See Ectopics)

Normally the sperm meets the ovum (egg) in the tube, and the resulting zygote (fertilized egg) travels down the tube toward the uterus, dividing itself over and over again. As it nears the uterus it forms a multicellular ball called the blastocyst, which implants around day six or seven in the specially prepared lining of the uterus called the decidua.

289

Q *What's happening about the time I miss my period and my urine pregnancy test is positive?*

A Your urine test cannot be positive until the blastocyst has attached to the wall of the uterus and the newly forming placenta has started making enough of the pregnancy hormone, human chorionic gonadotropin (HCG), to make the test positive. Usually this occurs no sooner than twelve days after conception. By the time you miss your period a true placenta is formed with little villi sticking into a pool of maternal blood in the uterine wall. This placenta is attached to the embryonic disc by what will soon become the umbilical cord.

At four weeks after ovulation, or six weeks from your last menstrual period, the gestational sac in the uterus is two to three centimeters in diameter, and the embryo is about four to five millimeters long. At approximately this time the heart begins to beat. Arm buds are also present by twenty-eight days after conception, or six weeks.

290

Q *I don't have my first obstetrical visit until ten weeks. What portion of my baby will develop before then?*

A Ten weeks is designated by most embryologists as the end of embryonic life and the beginning of fetal life. By eight weeks, or fifty-six days from conception (ten weeks by dates), essentially all of your baby's internal structural elements are formed. On average, the length of the fetus is about 40 millimeters, or an inch an a half.

While all of the internal structures are formed, they are by no means in their final states. The brain, spinal column, and nervous system are formed, but some neurologists believe new neural tissue is added until you've reached twenty-eight years of life. At this point, the fetal head is relatively huge compared with the rest of the body. The eyes are indentations still much too far apart to look human. The external ears, lips, and nose have not formed yet, but there are lumps suggesting where they will form. The gastrointestinal tract is formed, but the intestines for instance, are outside the body in the umbilical cord at ten weeks and are rotating into the position they will occupy for the rest of life. Limb buds have become true arms and legs and the fingers and toes are forming, but they have not yet distinctly separated.

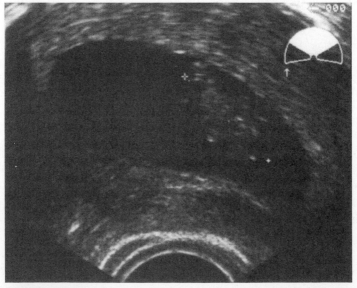

eighth week

The fetal tail is still present and won't completely reabsorb until about thirteen weeks. The embryo is shaped like the letter "C because its back grows faster than its front.

While the proper chromosomal codes to guide the growth of the external genitalia are present, the penis, scrotum, clitoris, and vagina are not yet developed at ten weeks.

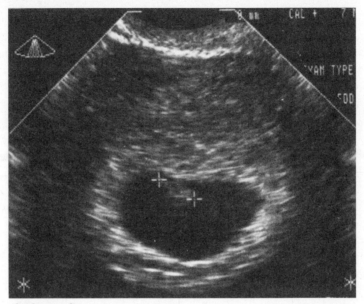

sixth week

291

Q *What can we learn from a vaginal ultrasound between eight and twelve weeks?*

A (See Section 2: Vaginal Ultrasound)
Unlike second trimester ultrasound, the information obtained from the early vaginal ultrasound is rudimentary with one exception. The measurements taken at this ultrasound will be more accurate at dating the pregnancy than any other information you can obtain without certain knowledge of the date of conception.

The standard error for this ultrasound examination is only plus or minus ninety-six hours. This sonogram should also confirm the number of fetuses, (which can be missed prior to eight weeks), the location of the gestational sac, the presence of the fetal heart beat, and the condition of the uterus and ovaries.

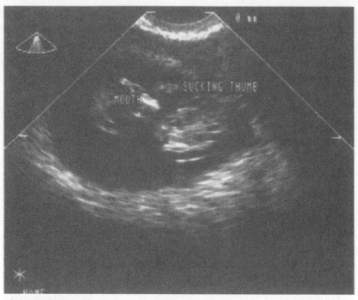

eleventh week

292

Q *What's happening right at the end of the first trimester?*

A The fetus is about 60 millimeters (two inches) long at twelve weeks. The amniotic sac contains about an ounce of clear, yellowish fluid. The brain, spine, heart, liver, stomach, intestines, kidneys, and bladder are completely formed, although the intestines are still partially out in the umbilical cord waiting until there is adequate room in the abdomen to return. The head is still disproportionately large, but the back begins to straighten by the end of the fourteenth week. The arms and legs have individual fingers and nails are beginning to grow. Nose, lips, and eyelids are just an early impression. External ears are forming, but they are lower and behind their final position. (The internal ear was formed by ten weeks.) The spine and ribs are rubbery, as yet without bone formation. The skin is transparent. Ovaries and testicles are beginning to form internally. External genitalia are within two weeks of being finally formed, but at this point look the same for boys and girls.

All that being said, as of June, 2005, a commercially available blood test which identifies fetal DNA in the mother's blood can reliably determine gender (sex) of the fetus by three weeks after conception, or 5 menstrual weeks! Researchers have discovered that "free fetal DNA" floats outside of cells in the mother's blood in miniscule amounts. This DNA can then be amplified and a simple test to look for the male "Y" chromosome can then be performed. The test, known as "Baby Gender Mentor" is marketed online. You can order the test online, put a few drops of your own blood from a finger stick in the test kit, and then mail it to Lowell Lab for processing, with 99.9% accurate results returned in 2-3 days.

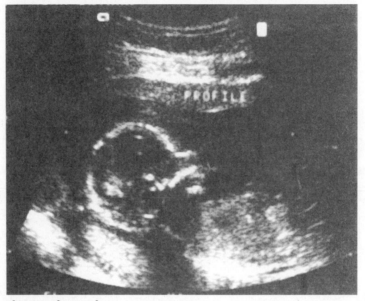

sixteenth week

Commercial use of the test raises several ethical questions however, since the results could theoretically be used to select the desired sex of a fetus, reject-ing the unwanted gender via early abortion. On the flip side, the technology used holds great promise for early diagnosis of genetic disorders such as Down's Syndrome and other genetic disorders. It could of course be used today when couples know that a certain sex linked disease can be present in only one gen-der. The same technology also has potential in terms of early testing for cancers such as ovarian, which also spill "free DNA" into the blood stream (Goldberg, Carey, "Test Reveals Gender Early in Pregnancy," *Boston Globe*, June 27, 2005).

SECOND TRIMESTER

293

Ⅱ *When can we tell the sex?*

A Without holding the fetus in your hand, about sixteen weeks is the ear-liest that doctors can reliably sex the fetus by ultrasound. Of course, sex can be determined by chromosomal testing, if indicated for other reasons, by as early as eleven to twelve weeks. (See Section 3: Amniocentesis and CVS) (See also answer to question 292.)

294

Q *When will I be able to feel my baby move?*

A Fetal movement is normally felt with a first pregnancy by around twenty to twenty-one weeks and is called "quickening." Movement may not be felt consistently, every day, until after twenty-five weeks, so relax if a day goes by without movement before this time. Many women with subsequent pregnancies can sense movement much earlier, as early as fifteen or sixteen weeks.

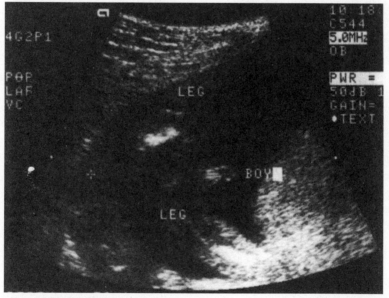

sixteenth week

295

Q *A woman in my Lamaze class says that her husband can see the baby move from all the way across the room. I never feel movement like that and I can hardly ever see movement at all. Is something wrong?*

A Ask your doctor to look on your ultrasound report and determine if your placenta happens to be in front rather than in back. Anterior placentas as they grow become a big fat couch pillow between you and your baby so that sensation of movements may be considerably muffled. Rarely, women claim to never have felt their baby's movements. Ultrasound examinations, during which movements can be witnessed, are reassuring for everyone in these cases. What is described above is, of course, different from a sudden decrease in fetal movement, which after twenty-five weeks can signal a problem. (See Section 3: Tests of Fetal Well-Being.)

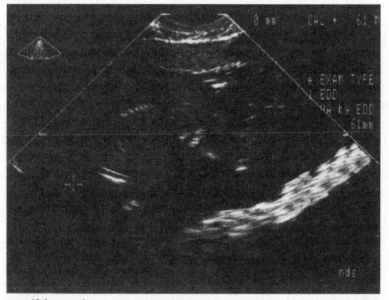

twelfth week

296

Q *What is the difference between a Level I ultrasound and a Level II ultrasound?*

A Level I and II ultrasound examinations differ according to the sophistication of the equipment used and the level of detail expected in terms of ruling out problems. Not everyone even uses the terminology Level I and Level II, but instead routine vs. targeted ultrasound. Both examinations will identify the number of fetuses, the position of the placenta, the amount of amniotic fluid, all the measurements appropriate to dating the pregnancy, the sex after sixteen weeks, the normal dimensions of the head and brain, a normal cross-sectional view of the heart that demonstrates that at least all the chambers are present, views of the spine adequate to rule out large open neural tube defects such as spina bifida, the presence of the stomach, kidneys, and bladder, and the site of the insertion of the umbilical cord on the abdominal wall of the fetus.

Targeted, or Level II, sonography is usually done with more sophisticated equipment and with a specially trained examiner, who may be a perinatologist (an obstetrician specializing in high-risk pregnancies), a radiologist, or a technician. It is ordered by your doctor if there is some specific reason to do so, whether that reason is your genetic history, drug exposure, or infectious history, or because of an abnormal routine sonogram.

297

Q *I know you can see a lot on the ultrasound at sixteen to seventeen weeks. What is it you look for developmentally?*

A That is a bigger question than you might expect and some people devote a lifetime of training to it just in order to know what to look for on such a sonogram. In short, the number of fetuses and, if there are multiple fetuses, the character of the membranes between them. The fetus may be sexed if you wish it. The amount of amniotic fluid and position of the placenta are noted. (See Section 8: Placenta Previa) Cross-sectional views of the brain, spinal cord, heart, liver, kidneys, bladder, and extremities are obtained and appropriate measurements taken.

Developmental Defects and Ultrasound

298

Q *What kind of problems can be diagnosed?*

A Many. Problem areas are detailed by system below. Placenta. (See also Section 8: Placenta Previa) The single most common abnormal finding is related to the position of the placenta. If the embryo implants very low in the uterus, the placenta may grow over the opening of the cervix. This is a placenta previa. If it completely crosses the cervical opening it is referred to as a total or complete previa. This occurs in only 1 to 3 percent of pregnancies and cannot be diagnosed with security until another sonogram is taken late in the third trimester. Partial previa usually resolves by about twenty-eight weeks. The placenta doesn't really move, of course, since it's implanted. However, the lower segment of the uterus stretches more than the upper and distance develops between the lower edge of the placenta and the edge of the cervix.

Often the extent of the previa cannot be diagnosed until the third trimester. Until that time, making love is usually prohibited. If the previa fails to resolve, it may even lead to bed rest after about thirty-four weeks or from the time of a bleeding episode until an amniocentesis for lung maturity can be done at about thirty-six weeks and subsequently a C-section performed.

Heart. Cardiac defects are the single most common category of anomalies identified in the second trimester with a liveborn incidence of about 8/1,000. Of those identified, about 1/3 will have chromosomal errors. By eighteen completed weeks, most major cardiac anomalies can be ruled out with a cross sectional view of the heart. An "echogenic focus" in the fetal heart valves is a frequent finding, which by itself, should not cause concern. When associated with other findings, it has a very weak association with Down Syndrome.

Recently, color flow Doppler is available on Level II or targeted ultrasound examinations and has been used to help identify abnormal flow of blood through the fetal heart.

Central Nervous System. Significant open neural tube defects (ONTD) may also be ruled out with greater than 95 percent certainty. (See Section 3: Ultrasound) These include absence of the upper skull and brain (anencephaly), which is incompatible with life; protrusion of part of the brain and cerebrospinal fluid through the back of the head (encephalocele), also associated with other anomalies frequently and usually incompatible with life; and protrusion of tissue through a vertebral defect in the lower back (spina bifida), the severity of which is very variable.

Hydrocephalus, or an enlarged head due to too much fluid in the chambers of the brain, can be identified by measuring certain ratios. The incidence of hydrocephalus is only 0.8/1,000, but about 85 percent of these fetuses have either additional malformations in the head and elsewhere or major chromosomal errors.

Choroid plexus cysts have recently been described and at least a couple of articles have associated them with increased risk of trisomies 21 and 18. Recent articles have refuted this and in our experience, the cysts always resolve by twenty-eight weeks, and do not appear to be associated with an increased risk of Down's syndrome. An isolated finding of choroid plexus cysts does not justify or indicate a need for amniocentesis.[1]

Gastrointestinal tract. Diaphragmatic hernia occurs in about 1/2,500 fetuses. It means that the intestines have protruded up into the chest through a defect in the diaphragm at the base of the lungs. It is associated with other major problems about half the time, and chromosomal abnormalities about 20 percent of the time.

Typically, neonatal surgery is required right after birth, and survival depends largely on the degree to which lung development was restricted by the herniation.

Abdominal wall defects include omphalocele and gastroschisis. The former is a defect in the abdominal wall that leads to the intestines remaining in the umbilical cord instead of the belly. The latter is another defect in which intestines, stomach, and, rarely, the liver are herniated into the amniotic fluid and float there freely prior to delivery. Both are usually treated surgically after birth with the exception of small omphaloceles. Not only can these defects be diagnosed by ultrasound, but amniotic fluid and serum AFP are elevated.

Esophageal atresia is a defect in which the esophagus (the tube from the mouth to the stomach) doesn't attach to the stomach, and may in fact partially attach to the trachea (breathing tube) instead. It is often associated with hydramnios (too much amniotic fluid) and lack of a stomach bubble on ultrasound. This is treated surgically soon after birth.

Duodenal atresia is a similar defect but further down the gastrointestinal tract. The duodenum is the part of the small intestine that attaches to the stomach. The classic "double bubble" sign may be seen on ultrasound due to distension of both the stomach and the first part of the duodenum before the blockage. This is treated surgically soon after birth, and is more common with Down's syndrome.

Genitourinary tract. Presence of the kidneys, a urine-filled bladder, and adequate amniotic fluid are reassuring that at least partial function exists.

Renal agenesis is a defect in which the kidneys fail to form at all. It occurs in about 1/4,000 births and is uniformly fatal. It is the primary feature of Potter's syndrome. When agenesis occurs unilaterally (on one side only) it may have no effect on the fetus at all.

Urinary tract obstruction in any one of several areas is the most common defect of the urinary tract. It leads to dilation of one or both ureters, and then to dilation of the base (pelvis) of the kidney. Mild forms may resolve on their own, but more severe ones may require surgery in the first months of life.

Cystic renal disease develops in response to severe obstruction. The cysts on the kidney may be extensive and essentially destroy it. When this occurs on both sides it may be fatal.

299

Q *What does the baby look like at sixteen weeks?*

A The fetus is about 12 centimeters (4 3/4 inches) long and now weighs no grams (about 4 ounces) at sixteen weeks. Almost all women will be showing by now. The fetus's body is now starting to grow much faster, and it is beginning to look a little more human as its proportions become familiar. The baby's external genitalia are identifiable on ultrasound. Eyebrows and lashes are present. Nails have begun to form. Teeth have begun to form under the gums even though they won't come out until months after birth. The baby can suck its thumb in a coordinated fashion. The ears have completed their external formation and have moved to the appropriate place on the side of the head. the baby's movements get more vigorous. Women having their second baby can often feel movement by this point.

300

Q *I've heard that 20 weeks has special significance. What's happening at this point?*

A This is the halfway point in your pregnancy. Legally in many states pregnancy losses beyond this point are classified as stillbirths and no longer are considered miscarriages, although the fetus is still more than a month away from being able to survive outside the womb in a Neonatal Intensive Care Unit (NICU). It weighs roughly 300 grams (3/4 of a pound). Crown-to-rump length is about six and a half inches, but measurements to the heel put the fetus at about a foot long. Downy hair, called lanugo hair, now covers the whole body. Scalp hair has begun to grow. The skin is becoming more opaque and less transparent.

Most first-time mothers feel the baby begin to move (quickening) from about twenty to twenty-two weeks.

301

Q *When will the baby begin to try and breathe?*

A At twenty-four weeks of gestation the fetus weighs about 630 to 650 grams (1 1/2 pounds). A fetus born at this stage will attempt to breathe, but even with hi-tech support, it will almost always succumb. The skin is now wrinkled, and fat is beginning to deposit beneath it. Eyebrows have formed.

THIRD TRIMESTER

302

Q *What's happening by the twenty-eighth week?*

A The fetus weighs about 1,100 grams (two and a half pounds). The skin is now covered with a cheesy, thick protective cream called vernix caseosa. Babies born after twenty-eight weeks usually survive today with intensive care support. The pupillary membrane which had been over the developing eyes disappears, and if babies are born prematurely at this stage they move, cry, and open their eyes.

303

Q *Why does my doctor say that 30 weeks is a big hurdle passed?*

A After thirty weeks, or about 1,500 grams, your baby would have a survival rate of over 85 percent if it were born prematurely into sophisticated NICU support. Still, between 25 percent and 50 percent of these babies will grow up to have some deficits in either cognition (thinking) or behavior. Preterm labor at this point will still be vigorously treated until about thirty-six weeks.

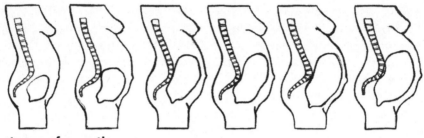

stages of growth

304

Q *What happens in the final eight to ten weeks to make the fetus ready for delivery?*

A To the naked eye, the baby simply puts on weight and gets longer, and by about thirty-seven weeks almost all will have figured which way is out and turned their head downward! Physiologically, however, your baby's lungs, liver, and intestines are still maturing.

FETAL PHYSIOLOGICAL DEVELOPMENT

Lungs

305

Q *When will the baby's lungs be ready to function on the outside?*

A Almost all babies are ready to breathe on their own by 37 weeks. Those who have trouble after birth usually require only minimal support, such as supplemental oxygen.

Babies born between thirty and thirty-four weeks almost always require considerable support, often including the use of a ventilator to breathe for the baby temporarily. Babies are underwater creatures until birth. The cells that line the air sacs (full of amniotic fluid in utero) prepare to function with air by producing surfactant. Surfactant is a compound secreted by these type II alveolar cells that overcomes the force of water tension. Water molecules have a tendency to stick together, or coalesce. Tiny air sacs out in the periphery of the lung cannot open and fill with air simply because of the water tension holding them closed. Surfactant acts to allow the walls of these air sacs to pull apart with ease.

By thirty-five weeks most babies have made substantial amounts of surfactant. This process can be stimulated by giving steroids either by injection or by mouth to the mother. Nonetheless, many babies under thirty-four weeks will require synthetic surfactant to be administered immediately after birth.

It is the absence of this surfactant that causes Premature Lung Disease or Respiratory Distress Syndrome (RDS). (See Section 8: Preterm Labor and Delivery)

306

Q *Is there a way to determine if a baby's lungs are ready to work yet?*

A Yes. Amniocentesis can be performed late in pregnancy to assess lung function, just as it can in early pregnancy when trying to make diagnoses of genetic defects. The fluid is analyzed for the L/S ratio.

The ratio of two compounds, lecithin and sphyngomyelin, or the L/S Ratio, can be determined from a small sample of amniotic fluid. Lecithin is the major agent of surfactant felt to be responsible for decreasing water surface tension in the little alveolar air sacs, which must open to allow lung function. Other tests to assess lung maturity on the fluid include phosphatidylglycerol, foam stability index, fluorescence polarization, optical density, and lamellar body counts.

Amniocentesis for lung maturity might be indicated in certain cases of preterm labor, placenta previa, preeclampsia, diabetes, or several less common conditions. (See Section 8: Obstetric Complications)

307

Q *My friend was told that her baby's lungs never developed because there was no fluid in them. Is that possible?*

A Amniotic fluid moving in and out of the fetus's lungs is essential to lung development. Premature rupture of membranes at a very early stage, usually at less than twenty-four weeks, for example, can lead to a baby born even months later with hypoplastic lungs. This condition is fatal, and when it occurs, unavoidable. There are other causes, such as Potter's syndrome, in which failure of the kidneys to develop results in lack of amniotic fluid, and thus lack of lung development. (See Section 8: Premature Rupture of Membranes)

Heart

308

Q *When does the fetal heart really start to function?*

A It really starts to function as soon as the circulatory system is a closed circuit and the heart begins to beat. On average this occurs at about twenty-six to thirty days after conception, or six weeks of gestation. The fetal heart is pumping the fetus's blood through the body and also through the placenta. The blood of mother and baby do not mix, but meet across thin membranes in the placenta to exchange gas and nutrients.

309

Q *What about the fetal heart? I've heard it is different from the adult heart.*

A The fetal heart is indeed different from the adult heart. Blood must flow through the heart differently because the oxygen comes from the placenta and not the lungs. There are connections between the right and left sides of the heart that must exist in the fetus to survive in the womb, and they must go away shortly after birth for the baby to survive in the outside world. The normal fetal heart rate is also in the range of 120 to 160 beats per minute, while for adults it is in the range of 60 to 90.

310

Q *How does the circulatory system switch over from fetal to newborn?*

A This is one of the miracles of childbirth. Shortly after the cord is clamped and cut, all sorts of pressure changes occur, and within the first couple of hours the foramen ovale (hole between left and right atrium) and the ductus arteriosus (connection between pulmonary artery and aorta) both close spontaneously. Sometimes they do not close correctly and persistent fetal circulation may occur, necessitating indocin, or sometimes even surgery, to close the ductus arteriosus. Conversely, with some cardiac defects such as tetrology of Fallot and transposition of the great vessels, the persistent fetal circulation, by allowing oxygenated blood to get out to the body, is all that keeps the baby alive.

Blood

311

Q *Where does my baby's blood come from?*

A Very early on, your embryo's blood is made in the yolk sac. This is the attachment to your placenta that is visible as a little ring next to the fetal pole. You can see this on the office ultrasound under ten weeks or so. After the baby's organs are completely formed, the liver takes over as the site of red blood cell production. Only near the end of pregnancy is the bone marrow beginning to take over, and it is here that blood will be produced for the remainder of life.

312

Q *How much blood does my baby have?*

A Not a lot. Near term, the newborn will have about 80 cc per kilogram. This means that a seven-pound baby will have only about 250 cc of blood. That's one juice box!

313

Q *Is it true that fetuses have a different kind of blood from us?*

A It is. Hemoglobin is the protein in the middle of red blood cells that allows them to carry oxygen. Fetal hemoglobin comes in three varieties all made very early on. Hemoglobin A, the molecule found in adults, is present as early as the eleventh week of gestation and gradually makes up a greater and greater percentage of the blood. Still, at term, only 25 percent of the hemoglobin present is of the A type. Fetal hemoglobin binds relatively more oxygen than Hemoglobin A. As a consequence, the fetus can extract oxygen from the placenta more efficiently.

314

Q *Other than red blood cells, what else is in the blood?*

A Immunoglobulins, which will be largely responsible for your newborn's ability to fight infection, are carried by the bloodstream. IgG,
one of the most important, is transported across the placenta from your
body. The vast majority of this immunoglobulin, however, is transported
to the fetus in only the final four weeks of gestation. Consequently, newborn preemies are poorly protected from infection. By term, the blood also
contains white blood cells that fight infection, platelets to help blood clot,
and a myriad of hormones.

315

Q *Is it true that breast-feeding is absolutely necessary to protect my baby from infection?*

A (See also Section 10: Breast Feeding)
Of course not. But after hundreds of studies on the topic, it does
appear to be true that breastfeeding is somewhat protective against gastroenteritis (diarrhea), and to a lesser extent, upper respiratory infections, in
the first year or so of life. This can be demonstrated with as little as two
months of breastfeeding.[2, 3]

Digestive System

316

Q *When does the fetus's digestive system begin to function? Does it only start with
feeding after birth?*

A Your baby is swallowing fluid, and the intestines are involved in peri-
stalsis (moving the contents along) by the end of the first twelve weeks.
The amount of amniotic fluid swallowed initially is tiny, but by the end
of pregnancy the amount swallowed has a substantial effect on amniotic
fluid volume.

317

Q *What is meconium, and why is it important?*

A Meconium is the sticky, dark greenish-black substance excreted shortly
after and occasionally shortly before birth. It consists of swallowed amniotic fluid, saliva, digestive enzymes, and desquamated (sloughed-off) cells
from the lining of the gut. Hypoxia (decreased oxygen) in later pregnancy or
in labor may stimulate the release of a hormone from the pituitary that causes

contraction of the colon and release of meconium into the amniotic fluid. This can lead to meconium aspiration in which the sticky material is breathed into the lungs, causing a severe chemical pneumonia and, very rarely, even neonatal death or stillbirth.

318

Q *When can the fetus eat if it is born prematurely?*

A In general, babies born after thirty-six weeks have little trouble eating. But trouble feeding can be related not only to the ability of the gut to handle food and digest properly, but also to the ability of the preemie to suckle. It takes strength and coordination to hold on to the nipple, suck, breathe nasally, and swallow.

But this is a critical question in neonatal medicine. While everyone knows that preemies may have trouble breathing, the public seems less aware that trouble eating may be very severe as well. In fact, a very premature gut, and especially one receiving less oxygen because of premature lung disease, may respond to feeding with necrotizing enterocolitis (NEC). NEC can be difficult to treat and even fatal. It is seen more commonly in preemies born before thirty-four weeks, and may be thought of as premature bowel disease. (See Section 8: Preterm Delivery)

319

Q *What kinds of problems could occur with the baby's liver and pancreas?*

A Probably the only thing you'll run into is that occasionally problems are accentuated and more likely with preemies. The newborn and especially the preemie newborn's liver cannot bind bilirubin well. Bilirubin is a breakdown product of red blood cells. In adults, bilirubin is chemically converted to a compound (in a process called conjugation) that the liver excretes into the bowel. In newborns, only a small percentage of bilirubin is handled this way. Because fetal red blood cells have shorter life spans, more bilirubin is produced. The immature liver cannot handle the load and unconjugated bilirubin can build up, causing newborn jaundice.

Jaundice itself is not dangerous, but it can be a warning of dangerously high levels of bilirubin. Very high levels of bilirubin deposit in the brain and can lead to a rare condition called kernicterus, which is associated with mental retardation, spasticity, and coordination problems.

Newborn jaundice is treated primarily with phototherapy. Babies are either exposed unclothed to ultraviolet light under warmers, or, nowadays, wrapped in pads containing fiber-optic cables; in this way, as much surface area as possible is exposed to the light. Light, through an unknown process, helps the liver conjugate bilirubin and also breaks down the compound by oxidation.

The fetal pancreas produces insulin at as early as eleven weeks of gestation. As pregnancy progresses, the pancreas releases insulin in a manner responsive to blood levels of glucose, just as it will after birth. However, the pancreas's digestive functions appear to be activated only around the time of birth.

Nervous System

320

Q *When can my baby sense things?*

A As early as ten weeks of gestation, the fetus may respond to local stimuli with squinting, mouth opening, partial finger closure, and flexion of the toes. Swallowing and breathing are present by fourteen weeks. By twenty-eight weeks the fetal eye is sensitive to light. Sound may be heard by as early as twenty-four weeks. Also at twenty-eight weeks, preemie newborns are known to respond differently to different tastes.

Viewed with ultrasound, the fetus can be seen to move its trunk by eight weeks of gestation. More coordinated movements develop as each area develops structurally. In other words, arms, toes, and fingers are moving before ten weeks of gestation.

There is definitive evidence from extremely premature infants that auditory response can be evoked at as early as twenty-four weeks of gestation. This means that at least theoretically, a baby should be able to hear its parents sing lullabies by five and a half months after conception, even though it is still four months before the delivery.

As with the other senses, data on fetal vision extrapolated from premature infants is helpful. We know that preemies at twenty-eight weeks of gestation respond to a light stimulus with pupillary constriction as well as with electrical signals from the retina to the back of the brain where vision is controlled. What they can see is harder to determine.

Premature infants as early as twenty-eight weeks clearly respond differently to different tastes. It is reasonable to assume that with overlapping neural pathways, smell could be functional at this point as well.

321

Q *When is the neural tube completely formed so that I can stop worrying about spina bifida?*

Believe it or not, the neural tube should be closed by day 28 of embryonic life, or by about six weeks from your last menstrual period. That is why drugs with increased risk of spina bifida formation have their effect often before you even know you are pregnant. It is also why the vitamin folic acid or folate is useful to prevent neural tube defects only if you are already taking it when you conceive and during the following month.

Urinary Tract

322

When do the baby's kidneys and bladder begin to function?

Fetal kidney function as defined by production of urine begins by twelve weeks of gestation. The full function of the kidneys, however, including excretion of concentrated waste products and control of urine pH (acid-base), remains immature even in fetuses that are close to term.

323

If kidney function is inefficient in the fetus, is it important for the fetus's survival?

It is important that the kidneys function in utero, but not for excretion of waste, as occurs after the baby is born. Amniotic fluid is largely made up of fetal urine in the second and third trimesters. If the kidneys fail to form or fail to function, severe oligohydramnios (decreased fluid) may result. Because the fluid is necessary for formation and function of the lungs, a fetus born with no renal function will be born with lungs that never developed.

Skeletal System

324

When do the baby's bones form?

By the tenth week, major ossification centers are formed and bones have started to grow. Initially, however, they are made of a cartilaginous matrix. Only months later will calcium actually be laid down into hard fetal bone. The spine grows faster than the front of the baby initially and accounts for the "C" shape of the former embryo, now fetus, at ten weeks.

325

Q *Don't the bones make the baby's blood?*

A Not initially. The yolk sac makes the first red blood cells. The fetal liver takes over at about ten weeks and only gradually relinquishes this function to the bone marrow. The bone marrow first forms and begins functioning at about fifteen weeks, but the liver continues to make red cells all the way through delivery.

326

Q *When do the joints form?*

A Arm and leg buds form as early as four weeks after conception (six weeks). The hands and fingers form somewhat earlier than the feet and toes. Fingers are still webbed at eight weeks and the feet are just nubs. By twelve weeks, however, the fingers and toes are distinct and little elbows and knees have formed. Hips can flex at this point and shoulders can rotate. By fourteen weeks, all the fetal joints appear to have virtually their full range of motion.

327

Q *What is the fontanel?*

A Otherwise known as the "soft spot," the fontanels are the intersections of the bony plates that make up the baby's skull. The larger, diamond-shaped "frontal" fontanel, and the triangular rear, or "occipital," fontanel are spaces that allow the skull to compress at birth. In concert with the "sutures" (linear spaces where the bony plates of the head butt up against each other), the fontanels also allow for growth of the brain after birth.

This is clearly another one of God's miracles of design. A baby whose head is considerably larger than the inside pelvic diameters of its mother may be born vaginally because of these fontanels and sutures. In short, when you push your baby out, its head may momentarily look like a banana, but it rounds up again quickly (See Section 7: Labor and Delivery)

Sexual Development

328

Q *What determines if my baby is a boy or a girl?*

Believe it or not, that question is not that easy to answer. Ultimately, the genetic gender of your baby is determined by the sex chromosome that the father contributed in the sperm—Y for male and X for female. Thus, a chromosome type with 46 chromosomes (two sets of 22) plus XX is female; a type with two sets of 22 plus XY is male. This is expressed as 46xx or 46xy.

The question gets complicated because the development of the external genitalia or sex organs is not simply determined by the chromosomes. This means that while your baby could have 46xy chromosomes, it could have female external genitalia. The converse can be true as well.

329

If it is not the chromosomes, then what determines whether my baby's genitals look male or female?

Male hormone, plain and simple. Prior to eight weeks of gestation, the genital tracts of both male and female are identical. In the absence of male hormone, all fetuses would develop external genitalia of the female. (Tough for a guy to admit, but without hormonal intervention, all human fetuses are destined to become female.) Normally, if the chromosomes are XY, testes develop, they make testosterone, and the response is the development of the penis and scrotum and the descent of the testicles. In the normal female, with testosterone absent, the external structures become the clitoris, labia, and vagina instead.

If the male fetus is either missing male hormone receptors, or the female fetus is exposed to too much male hormone from the adrenal gland, the ambiguous genitalia result. The condition is called either male or female pseudohermaphrodism and is luckily quite rare.

PLACENTAL DEVELOPMENT

330

What exactly is the placenta?

The placenta, commonly called the "afterbirth," is a living organ whose normal function is absolutely essential to the growth, development, and survival of the fetus. It is responsible for providing your fetus with oxygen and nutrients as well as for disposing of carbon dioxide and waste products. You can visualize the placenta as a sponge, attached to the fetus by the umbilical cord, that soaks in a pool of maternal blood located in the wall of the uterus. This is a gross oversimplification, for the placenta is a hormonally active, immunologically essential, extremely complex biochemical interface between you and your baby.

331

Q *Where is the placenta?*

A The placenta is attached to the inner wall of your uterus exactly where the blastocyst implanted about six to seven days after conception. It then grows as the baby grows and will eventually weigh about one-sixth of the weight of your baby at term.

At just seven to eight days after implantation, the blastocyst consists of cells that will become the baby. These are called the inner cell mass, and cells that begin to form the placenta are called trophoblasts. Fetal blood and maternal blood never mix, but exchange gas and chemicals across the one-cell-layer thick walls of the placental villi.

332

Q *How about the membranes?*

A Two types of membrane evolve around the pregnancy. The inner membrane is called the amnion and the outer one is called the chorion. By twelve weeks, the two membranes are fused together to form a sac, and the sac has grown so that the chorion is fused all around to the inside wall of the uterus. Just as the placenta transfers gases and biochemical compounds across the surface of the villi, the membranes are actively involved in transport of fluid in and out of the amniotic sac. The membranes normally stay intact, containing the amniotic fluid, until labor occurs after the 38th week. Spontaneous rupture of the membranes occurs sometime during labor about two-thirds of the time and before the onset of labor about one-third of the time.

333

Q *Can the membranes tell you something about what kind of twins one might have?*

A (See also Section 8: Multiple Gestation)
Yes and no. Twins may be identical (monozygotic—from one egg) or fraternal (dizygotic—from two eggs). If there is one placenta, one chorion, and one or two amnions, the twins are monozygotic identical twins. A pregnancy with one placenta, two chorions, and two amnions may be either monozygotic or dizygotic. A pregnancy with two placentas, two chorions, and two amnions is likely to be dizygotic, but may be monozygotic if division occurred within the first seventy-two hours after fertilization.

This undoubtedly seems confusing. All that you need to remember is that unless there is only one placental disc and one chorion (in which case the twins are identical), no one can be sure whether they are identical or fraternal. (Of course, if one baby has a penis and the other doesn't, that's a hint that they are dizygotic, and therefore, fraternal.)

334

Q How about the umbilical cord?

A The umbilical cord has a complex origin. Suffice it to say that it has something to do with the disappearing yolk sac, as well as formation and rotation of the intestines, and that by about ten weeks the umbilical cord is finally formed. Normally the cord has three vessels—two arteries and one vein. Recall that in the fetus the vein carries the oxygenated blood to the fetus, and the arteries carry deoxygenated blood away from the fetus and back to the placenta (opposite to the way adult arteries and veins work).

The umbilical cord is full of fetal blood only. This blood carries the gases, nutrients, and wastes back and forth to the placental interface. Therefore, the umbilical cord must not be occluded, or fetal injury and/or death could occur. Wharton's jelly is a thick, rubbery, clear proteinaceous substance that surrounds the vessels of the twisted cord and helps to prevent compression.

335

Q What kind of problems can there be with development of the cord?

A Several variations of the cord's connection to the body of the placenta may occur.

Attachment Problems

Velementous insertion of the cord occurs about 1 percent of the time with singletons, but much more with multiple pregnancies. It means that the vessels of the cord insert and traverse a distance across just the amnion, substantially away from the edge of the placental disc. This exposes them more readily to compression, or even transection with membrane rupture or during labor.

Marginal insertion of the cord means that the cord vessels insert right at the edge of the placenta; this is slightly less dangerous than velementous insertion.

Vasa previa occurs with velementous insertion when the vessels actually cross over the cervix on their way to the placenta. This can lead to a lethal loss of fetal blood should those membranes rupture with labor, whether preterm or not. (See Section 8: Previa)

Cord Problems

Knots in the cord may be false knots, which are really just kinks, or true knots, in which the actually passed through a loop of cord early on. True knots occur only about 1 percent of the time, but lead to 6 percent of stillbirths or newborn deaths. Nuchal cords (cord around the neck) occur with about one-third of all deliveries. Contrary to popular belief, they are rarely associated with stillbirth. They are, however, associated with fetal heart rate changes as the baby descends the birth canal in labor. These changes may on occasion be severe enough to warrant cesarean section.

Torsion (twisting) of the cord occurs normally with fetal movement. In rare instances, it may be so severe as to seriously compromise blood flow. With monamnionic (one inner sac only) identical twins, cord twisting and entanglement leads to a fetal death rate during the pregnancy of 50 percent.

Single umbilical artery is a frequent anomaly where one of the vessels leading *away* from the fetus is absent. It is occasionally associated with chromosomal defects such as Down's syndrome, but more often is isolated and only rarely is of any clinical significance. When present, more frequent ultrasound to rule out IUGR is appropriate.

336

Q *What is cord blood stem cell collection?*

A This is the process wherein a sterile sample of cord blood is extracted with a needle immediately after delivery, specially packaged, and mailed to a company that then freezes the sample until such time as it might be needed to treat your baby, a sibling or even you or your partner in the future when faced with a myriad of life threatening diseases. Stem cells are building blocks with all the genetic material to become any cell in the body! There are over 70 diseases currently treatable in 2011 with cord blood stem cell transplant and the chances of a family member utilizing them for this reason is about 1 in 200. These diseases include leukemias, lymphomas, Hodgkin's, multiple myeloma, brain tumors, Ewing sarcomas, testicular cancer, storage diseases, immune deficiencies, Tay Sachs, Lesch-Nyan, and many many more.

337

Q *If these diseases are so rare, is there any other reason to collect stem cells?*

A Research through 2011 is clearly showing that the major use for both cord blood and recently cord segment stem cells will be regenerative medicine. Already stem cells have restored normal heart function, corneal function, cured sickle cell, vastly improved children with cerebral palsy and traumatic brain injury, and there are ongoing trials with regard to diabetes, spinal cord injury, autoimmune diseases, burn patients, joint damage, Alzheimer's, ALS, Parkinson's, stroke, liver and kidney failure and many others. Now estimates a family member using their stem cells has risen to 1 in 4! (www.cordblood.com)

338

Q *Should all pregnant women plan on stem cell collection and how do we arrange it?*

A In my opinion, stem cell collection should become standard of care reimbursed by insurers across the nation. You can get more information on stem cell collection at www.cordblood.com. There are over 20 companies which offer these services, but CBR has done collections for the longest. Simply notify your doctor that you are interested before 37 weeks or so, and he will head you in the right direction.

339

Q *What does placental calcification mean?*

A As the placenta ages, especially after forty-one weeks of gestation, calcification forms throughout. The degree of placental calcification only correlates very roughly to the age of the placenta and to decreasing function. In other words, calcification is a normal process over time. Occasionally, if a large degree of calcification is seen before thirty-six weeks on ultrasound, it may be a soft indicator of a placenta whose function is failing. It may also accompany chronic disease such as hypertension or diabetes.

SUGGESTED READING

For great pictures of your developing gymnast:

Bryan, Terry. 1995. *The Miracle of Birth: A Fascinating See-Through View of How a Baby Develops.*

Curtis, Glade. 1997. *Your Pregnancy Week by Week*, 3rd Ed. Tucson, AZ; Fisher Books.

Nilsson, Lennart, Text by Lars Hamberger. 1990. *A Child is Born*. New York, NY: Delacorte Press/Seymour Lawrence.

Nilsson, Lennart. *The Miracle of Life,* 60 min. First part of Emmy Award Winning NOVA series chronicles development from conception to birth with actual video footage.
To Order Call: 1-800-299-3366 ext. 287. Childbirth Graphics. Div. of WRS Group Inc. Ask for item #HX46632.
Web Site: http://www.childbirthgraphics.com
E-Mail: Sales@wrsgroup.com

WEBSITES

Cord Blood Banking
http://www.cordblood.com

Fetal Development
http://www.babycenter.com/fetaldevelopment/
http://www.nlm.nih.gov/medlineplus/ency/article/002398.htm

Section Five

Drugs in Pregnancy

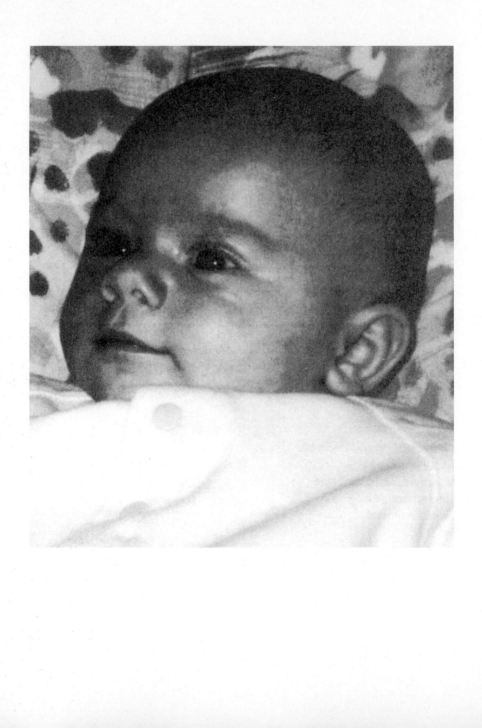

INTRODUCTION

If you happen to be reading this information straight through, then this particular section, perhaps above all others, deserves a brief introduction. The use of drugs in pregnancy, whether illicit, over-the-counter (OTC), or prescription, is widespread. Just deciding that no medicines should be taken in pregnancy is neither practical nor wise. Many OTC medicines are felt to be completely safe in pregnancy and alleviate considerable suffering. Many prescription medicines are required for controlling diseases that, untreated, would be much more harmful to the pregnancy than the effect of the medications. This is often true even when the medicine is known to slightly increase the risks of some birth defects.

However, one sweeping caveat is appropriate. Try to avoid OTC medicines until you've completed your tenth week of pregnancy! That includes avoiding them when trying to get pregnant, since many critical organ systems form from twenty to fifty days after conception, when you may not even be aware of your pregnancy. If you have read the section on fetal development, you are now aware that virtually all critical structures have been formed by the completion of the tenth week from your last menstrual period. Some organogenesis, notably of the external genitalia, is not complete for several weeks after that.

However, avoiding OTC medicines during the first trimester will eliminate the huge majority of risk associated with drugs in pregnancy. If you wish to use this volume to research an OTC medicine, be sure to evaluate all of the ingredients individually, since each of hundreds of compounds has different combinations of drugs. Of course, adhere to your doctor's advice. Many drugs are completely safe even prior to ten weeks, and if advised to use them by the doctor you trust, you should certainly consider it. Likewise, even if the description in this volume is reassuring, your doctor's advice takes priority, since he or she knows your individual circumstances.

Prescription medicines should be discussed with your doctor before you get pregnant. If that is not possible, at least read the package inserts and/or ask your pharmacist about potential problems early in pregnancy. Do not stop any prescription medicine for a potentially life-threatening chronic condition without first discussing it with your doctor, even if you know you have just conceived.

TERATOGENS IN GENERAL

General Understanding

340

Q *What is a teratogen?*

A A teratogen is an agent, which when exposed to a developing fetus at some point, has the potential to cause a birth defect. This agent may be a drug, a chemical, an environmental exposure, or even an infection.

It's not as easy as you might think to prove that a drug is a teratogen. First, there must be proof that the exposure actually occurred and at what times in gestation. Next, there must be consistent findings from more than one epidemiological study (a study that looks at a whole population in which the thing you are looking for occurred), which have sufficient numbers to be statistically significant, and which control for confounding factors—that is, rule out things other than the suspected agent that could have led to the outcome. Prospective studies (forward-looking) with case controls proving relative risk (increased) of more than sixfold are adequate, to prove that an exposure is truly teratogenic. But these type of studies are exceedingly rare in humans since pregnant women are unwilling to volunteer for a placebo-controlled trial to see if a certain drug causes a birth defect. Finally, the potential causal relationship between drug and birth defect should make biological sense. In other words, there should be a plausible mechanism to explain how the teratogen causes the birth defect.

341

Q *How often are babies born with defects?*

A Major birth defects occur in about 3 percent of all births. Over time, more subtle defects become apparent, and the defect rate climbs to 4.5 to 5 percent by age five. Less than 50 percent of the time is the exact cause or mechanism ever identified.[1]

342

Q *My friend just read in a magazine that taking _____ can cause a problem. Everybody I know has taken that! How do I know if it can really cause a problem?*

A First, talk with your doctor. Magazines write articles to sell magazines, not unlike the rationale for the choice of guests and topics on TV talk shows. Unfortunately, even well-meaning authors misinterpret animal studies, or draw inappropriate conclusions from observational studies. For example, if a study found that 50 percent of people seen playing tennis this spring had symptoms of gallstones, a false conclusion would be that tennis should be avoided, since it could be the cause of these gallstones.

In short, if 3 to 5 percent of all children exhibit some type of birth defect and more than 95 percent of the population uses over-the-counter medicines, someone is bound to conclude that simply because you were taking the medicine during the pregnancy that it was the cause of the defect. Association and causation are two very different things as any scientist, doctor, or attorney understands.

343

Q *Why not just avoid all medicines when you're pregnant?*

A Overall, that's not a bad idea. However, many prescribed medicines for controlling chronic illnesses may be essential to your baby's health if they are essential to yours. You wouldn't have a diabetic stop her insulin, a hypertensive stop her blood pressure medicine, or an asthmatic stop her inhaler unless she discussed discontinuing the medication with her doctor.

As for over-the-counter (OTC) medicines, studies show that over 90 percent of American women take such medicines while pregnant, even if the medicine was taken before the women knew they were pregnant.[2] If possible, avoiding all OTC medicines in the first ten weeks of pregnancy would be prudent and by definition the safest course of action.

There are isolated reports of potential birth defects with almost all OTC medicines. But these reports do not establish cause and effect. Remember that most of these medicines are used for headache, fever, runny nose, coughing and sneezing—symptoms of the common cold or the flu. In short, OTC medicines are often used in the first trimester for viral illnesses and there is no way to separate the effect of the virus from the effect of the drug (See Cold and Flu Remedies below)

344

Q *How can I know which drugs are safe and which aren't?*

A The simple truth is that you can't. The best thing to do is trust your doctor's opinion. Drug effects are dependent on many factors. Exactly when in gestation you were exposed, the dosage taken, other medicines involved, the metabolic and digestive changes of pregnancy—all may affect the likelihood of a problem. Your doctor is trained to evaluate these variables, and has access to the necessary references.

Agent	Effect	Comment
1. Alcohol	Growth restriction, mental-retardation, unusual facial features, small head, heart and kidney malformations	Confused by nutritional deficiency, smoking, other drugs.
2. Male hormone derivatives **(Testosterone; Danazol)**	Virilization of female fetus, advanced genital development in males	Brief, incidental exposure not too worrisome
3. ACE class of blood pressure medicines **(Enalapril, Captopril)** *(anti-clotting drugs)*	Oligohydramnios, kidney defects; bone defects in skull; growth restriction	30 percent of fetuses affected; worse in second and third trimesters
4. Cousmarins **(Warfarin, Coumadin)** *(anti-clotting drugs)*	Bone and cartilage problems; short hands and fingers; eye problems; growth restriction; anomalies, abruption, fetal bleeding central nervous system problems	Worst at six to nine weeks; Later associated with still birth
5. Folic acid antagonists **(Methotrexate, aminopterin)** *(chemotherapy agents)*	Increased risk of miscarriage assorted malformations;	30 percent malformation rate if exposed during first trimester
Antiepilectics		
6. Carbamazepine **(Tegretol)**	Neural tube defect; small head, growth restriction, developmental delay	1-2 percent risk of spina bifida if given alone in first trimester
7. Phenytoin **(Dilantin)**	Phenylhydantoin Syndrome with mental retardation, small head, slowed growth, abnormal facial features, and heart defects	Only 10 percent have syndrome, but 30 percent have some problem
8. Valproic acid **(Depakene)**	Spina bifida and minor facial defects	1 percent affected; exposed before six weeks
9. **Trimethadione**	Cleft lip and plate; heart defects; small head; mental retardation; eye, limb, and genitourinary defects; facial abnormalities	65 percent affected if used in first trimester
Antibiotics		
10. **Tetracycline**	Permanent discoloration of teeth	No effect unless exposure is during second or third trimester
11. **Streptomycin; Kanamycin**	Hearing loss	Related **gentamicin** and **vancomycin** safe
12. **Cocaine**	Defects of heart, face, limbs, genitourinary tract; bowel atresia, cerebral infarcts	Maternal complications include sudden death and placental abruption
13. **DES**	Clear cell cancer of the vagina and cervix, abnormalities of the cervix and testes	Actual cancer risk low; reproductive abnormalities associated with infertility and second trimester loss
14. **Lithium**	Heart defects; esp. Ebstein anomaly	Risk lower than once thought; late-effect toxicity for kidney; thyroid, and muscles
15. **Thalidomide**	Limb defects, heart and genitourinary defects	20 percent affected if exposed between days 35 and 50
16. **Lead**	Abortions; stillbirths	Fetal central nervous system may be affected
17. **Mercury**	Seizures; blindness; retardation; spasticity	Cerebral palsy with third trimester exposure; found in fish contaminated with methyl mercury

*Adapted from *Teratogens*, ACOG Educational Bulletin, No. 236, April, 1997

345

 What about drugs I took before I even realized I was pregnant?

A In women with regular menses, the missed period occurs about fourteen to sixteen days after conception. Anything taken during this time is extremely unlikely to cause a problem. In fact, anything taken prior to five weeks of gestation, or about three weeks (twenty-one days) after conception falls into the "All or None Category." This means that any insult to the developing fetus is likely to have either no effect or, very rarely, cause a miscarriage, but it will not cause a birth defect In short, you could sit on top of a malfunctioning nuclear reactor and it wouldn't cause a birth defect under five weeks. Any exposures in this time frame would be much less likely to cause a birth defect than just one or two weeks later. (Prominent exceptions would be drugs known to affect closure of the neural tube and increase the risk of spina bifida, such as carbamazepine, methotrexate, aminopterin, and valproic acid, which can cause problems as early as twenty days after conception.)

346

Q *Do we know which drugs can cause birth defects?*

A Of the hundreds of thousands of drugs available commercially, whether prescription or over the counter, only a very few have actually been shown to cause birth defects in humans. In fact, as of this writing, there are only seventeen drugs or categories of drugs absolutely known to be capable of causing birth defects. Even these affect only some pregnancies and only under certain circumstances. For example, thalidomide, a widely available sleep aid in the 1950s, caused hundreds of thousands of babies to be born with limb defects. However, it only caused problems when taken between days 35 and 50 of gestation (six and a half and eight weeks) and even then, only 20 percent of fetuses were affected.

Remember that even drugs that have been proved to cause birth defects don't do so in every pregnancy. Their chances of causing a problem are related to timing and dosage among other variables.

On the left are the eighteen drugs and chemicals that have been proved to increase the risk of birth defects.★ If you are taking these drugs or have taken one of them recently, you should discuss the risks and benefits with your doctor.

FDA Classification

347

Q *Isn't there an FDA classification system in place to help out?*

A There is a classification system for prescription drugs based on reasonably recent research available to the Food and Drug Administration (FDA). The primary usefulness of the FDA Classification, however, is in identifying drugs that are either absolutely to be avoided under all circumstances, or that are known to increase the chance of birth defects but whose benefits may outweigh their risks, such as with certain seizure medicines.

There are five FDA categories, A, B, C, D, and X. They are defined by the FDA and used by manufacturers to label their products with respect to their use in pregnancy. These categories accompany listings in the *Physician's Desk Reference* (PDR).

Category A: Safe

Controlled studies in women fail to demonstrate a risk to the fetus in the first trimester, and there is no evidence of risk in later trimesters. Possibility of fetal harm seems remote. (Not many drugs other than vitamins fall into this category, and as mentioned under Dietary Guidelines, even some vitamins may be toxic if taken to excess.)

Category B: Very probably safe

Either animal reproductive studies have not demonstrated risk but no controlled studies in women exist, or animal reproductive studies have shown an adverse effect that was not confirmed in controlled studies in women in the first trimester.

Category C: May be safe

Either studies in animals have revealed adverse effects on the fetus but no controlled studies in women exist, or studies in women and animals are not available. Drugs should be given only if the potential benefit outweighs the potential risk to the fetus.

Category D: Safe only in rare instances

Positive evidence of human fetal risk exists, but the benefits from use in pregnant women may be acceptable despite the risk. In other words, if the drug is required for treatment of disease which untreated would itself be a serious risk, then the doctor and patient may judge the benefit to outweigh the risk.

Category X: Never safe

Studies in animals or human beings have demonstrated fetal abnormalities, or evidence exists of fetal risk based on human experience, or both. The risk in pregnant women clearly outweighs any possible benefit. These drugs are contraindicated in women who are pregnant or planning pregnancy.

348

Q *Are all eighteen substances known to cause birth defects classified as Category X?*

A Absolutely not. Many of the drugs known to cause defects do so only in a very narrow time frame with respect to the developing fetus. Tetracycline is a good example. Everyone knows not to use this antibiotic in pregnancy, and yet it causes no harm until *after* the first trimester. The antiseizure medicines listed as teratogenic may be essential to the health of the mother even though they carry some finite risk of birth defects. They aren't Category X either, although they may be Category D.

349

Q *Aren't there infections that can cause birth defects as well, such as rubella?*

A There are six commonly cited infections associated with birth defects. These include rubella (German Measles), cytomegalovirus (CMV), varicella (chicken pox), syphilis, toxoplasmosis, and primary herpes simplex. Parvovirus 19 (Fifth's disease) has not been associated with defects, but with fetal anemia and in utero heart failure. All of these are discussed in more detail in Section 8: Obstetric Complications (Infections).

COMMON OVER-THE-COUNTER DRUGS

Nausea Remedies

350

Q *Can I take something for this nausea?*

A First, follow the suggestions under "Morning Sickness" in Section 2. Nestrex is a commercial OTC preparation of pyridoxine (vitamin B6) and glucose. It is considered perfectly safe in pregnancy. Vitamin B6 was one of the active ingredients in Bendectin, one of the most studied drugs ever. Thirty-three million women used it from the late 1950s to the late 1970s, when the manufacturer discontinued production because of an onslaught of litigation. The other active component of the drug in the 1970s was doxylamine. (See NyQuil below, also Unisom.) An earlier ingredient was removed because it was felt to be ineffective.

There was never scientific proof that Bendectin caused any birth defects. Several studies showed minimal associations with individual anomalies, but none with statistical significance adequate to establish a cause-and-effect relationship. In fact, "the evidence indicating that doxylamine-pyridoxine is safe in pregnancy is impressive."[3]

Doxylamine is available over the counter as Unisom (Category B). Pyridoxine (Category A) is also available alone or in Nestrex as an OTC medicine. Using Unisom and Nestrex in combination is a very effective measure to combat morning sickness.[4]

However, because of the controversy and litigation that surrounded Bendectin, it would be prudent to confine the use of this combination to later than the completion of week nine from your last menstrual period. NOTE: This advice is not consistent with the product labeling. The manufacturer feels that despite its Category B status, Unisom should not be used in pregnancy. From a scientific standpoint this prohibition is not justified, although it might be justified from a legal standpoint. (See Morning Sickness under Prescription Drugs for additional information.)

Artificial Sweeteners

351

Q *What about Nutrasweet? Aren't artificial sweeteners dangerous?*

A Nutrasweet (Category B) is aspartame, a chemical compound made of two naturally occurring amino acids, L-aspartic acid and L-phenylalanine. It is one of the most studied compounds ever approved by the FDA. Aspartame does not pose a risk to the fetus, and pregnant women may consume foods with this additive or use artificial sweeteners, such as Equal, that contain it.

However, women who have phenylketonuria (PKU) should probably avoid aspartame. PKU affects one in fifteen thousand people; the heterozygous state (one of the PKU genes instead of two) affects one in fifty people. Those who have PKU are missing an enzyme that converts phenylalanine to tyrosine, and phenylalanine can then build up to toxic levels. Babies born to women with PKU who were not on controlled diets may be affected with heart defects, mental retardation, low birth weight, and microcephaly. In reality, however, aspartame provides so tiny a change in blood levels that it is safe even for those with PKU.[5]

The American Academy of Pediatrics considers breast-feeding safe while using aspartame, but patients who have PKU should keep track of their intake.

You should probably not use saccharin (Sweet'N Low). Aspartame (Nutrasweet, Equal) is a better choice in pregnancy than Sweet'N Low. However, saccharin (Category C) may be unjustly accused with respect to pregnancy. There is no animal or human data to support the belief that saccharin is a teratogen. So if you've used it by mistake, don't worry. Concern about saccharin focuses around findings of increased risk of bladder cancer in laboratory animals. Even increased risk of bladder cancer has never been demonstrated in humans. Splenda (maltodextrin, dextrose, and sucralose) poses no risk whatsoever in pregnancy.

Headache, Cold, and Flu Remedies

352

Q *My friend's doctor put her on a baby aspirin a day because she's had lots of miscarriages. I usually use aspirin for headaches, but isn't it dangerous in pregnancy?*

A Aspirin (a type of salicylate) is classified as Category C. Aspirin readily crosses the placenta to the fetus. In studies totaling more than fifty-four thousand patients, about 61 percent remembered taking aspirin during their pregnancy. It is widely consumed and often a component of other OTC medicines without the patient realizing it. (Aspirin is an ingredient in some Alka-Seltzer, Bayer, Bufferin, Ecotrin, Cama, Excedrin, Vanquish, and Ascriptin products.) Aspirin's effect on pregnancy is extremely dose-dependent; full-dose aspirin (2502,000 milligrams per day) is classified as Category D in the third trimester, since it may cross the placenta and cause bleeding problems in the newborn.

Low-dose aspirin therapy (82 milligrams per day) is entirely different. One of its biochemical effects is to decrease the concentration of a certain prostaglandin (Thromboxane A2) and increase the concentration of prostacyclin. This has the effect of allowing greater blood vessel dilatation, which might be helpful in preventing preeclampsia. In combination with heparin, another blood thinner, aspirin has been found to reduce the incidence of recurrent miscarriage in some habitual aborters.

Full-dose aspirin (250 to 2,000 milligrams per day) should not be used in the third trimester. Not only might it cause bleeding in the fetus or newborn, but it has the effect of prolonging gestation or inhibiting the onset or progress of labor.

The Collaborative Perinatal Project looked at 50,282 pregnant women, of whom 32,164 used aspirin, 14,864 of whom used it in the first trimester. They found no evidence of increased birth defects.[6]

The American Academy of Pediatrics advises cautious use of aspirin while breast-feeding, noting that it is excreted in breast milk only in extremely small amounts and would usually be safe.[7]

353

Q *Can I use nonaspirin pain relievers, like Tylenol?*

A Acetaminophen (Tylenol) (Category B) is used frequently by pregnant women for pain relief and to reduce fever. In usual doses (250 to 2,000 milligrams per day), acetaminophen has not been suspected of causing birth defects even in the first trimester. Unlike aspirin, acetaminophen does not affect platelet function and poses no risk of bleeding in mother or fetus. Even when it was taken with a narcotic, such as codeine (Tylenol #3) there were no adverse affects from first trimester exposure.[8] Acetaminophen is found as an ingredient in these products, as well as others: Actifed, Alka-Seltzer, Allerest, Bayer Select, Comtrex, Contac, Coricidin, Drixoral, Excedrin Extra Strength and PM, Percogesic, Sinarest, SineAid, Sinutab, Sudafed Severe Cold, TheraFlu, and DayQuil/NyQuil.

The American Academy of Pediatrics considers it safe to breast-feed while using acetaminophen.

While ibuprofen (in Advil products, Bayer Select Ibuprofen, Motrin IB, Nuprin, and an ingredient in Dimetapp Sinus, Sine-Aid IB), like Tylenol and aspirin, is a common pain reliever, it has its own special risks. Ibuprofen is classified as Category B except for the third trimester, where it has been classified as Category D. The Michigan Medicaid Recipient Study looked at 3,178 first trimester exposures between 1985 and 1992 and found no data to support ibuprofen as causing an increased incidence of birth defects.[9]

However, if it is used in the third trimester, ibuprofen has been shown to increase the risk of prolonged gestation, prolonged labor, and, rarely, can cause persistent pulmonary hypertension in newborns. Another concern is that all prostaglandin synthetase inhibitors (for example, ASA, ibuprofen, and indocin) taken in the third trimester run the theoretical risk of closing the ductus arteriosus in utero. This connection between the pulmonary artery and the aorta must stay open for the fetus to survive. (See Section 4: Fetal Development)

Antihistamines

354

Q *I've taken Benadryl frequently in the past. Can I use it in pregnancy?*

A Diphenhydramine (Category C) (Benadryl—all combinations; Actifed Allergy Nighttime Caplets; Contac Cold/Flu Night Caplets; Tylenol Maximum Strength Nighttime products) has been widely used in pregnancy and even more so since it has become available over the counter. It is used to relieve allergies, colds, itching, and sleeplessness, often in combinations with other ingredients. The Collaborative Perinatal Project monitored 50,282 pregnant women, 595 of whom were exposed during the first trimester and 2,948 who were exposed in any trimester. They found no evidence to suggest a causal relationship with birth defects. Benadryl is categorized as "C" because of several isolated defects reported with questionable statistical significance. Consequently, it is recommended that Benadryl be avoided during the first trimester.[10]

While levels of Benadryl have not been reported in human breast milk, the manufacturer says it is contraindicated in breast-feeding because of the increased sensitivity of newborns to antihistamines.

355

Q *What about the common antihistamines like brompheniramine, chlorpheniramine, triprolidine, and cyproheptadine, which are found in cold and allergy medicines?*

A Brompheniramine (Category C) (Dimetapp, Alka-Seltzer Sinus™, DayQuil) has been found in the Collaborative Perinatal Project to have a slightly increased risk of defects when taken in the first trimester. The risk did not apply during the other trimesters. Combinations including brompheniramine should be avoided in the first trimester.

Chlorpheniramine (Category B) (Contac, Allerest, Alka-Seltzer Cold™), unlike brompheniramine, has no reports of defects, even in the first trimester, according to the Collaborative Perinatal Project. However, these medicines often occur in combination with decongestants, as do those indicated above, and all OTC cold medicines should be avoided in the first trimester.

Triprolidine (Category C) (Actifed) has not been found to be associated with birth defects in any study to date. However, in the Collaborative Perinatal Project only sixteen exposures were documented. Presumably it is categorized as "C" because of the lack of data.

Cyproheptadine (Category B) (Periactin) has been used to treat Cushing's Syndrome as well as common allergies. The Michigan Medicaid Recipient Study reviewed 285 first trimester exposures and found no increase in the expected number of birth defects.

The American Academy of Pediatrics considers the first three of the above antihistamines to be safe in breast-feeding. There is insufficient data on the fourth. The prescription antihistamines used for allergic rhinitis, Claritin, Allegra, and Zyrtec are all considered safe in pregnancy after 9 weeks gestation, including the "D" variants, which contain pseudoephedrine as a decongestant.

356

Q *Don't most of the OTC cold medicines often contain a decongestant along with the antihistamines?*

A Yes. The most common one is pseudoephedrine (Category C). Phenylpropanolamine was at least as common, but removed from the market by the FDA in 2001 due to concern over the risk of stroke.

Pseudoephedrine is found in some formulas of Actifed, Alka-Seltzer, Allerest, Advil Cold and Sinus, Benadryl Allergy Decongestant, Benylin, Comtrex, Contac Cold/Flu, Dimetapp Sinus, Drixoral Cough/Congestion LiquiCaps, Motrin IB Sinus, Novahistine DMX, Robitussin Cold & Cough, Robitussin Maximum Strength Cough & Cold, Sine-Aid, Sinarest, SineOff, Sinutab, all Sudafed products, TheraFlu, Triaminic, Tylenol MultiSymptom, Vicks 44 and NyQuil/DayQuil.

Both phenylpropanolamine and pseudoephedrine are members of the class of sympathomimetic amines that function by constricting small blood vessels and thus drying up nasal passages. They have been weakly associated in the first trimester with non-life-threatening, and nonmajor cosmetic defects, including inguinal hernia and clubfoot. Phenylephrine is in this same category.

Because of the small first trimester risk, OTC cold medicines should be avoided in the first trimester if possible. Note that phenylpropanolamine is also found in Dexatrim and Acutrim appetite suppressants. These medicines should not be used in pregnancy.

The American Academy of Pediatrics considers it safe to breast-feed while taking these medicines.

357

Q *What about NyQuil LiquiCaps?*

A NyQuil (Category C) is a combination of acetaminophen, pseudo-ephedrine, doxylamine, and dextromethorphan. Unlike some other formulations, the LiquiCaps do not contain any alcohol.

The first two ingredients are addressed elsewhere. Doxylamine (NyQuil LiquiCaps, also in Alka-Seltzer Plus Nighttime Cold, Unisom, and Nytol Maximum Strength) was one of the two active components in the drug Bendectin used by 33 million American women before it went off the market due to litigation. Despite this, no scientific proof was ever available to show a causal relationship between Bendectin and birth defects. The other active component in Bendectin was vitamin B6. There are over sixteen large studies indicating that doxylamine is safe in pregnancy in all trimesters.[11] There is little or no evidence to implicate doxylamine as a problem.

Dextromethorphan is a narcotic-derived cough suppressant with no addictive and no teratogenic properties. Even its analgesic, addictive isomer, levorphanol, is classified as Category B. There is no reason to believe that dextromethorphan has a causal relationship with any birth defects.

In short, NyQuil LiquiCaps may be one of the safest combination cold medicines that there is for pregnancy. It should be considered Category C only due to the very minimal risk posed by pseudoephedrine. (See pseudoephedrine) As such, as with most OTC medicines, if possible it should be avoided in the first trimester. They should be avoided in the first trimester.

358

Q *What else has dextromethorphan in it?*

A Dextromethorphan is a narcotic-derived cough suppressant that has no addictive or teratogenic properties. It is not only found in NyQuil, but as an ingredient in the following: Alka-Seltzer Cold & Cough, Benylin products, Comtrex MultiSymptom, Contac Cold/Flu, Dimetapp DM, Drixoral Cough, Novahistine DMX, Robitussin products M, CF, and Maximum Strength; Sudafed Cold & Cough, TheraFlu, Triaminic, Tylenol Multi Symptom Cold.

Many of these medicines have combinations of both Category B and Category C drugs, and all of the components should be considered before deciding if you want to use them. They should be avoided in the first trimester.

359

Q *Can I use Robitussin for a cough?*

A Guaifenesin (Robitussin products, Benylin, Sudafed Cough Syrup, DayQuil LiquiCaps, Triaminic Expectorant) (Category C) is an expectorant often found in combination with other components such as the narcotic derived cough suppressant dextromethorphan (Robitussin DM), or codeine in the prescription version (Robitussin AC). Guaifenesin is listed as category C only because of a few isolated instances of inguinal hernia. The Michigan Medicaid Recipient Study looked at 1,479 first trimester exposures to guaifenesin and the general class of expectorants and found no increased risk of birth defects.

Robitussin can probably be used safely in all trimesters, including AC, DM, and CF variations. As with all OTCs any minimal concerns could be eliminated by avoiding its use in the first trimester. (See this section: Prescription Drugs-Asthma)

360

Q *What about expectorants other than Robitussin, such as Tussi-Organidin?*

A All OTC medicines, such as combination cough preparations that have as an ingredient iodide or iodine, should be avoided. These medicines have the capacity to cause fetal hypothyroidism, and goiter in the newborn. Note also that the use of vaginal douches such as povidoneiodine have been associated with newborn goiter.

Nasal Sprays

361

Q *I've heard I can't use nasal sprays such as Afrin for congestion. Is that true?*

A Oxymetazoline hydrochloride (Afrin; Neo-Synephrine; Sinex) Category C) is another sympathomimetic amine designed to constrict small blood vessels and thus dry up nasal secretions. There are no reports linking oxymetazoline to congenital defects. Studies indicate that the theoretical risk of uterine blood vessel constriction is not valid unless the medicine is overdosed, but this accounts for its "C" categorization. When used as directed with one squirt per nostril only every twelve hours there is probably no risk at all.[12] (See Prescription Drugs for Steroids and Cromalyn Nasal Sprays)

Caffeine

362

Q *I've heard that caffeine can be dangerous. Do I need to avoid all caffeine in pregnancy?*

A Caffeine (Category B) is the most commonly consumed drug in the world and is found in coffee, tea, and sodas, in many OTC medicines for headache, colds, and flu, and is also added to many foods. A cup of coffee has about 100 milligrams of caffeine, a cola about 50 milligrams, tea about 25 milligrams, and decaf coffee about 5 milligrams.

Caffeine crosses the placenta quickly and completely. Once again, the Collaborative Perinatal Project evaluated 50,282 pregnant women, and found 5,378 first trimester exposures and 12,696 overall. They found no relationship with birth defects. Because of a purported increased relative risk of a few isolated defects, follow-up studies were performed, and they reconfirmed the lack of a relationship between caffeine and birth defects.[13] Caffeine and its effect on pregnancy has been thoroughly reviewed and found not to be associated with birth defects in multiple other studies as well.[14]

It is true that more than 500 milligrams per day (about five cups of coffee or ten colas) has been associated with a higher incidence of maternal cardiac arrhythmias (palpitations). High caffeine intake of more than 500 milligrams per day in combination with smoking has been associated with infants of lower birth weight than infants born to smokers alone.

The American Academy of Pediatrics also feels that usual caffeine use, meaning less than 500 milligrams per day, is safe in breast-feeding.[15]

Topical Remedies

363

Q *Is it okay to use topical antibiotics such as Bacitracin, Cortisporin, Neosporin, and Metrogel?*

A In general, there is almost no evidence to link topical antibiotic treatments with birth defects. Bacitracin (Category C) has never been associated with defects, but little information is available. Cortisporin and Neosporin are combinations of Polymyxin B, Bacitracin, and Neomycin and are Category C. While no information exists linking Neomycin to any birth defects, its close relatives Streptomycin and Kanamycin have been linked after oral use to deafness in newborns; thus its "C" categorization.

Metrogel is a newer topical metronidazole indicated for acne, but also for Gardnerella vaginalis (bacterial vaginosis). Metronidazole is classified as Category B, but there have been years of conflicting reports with respect to oral dosages. Currently, the topical version is considered safe in all trimesters.

There is no reason to believe that small amounts of topical antibiotics pose a significant risk in any trimester.

364

Q *Is it safe to use topical steroids?*

A Topical steroids are available over-the-counter in many forms and combinations. They are most commonly used to treat itching, whether of the skin or that associated with hemorrhoids. The most common of these is hydrocortisone (Cortizone-5&10, Preparation H Hydrocortisone 1%, Cortaid Spray, Bactine Hydrocortisone Anti-itch Cream, and Caldecort Anti-itch Spray) and its variant hydrocortisone acetate (Anusol HC, Caldecort Anti-itch Cream, Cortaid Cream, Lotion & Ointment, and Nupercainal Hydrocortisone 1%).

Topical hydrocortisones achieve systemic doses far less than those achieved, for example, with inhaled steroids for use in asthma. There is no data to support a causal relationship between topical steroids and congenital defects in any trimester. Like all OTC medicines, however, avoid first trimester use if at all possible.

Eyedrops containing corticosteroids may be used safely in all trimesters of pregnancy under the supervision of an ophthalmologist. All of the steroid-containing eye preparations are available by prescription only at this time.

365

Q *Can I use eyedrops such as Visine and Murine just for irritation and redness?*

A Oxymetazoline (Visine) and tetrahydrozaline (Murine) may both be used safely in pregnancy. As discussed under oxymetazoline (Afrin), the concentrations achieved systemically with eyedrops are inconsequential and there is no reason these products need to be avoided in pregnancy when used in the appropriate dosages.

366

Q *Can I use sunscreens? They seem to have an awful lot of ingredients.*

A All of the OTC sunscreens are considered safe in pregnancy. In fact, in order to avoid unsightly concentrations of pigment around the lips, cheeks, eyes, and forehead (mask of pregnancy or melasma), it is advisable for pregnant women to use sunscreens with an SPF of at least 15 when in the sun for prolonged periods.

If you haven't worn sunscreen or what you did wear still allowed you to get a painful sunburn, you can use OTC sprays and creams such as Americaine, Nupercainal, Solarcaine, Benadryl, Cortaid, Cortizone-5, 10, Rulagel, and Dermaplast. (See also question 385.)

367

Q *I got into a red ant pile when I was gardening. What can I use on the bites?*

A Itching and swelling around insect bites can be treated with all the usual OTC creams and sprays. Those listed for sunburn may be used, including spray Benadryl and Cortaid. In addition, calamine lotion combined with Benadryl (Caladryl) is safe and effective in pregnancy.

368

Q *Can I use my medicated shampoo, Tegrin?*

A Coal tar shampoo (Tegrin) and shampoos containing selenium (Head & Shoulders; Selsun Blue) may both be used safely in pregnancy for the treatment of dandruff and psoriasis. All other OTC shampoos are thought to be safe in pregnancy as well.

Heartburn Remedies

369

Q *My heartburn has been terrible and antacids just don't seem to cut it. Can I use OTC medicines such as Tagamet, Zantac, and Pepcid AC?*

A Cimetidine (Tagamet) (Category B) is one of the most widely used drugs in the world. It is an H2-receptor antagonist that inhibits gastric acid secretion. Data from the Michigan Medicaid Recipient Study looked at 460 pregnancies with first trimester exposure and did not support any association with increased birth defects.[16]

Ranitidine (Zantac) (Category B) has not been found to have a causal relationship with birth defects.

Famotidine (Pepcid AC) (Category B) has not been found to have a causal relationship with birth defects, but data is lacking to draw conclusions.

Prilosec (Category C) went over the counter in 2003. While an effective new class of histamine blocker, it should be avoided in the first trimester due to chromosomal mutations found in animal studies.[17]

Protonix (Category B) and Nexium (Category C) are newer proton pump blocker antacids. Both Protonix and Nexium are widely used after the first trimester. Some retrospective data base studies in 2010 suggest an increased risk of cardiac defects only with first trimester use, but these are not confirmed with controlled studies.

The American Academy of Pediatrics recently reclassified cimetidine as compatible with breast-feeding. Zantac and Pepcid AC use while breast-feeding should be discussed with your doctor.

The prescription gastric acid inhibitor, misoprostol (Cytotec) (Category X) causes uterine contractions and bleeding, and induces miscarriages. It is prohibited in the first two trimesters of pregnancy. At the end of the third trimester, Cytotec may be administered orally or vaginally to induce labor. It should never be self-administered, but given under the direction of your physician.

370

Q *Which antacids are safe to use for heartburn and acid reflux?*

A Mylanta, Mylanta II, Maalox, Gaviscon, Gelusil, and Tums are all safe to use in pregnancy. Both the calcium Tums and Mylanta Gelcaps (calcium carbonate and magnesium carbonate) avoid sodium and may also serve as an extra source of calcium. Mylanta liquid is magnesium hydroxide and aluminum hydroxide combined, and while it has no source of calcium, it is low in sodium. Maalox liquid is similar to Mylanta, but its Heartburn preparation has more sodium. Gaviscon and Gelusil are similar to both Maalox and Mylanta and are also now very low in sodium.

Many variants of these products also contain simethicone, which is intended to reduce gas and flatulence, although recent evidence suggests this is of doubtful effectiveness. In any event, the addition of simethicone is harmless.

Remember, if your heartburn symptoms are severe, use the antacids multiple times during the day rather than just when you feel the symptoms. Usually, they will work better preventively than therapeutically.

Diarrhea Remedies

371

Q *I usually use Pepto-Bismol with diarrhea. Is it safe in pregnancy?*

A Pepto-Bismol (Category C) is bismuth subsalicylate. While no data exists to implicate bismuth or its salts as teratogenic, considerable data exists about salicylates. (See Aspirin) Because of potential problems in the third trimester such as bleeding, fetal or neonatal bleeding, prolonged pregnancy, and prolonged labor, use of Pepto-Bismol for diarrhea should be confined to the second trimester.

Pepto-Bismol should not be used while breast-feeding. If you can't use Pepto-Bismol, you may wish to consider alternatives. Imodium A-D (loperamide) (Category B) has not been associated with birth defects in any trimester in any published reports. It currently is considered safe, but should be avoided in the first trimester if possible.

The American Academy of Pediatrics considers loperamide use compatible with breast-feeding.

Kaopectate (Category C) has not been linked with adverse fetal outcome. However, prolonged use over weeks could be associated with iron-deficiency anemia and hypokalemia (low potassium), and therefore, Kaopectate should be used sparingly and for brief periods only.

There is no reason to believe Kaopectate is a risk for the breast-feeding infant.

Constipation Remedies

372

Q *Can I use milk of magnesia for constipation?*

A Milk of magnesia is primarily magnesium hydroxide. Magnesium has been used in the form of sulfate for many years in the treatment of both preterm labor and preeclampsia, primarily in the third trimester. The amount of magnesium absorbed from milk of magnesia is not considered a fetal danger. In fact, most of the magnesium stays in the bowel and draws water in accounting for its effectiveness in constipation.

However, milk of magnesia in its flavored forms, such as mint, also contains saccharin. As mentioned above, saccharin is classified as Category C although its true risk is probably minimal and has never been related to teratogenicity—only bladder cancer in laboratory animals.

Like almost all OTC medicines, milk of magnesia should be considered safe when used in accordance with its labeling, but best avoided in the first trimester.

Bulk laxatives such as Metamucil and Fibercon contain inert ingredients that stay within the bowel and pose no known risk to the fetus. They may be used safely while pregnant or while breast-feeding.

Stool softeners such as docusate sodium (Colace) and docusate calcium (Surfak; Doxidan) are also inert and may be used safely in pregnancy. Casanthranol (Category C) and docusate sodium (Pericolace), on the other hand, contain a cathartic that at least theoretically could stimulate the smooth muscle of the uterus and precipitate preterm labor; therefore, it should be avoided. There is no evidence of any link between casanthranol and fetal malformations. Similarly, Ex-Lax which contains phenothalin and is a cathartic, should be avoided.

Water is still the best medicine for constipation. At least ten to twelve ten-ounce glasses per day will usually eliminate any problems of constipation.

Castor oil (Category B) is felt to be safe in pregnancy; however, because of its tendency to stimulate the smooth muscle of the bowel, and consequently the potential for stimulating preterm labor in susceptible pregnant patients, it is advisable that its use be avoided between twenty and thirty weeks.

Hemorrhoid Remedies

373

Q *What can I do for hemorrhoids?*

A Hemorrhoids in pregnancy are simply dilated anal veins, worsened due to compression by the growing uterus. The best thing you can do is avoid constipation by increasing water intake. However, when hemorrhoids are particularly swollen and tender, Preparation H and Tronolane are both topical ointments (also available as suppositories) that may be used safely throughout pregnancy.

Formulations with steroids in them are available by prescription and may also be used under your doctor's guidance.

Yeast Infection Remedies

374

Q *Are the OTC medicines for vaginal yeast infections considered safe?*

A For many women yeast infections are more common during pregnancy than any other time. Recognize that self-diagnosis of yeast vaginitis in pregnancy is not always easy, since normal vaginal discharge may mimic it. However, severe itching, redness of the labia, a thick, white discharge, and little or no odor are in all probability indicators of a yeast infection.

All of the OTC yeast preparations are safe in all three trimesters. Clotrimazole (Gyne-Lotrimin; Mycelex), miconazole (Monistat), and butoconazole (Femstat) may all be used interchangeably, Vagistat is also considered safe. If you're not familiar with yeast infections from previous experiences, or you're not absolutely sure of the diagnosis, see your doctor before treatment.

ILLICIT DRUGS

375

Q *I used to smoke a little pot now and then. Is marijuana dangerous in pregnancy?*

A Delta-9-tetrahydrocannabinol, or marijuana, may be used by as many as 15 percent of pregnant American woman. While marijuana use is illegal almost everywhere in the United States, there is no confirming evidence of any link to birth defects. In fact, there is fairly strong evidence to support the statement that there are no known adverse effects to marijuana use with respect to the fetus.[18]

Because of the mind-altering effects of cannabinols and the propensity to combine its use with alcohol or other recreational drugs that also alter judgment and reaction time, doctors advise against the use of marijuana during pregnancy.

376

Q *I took dextroamphetamine to lose weight in the past. Will it cause birth defects if taken in pregnancy?*

A Dextroamphetamine (Category C) is not known to be a teratogen. As with all drugs of potential abuse, studies are clouded by multiple drug use. The Collaborative Perinatal Project reviewed 671 first trimester exposures and 1,898 exposures at any time during pregnancy and found no statistically significant evidence to link amphetamines to birth defects.

There are some isolated reports of an amphetamine withdrawal syndrome in newborns characterized by shrill crying, irritability, jerking, and sneezing but these findings were all confounded by possible concurrent hidden narcotic addiction in the mothers. There is also mixed evidence of slowed growth, prematurity, low birth weight, and possible increased risk of bleeding into the brain in babies of illicit users.

In short, amphetamines do not pose a risk of congenital anomalies, but may pose other risks to the fetus with possible long-term consequences; they should therefore be avoided in pregnancy.

Metamphetamine (Category C) is used legitimately to treat obesity, narcolepsy, and attention deficit disorder in children. It is also available on the street in an intravenous form known as Ice or Blue Ice. In a large 1976 cohort study there was found no increased risk of major or minor congenital defects compared to controls.[19]

However, others found in 1987 that there was a distinct fetal withdrawal syndrome demonstrated by tremors, abnormal sleep patterns, poor feeding, and muscle spasticity. Users also had babies with lower birth weight, prematurity, slowed growth, and evidence for increased bleeding into the brain and subsequent brain damage.

In short, metamphetamines do not pose a risk of congenital anomalies, but may pose other risks to the fetus with possible long term consequences. These drugs should not be used in pregnancy.

Adderall (amphetamine and destroamphetamine) (Category C) is legitimately prescribed to treat ADHD in adults. It should be avoided in pregnancy if possible for the reasons above.

377

Q *What can cocaine do?*

A Cocaine (Category C by prescription; Category D by abuse) is one of the most dangerous drugs that can be used in pregnancy. As a medicine, cocaine has a role as an extremely effective topical anesthetic; however, used in uncontrolled dosages via snorting or via smoking in the form of crack, the drug can quickly be lethal to pregnant women and their fetuses. It is also known to be extremely addictive.

The American College of Obstetricians and Gynecologists (ACOG) reported in 1990 that cocaine could lead to heart attack, arrhythmias, aortic rupture, stroke, seizures, rapid lethal temperature rise, and sudden death.[20]

Abruptio placentae (premature placental separation) is caused by cocaine use. It frequently leads to the death of the fetus and, rarely, to the death of the mother as well. Cocaine is known to raise blood pressure and constrict blood vessels, which may cause the placenta to tear away from the wall of the uterus. Cocaine use in pregnancy has also been associated with increased risk of miscarriage, premature delivery, growth retardation, meconium-stained fluid, and even a stroke in the fetus.

Multiple birth defects have been associated with cocaine use, including those affecting the brain, intestines, arms and legs, and kidney and bladder. Cocaine should not be used in any trimester of pregnancy.

378

Q *Does heroin harm the fetus?*

A Heroin (Category B; Category D in the third trimester) is an opiate narcotic, and like all the narcotics, it has not been linked causally to congenital defects in large studies. There is one cohort study from 1979 that looked at 830 addicted mothers and found increased incidences of some malformations, but it is unconfirmed by other studies.[21]

This does not, however, make it safe in pregnancy. The incidence of growth retardation, perinatal death, and stillbirth is increased in the addicted population. There are also some reports of developmental delay in these children. All investigators agree that 85 percent of the newborns of addicted mothers experience withdrawal for from two to six days. Symptoms include diarrhea, vomiting, fever, tremors, irritability, and sneezing, and seizures in some.

A perinatal death rate was as high as 39 percent in one review.[22]

Methadone (Category B; Category D in third trimester), which is used almost exclusively to treat heroin addicts, may be considered to have the same risks as those for heroin. It does not, in itself, cause any congenital birth defects.

Codeine and hydroxycodone (Vicodin; Lortab; Lorcet; Tylenol #3) (Category B), as well as Demerol and morphine (Category B) are prescription drugs that are often abused, and may therefore become illicit in the way they are used. They have all of the addictive characteristics of the other opiates and all of the potential complications. However, used in prescription dosages for brief periods of time for specific indications, they do not pose a significant risk to the fetus.

379

Q *I know some people who are doing LSD. Does it cause birth defects?*

A Lysergic acid diethylamide (LSD) (Category C) is used for its halluci-nogenic properties. It may not be prescribed legally in the United States and it is often bought on the street cut with a variety of other drugs. The data on LSD is extremely confusing, with literally hundreds of different defects reported in small numbers, which do not reach statistical significance. Available data does not support LSD as a causative agent of birth defects, miscarriages, or chromosomal abnormalities. However, there is no long-term follow-up study available.[23]

Because of LSD's hallucinogenic effects, it poses a definite indirect risk to the fetus. As with other mind-altering substances, potential injury or death to the mother must be considered the greatest risk to the fetus, and LSD should never be used in pregnancy.

380

Q *What about PCP?*

A Phencyclidine (PCP) (Category X) is another illicit hallucinogen. While initial studies showed causal relationship to birth defects, more recent studies have shown PCP not be a direct neurotoxin as originally believed. Since the drug could theoretically have serious adverse effects on the fetal central nervous system, it has been categorized as "X."[24]

CHEMICALS

381

Q *What can cigarette smoking or nicotine really do in pregnancy? Seems like all our parents smoked during pregnancy!*

A First of all, not all of our parents smoked when they were pregnant. Unfortunately, despite the wealth of evidence condemning smoking as harmful to health, Americans, and especially young women, continue to smoke in record numbers, with roughly 30 percent of women of reproduc-tive age still smoking regularly.

Cigarette smoke contains not only the addictive drug nicotine, but also over 580 other compounds known to be carcinogenic (cancer-causing) or neurotoxic (poisonous to the nervous system). Babies born to smokers are known to have lower birth weights than those born to nonsmokers. Smokers also have babies with higher perinatal death rates (stillbirth and death soon after birth). Evidence suggests higher miscarriage and placental abruption rates as well.[25]

There are several possible explanations for these findings, including carbon monoxide's effect on fetal red blood cells; the constricting effect of nicotine on small blood vessels such as those found in the placenta; reduced appetite and therefore decreased caloric intake; and decreased maternal blood volume.[26]

In short, women *should not smoke* during pregnancy under any circumstances.

382

Q *Okay, Okay! I'm going to quit smoking! Can I use the patch in pregnancy?*

A The transdermal nicotine patches (Nicotrol; Habitrol; Prostep) (Category D) deliver a constant dose of nicotine everyday. It's hard for a doctor to purposely give you a drug that is teratogenic in animals, known to be a carcinogen in humans, and is associated with growth retardation, low birth weight, placental separation, and an increased rate of stillbirth. If you are sincere about wanting to stop smoking, follow your doctor's advice about whether the benefits of the patch outweigh the risks.

Zyban (bupropian) is an oral medicine to help stop smoking and is considered safe in pregnancy. (See Antidepressant: Wellbutrin)

383

Q *What are the real effects of alcohol on my pregnancy?*

A There is no question that alcohol is a teratogen; that is, it increases the risk of certain birth defects. These include the fetal alcohol syndrome, characterized by mental retardation, typical alteration of facial features, microcephaly (small head), kidney and heart malformations, and slowed growth both in and out of the uterus. It was first described in 1973, but has subsequently been confirmed by many others. Data is weak for one to two alcoholic drinks per day. Women who drink more than six drinks per day are at a 40 percent risk of their fetus developing the syndrome.[27]

There is, however, no established safe level of alcohol consumption, and the best advice is to drink no alcohol in pregnancy.

If you drank alcohol before you knew you were pregnant, remember the "all or none effect." It is thought to be essentially impossible to cause a birth defect in the first eighteen days after conception. That means that quitting alcohol when you miss your period and your pregnancy test is positive is very likely to be safe enough.

384

Q *I've heard that it's not safe to color or perm my hair. Is that true?*

A As mentioned previously, we would try to avoid all drugs and alcohol in the first trimester. After twelve weeks, there is no evidence to support the type of dyes being used today for hair coloring as dangerous for the pregnancy. Remember the "all or none effect" as well; that is, if you colored your hair before six weeks and didn't know you were pregnant, don't worry about it.

Avoid perming your hair and all chemicals or drugs in the first trimester. After twelve weeks there is no worrisome evidence of any problems associated with perming your hair.

385

Q *I can't tan the back of my legs because I can't lie on this huge belly. Is it safe to use tanning lotions?*

A Tanning lotions in general have a large number of chemical components. For example, Banana Boat Sunless Tanning Creme has twenty-six ingredients in addition to purified water, none of which is even a sunscreen. While none of these ingredients is known to be a teratogen when the cream is applied topically, doctors recommend avoiding the usage of tanning lotions at least during the first trimester. Tanning lotions tend to be used over large surface areas, and at least theoretically, significant absorption could occur.

386

Q *What can exposure to lead or mercury do?*

A Lead is a known teratogen. Exposure to high levels, whether from inadvertent ingestion of water contaminated by older pipes or from exposure to lead in cookware, can affect the development of the fetal nervous system. High blood levels of lead in pregnant women are also associated with increased abortion rates and with stillbirth. Lead levels can be drawn in those at risk prior to pregnancy to determine specific risk.

Likewise, your own water can be tested for lead levels. This may be relevant if you have a house built before about 1955, and contacting the Environmental Protection Agency (EPA) or your local Health Department is all that's required to find out how to have your water tested. If you live in an older apartment in a big city, and you are unsure about the lead content of the water, try running the tap for several minutes before using the water for drinking or cooking. Specifically avoid drinking or cooking with water from the hot tap. Cold water is less likely to draw lead from the pipes into the water. Use only glass or plastic containers to store liquids such as juices and water.

Mercury is another known teratogen. Fish and grain may, rarely, be contaminated with methyl mercury. Some latex paints may also have unacceptable levels of mercury. Cerebral atrophy (wasting), spasticity, seizures, blindness, and cerebral palsy may all be caused by mercury. Recommendations came out in 2001 limiting tuna and salmon intake to only 1–2 servings per month due to mercury risk.

387

Q *I'm a dental hygienist and work around anesthetic gases. Can they cause birth defects?*

A There is no reliable data to suggest that anesthetic gases increase the risk of congenital birth defects. There is conflicting data about whether or not anesthetic gases in common use may be associated with a slight increase in the miscarriage rate.

There is, however, general agreement that passive exposure to these gases (when the pregnant woman in question is not the patient inhaling these gases directly) is associated with negligible risk. The specific chemicals benzene, formaldehyde, and ethylene oxide are thought to increase the risk of miscarriage.[28]

388

Q *We're remodeling our house and I need to do a lot of painting. Are paint fumes teratogenic?*

A Paint fumes (from oil-based paint) are primarily petroleum distillates. This means that there are many different compounds all mixed up together that have been derived from crude oil by the refinery process. Many of these can be dangerous to both you and the fetus. Use of latex (water-based) paints is preferred whenever possible, although even some of these were found in the late 1980s to have unacceptable mercury levels. (The FDA mandated organic mercury be removed from such paints and a check of the labeling should reassure you if this is still the case.) Glossy trim paints are now available in latex-based as well as oil-based forms. You should always keep any room you are painting well ventilated, take breaks every fifteen to thirty minutes, avoid oil-based paints such as those used for trim and wood-work, and avoid any paint fumes during the first trimester.

A good general rule would be to avoid indoor painting in the first and second trimesters. In particular, consider asking your husband to paint the nursery while you add helpful, loving direction from the lounge chair in the living room, sipping your lemonade, with the windows open and the fan blowing. If you must be directly involved, follow the guidelines above.

389

Q *Can I apply insect repellents such as 6-10™, Off™ and Cutter's™ while I'm pregnant?*

A The risk of disease from an insect bite far outweighs the potential for a problem from a topical repellent. Insect repellents may be used without concern in all trimesters.

Avoid chemical exposures in the first trimester. If you are seeing enough cockroaches to consider having an exterminator come, you may safely have your house exterminated in the later trimesters, but if aerosol bombs are used, leave the house for the recommended amount of time, or at least several hours. You can be fairly sure you have been gone long enough if you can't smell any chemicals on your return. Be sure to put away all food, plates, and utensils before the extermination. Have someone else wash off kitchen counters and the stove after the process is complete. Liquid applications along the floorboards may be done without concern.

Insecticides are potentially dangerous, especially early in pregnancy. Some would in fact argue that the insecticides in common use are more dangerous than the roaches, ants, moths, gnats, and spiders that you may wish to have out of your house or apartment. If your landlord is having your apartment exterminated along with the rest of the building, simply ask that your apartment be skipped. You can safely use insect traps such as "Roach Motel" or Combat products.

RADIATION

390

Q *I work at a CRT all day long. Is it true that they can be dangerous?*

A There is no conclusive evidence to implicate the electromagnetic fields emanating from video display terminals (VDT) or other cathode ray tubes (CRT) with birth defects or increased incidence of abortion. Interestingly, much more radiation emanates from the rear of these units. If you are concerned at work, configure your space so as not to be close to the rear of someone else's unit.

391

Q *I'm an ultrasound technician. Is it safe for me to be around ultrasound all day long for months?*

A There is no evidence to support a contention that ultrasound, whether diagnostic or therapeutic, increases the risks of abortion or birth defects.[29]

392

Q *I've got a lump in my breast and my doctor wants me to get a mammogram. Am I right to worry that the X-ray might harm the baby?*

A Radiation is a known teratogen. Excessive X-ray exposure has been linked to microcephaly and mental retardation. What few people realize, however, is that the doses used in common diagnostic radiology are nowhere near high enough to cause birth defects. Five rads (or 0.05 Gray) is believed to be the *minimum* exposure compatible with significant fetal risk. To put this in perspective, estimated fetal exposures are:

Dental	less than 0.02 rads
Chest X-ray(2 views)	0.02-0.07 rads
Abdominal view	0.10 rads
IVP	less than 1 rad
Hip film	0.20 rads
Mammogram	0.02 rads
CT Scan Head/Chest	1 rad
CT Pelvimetry	0.25 rads

None of these procedures is felt to pose any risk to the fetus in any trimester.

A very few procedures expose the fetus to enough ionizing radiation to make us nervous. In general, these are the moving picture X-rays such as Barium enemas (4 rads) and small bowel series (4 rads). Studies with multiple exposures of the abdomen such as abdominal CT (3.5 rads) deliver more than ten times the radiation of simple X-rays such as those of the chest, abdomen, or hip, or a mammogram.

With a threshold of 5 rads, the barium enema and abdominal CT get close enough to merit warning signs to patients in radiology suites.

Doctors know what levels are not safe and what their effects can be. There is no *proven* fetal risk at less than eight weeks or more than twenty-five, but from eight to fifteen weeks, the risk of central nervous system damage and mental retardation are increased in studies of pregnant women who survived the atomic bomb blasts.

There are multiple studies confirming the lack of fetal risk at exposures less than 5 rads.[30]

The evidence for carcinogenesis as a result of in utero exposure to X-rays or any other form of ionizing radiation is slim at best. One estimate is that in utero exposure could lead to a risk of childhood leukemia of 1 in 2,000 when the normal risk of leukemia is 1 in 3,000.[31] In short, abortion should never be recommended because of diagnostic radiation exposure.

393

Q *Is it safe to have imaging with MRI?*

A Magnetic Resonance Imaging (MRI) does not involve any ionizing radiation, but only exposure to electromagnetic fields. It is these fields that realign hydrogen atoms differently in different tissues and allow the possibility of a computer-generated image. It is an excellent method for visualizing the pelvis and potentially for studying the fetus There have been no reported adverse fetal effects with MRI; however, the National Radiologic Protection Board arbitrarily ruled out use of MRI in the first trimester.

394

Q *Can Nuclear Medicine Imaging be done safely in pregnancy?*

A Nuclear medicine techniques are used primarily to study the heart, lungs, thyroid, bones, and kidneys. These techniques work by "tagging" certain chemical agents with a radioactive isotope, which is then inhaled or injected.

Technetium Tc 99m is a radioisotope whose use for brain, bone, kidney, and heart imaging results in less than 0.05 rads exposure to the fetus. Tc 99m is used in pregnancy to rule out pulmonary emboli (blood clot to the lungs), when it is injected to visualize the lung vessels, and xenon gas (127XE) is inhaled to visualize the air spaces in the lung. Use of these in pregnancy is considered safe.

Radioactive iodine (I-131) readily crosses the placenta and can severely affect the fetal thyroid if used *after* twelve weeks of gestation. Therefore, I-131 is contraindicated in pregnancy.

395

Q *I work as a flight attendant and regularly find myself at thirty thousand feet. I've heard that repeated exposure to ambient (all-around) radiation at high altitude with thin atmosphere is dangerous to my fetus. Is that true?*

A There is no statistically significant evidence to link pressurized high-altitude flight to birth defects. All of the concerns are theoretical and there exists at least forty years of experience worldwide to date to indicate that those concerns are unfounded in reality. Flight attendants do not have a higher birth defect rate than nonattendants. Some have suggested that since radiation levels are highest at higher altitudes and nearer the pole where the atmosphere is thinner, that pregnant pilots and attendants be reassigned to lower-altitude, shorter flights nearer the tropical latitudes. This is an interesting suggestion, but it is probably hard to support from the available literature.

Airlines typically have their flight attendants removed from flight status at twenty-eight weeks because of their altered body mechanics, which make it impossible or unsafe for them to operate heavy emergency doors, chutes, and carts.

396

Q *I've heard that the electromagnetic fields from heating blankets can be dangerous in pregnancy. Is that true?*

A Studies suggesting that electromagnetic fields (EMFs) might be dangerous in pregnancy are relatively recent. EMFs come from power lines, household electrical wiring, household appliances, and electric blankets. Only the latter provides prolonged continuous exposure. EMFs have never been associated with birth defects, but some studies have suggested increased risks of later childhood leukemias for those children living directly below high-power line distribution towers. While the increased risk suggested is small, it might be advisable to avoid electric heating blankets and electrically heated water beds during pregnancy.

397

Q *We live right underneath high-tension power lines. I've heard that they can cause an increased risk of cancer later on in the baby I am carrying now. What's the current feeling on this?*

A Electromagnetic fields from high-voltage power lines and their potential adverse effect on health have been a source of controversy and debate in recent years. In 1997 a widespread study coordinated by the National Cancer Institute found no evidence that power lines increase the risk of childhood cancers.[32] While there are many people who dispute these findings, there does not seem to be enough evidence to justify changing where you live due to potential exposure during pregnancy or early childhood. A similar Norwegian study reached the same conclusions in 1997.[33]

398

Q *Can I continue to use a tanning bed while I'm pregnant?*

A Tanning salons use many different types of tanning beds, benches, and booths, all of which have differing amounts of UV-A and UV-B wavelength exposure. While many tanning salons will tell you that you have no risk of "burning" because there is no UV-B (short-wavelength UV) produced by their lights, this is often not the case. Similarly, skin cancers can be promoted by sun exposure and artificial tanning. However, there is some argument that predominantly long-wavelength UV-A tanning may be somewhat protective from actual sun exposure carcinogenesis.[34]

There is almost no data on tanning beds and pregnancy. As a consequence, their use should be avoided until at least ten weeks of gestation. After ten weeks, a towel over your lower abdomen will protect your fetus from any ultraviolet (UV) exposure.

PRESCRIPTION DRUGS

Introduction

The discussion of over-the-counter drugs in this volume is extensive primarily because the consumer often makes her own decision about using these medications. Chemical and radiation exposures can be inadvertent and are covered in some degree of detail above, in the hope of preventing accidental dangerous exposures.

Prescription drugs, however, should be controlled by your physician. It is a good idea to let your obstetrician coordinate all of your medications, even if they are prescribed by another specialist. The questions below are ones that are commonly asked about prescription drugs used to treat common pregnancy complaints, or relatively common chronic disease states complicated by pregnancy. This section is by no means exhaustive. Your obstetrician should be the one with whom you discuss the relative risks and benefits of the drugs you receive. Remember that even if a drug has been associated with slightly increased risks of certain birth defects, the disease state for which it is being prescribed, if left untreated, might be much more harmful than the drug itself.

Vaccines and Immunizations

399

Q *Which vaccines are safe and which are not in pregnancy?*

A Vaccines are broken into groups; some contain a live but weakened virus, some contain an inactive virus, some are inactivated bacteria, some are toxins, and others are immune globulins. The following live virus immunizations are not safe in pregnancy: measles (rubeola), mumps, German measles (rubella), BCG, vaccinia, zoster, and chicken pox (varicella).

Polio and yellow fever vaccines also contain live viruses and can only be given in pregnancy if the benefits far outweigh the risks.

Recommendations for flu vaccine changed in 1997 and again in 2000. CDC now recommends flu vaccine for *all* pregnant women in the 2nd & 3rd trimesters. It is an inactivated viral vaccine and is considered safe in pregnancy.

ACOG recommends vaccination for diphtheria, tetanus and pertusis with TDap before pregnancy or immediately after pregnancy, even if breast feeding, if you have not been vaccinated in the previous 2 years.[35]

Rabies vaccine, indicated only for those exposed because of the bite of a suspected rabid animal, contains an inactive virus. It may be used in pregnancy safely. The rabies hyperimmune globulin is also safe in pregnancy and should be given when suspicion of infection occurs.

Hepatitis B vaccine is an inactive virus vaccine. The entire series of three shots may be given safely in pregnancy for those at high risk of exposure—women who work at blood banks, for example. The hepatitis B hyperimmune globulin is also safe in pregnancy and should be used after exposure along with the vaccine, then separately at one month and at six months.

The pneumovacc is an inactivated bacterial vaccine. It may be safely used in pregnancy in those with chronic underlying lung or heart disease as advised by the woman's doctor.

The other inactivated bacterial vaccines protect against cholera, plague, and typhoid; vaccines for these diseases may be used in pregnancy as indicated.

400

Q *Can I get a tetanus shot in pregnancy if needed? And what is this I hear about whooping cough and a vaccine in pregnancy?*

A Tetanus toxoid may be used safely whenever indicated in pregnancy. It is usually given with diphtheria and pertussis vaccines, both of which are safe in pregnancy, called TDap. The CDC now recommends all women be vaccinated for pertusis (whooping cough) immediately after delivery, even if breast feeding, if not vaccinated in the previous 2 years with the older Td vaccine. It also says pregnant women in the second and third trimesters may receive TDap if exposure warrants it. Tetanus hyperimmune globulins are also safe to give after possible exposure.

401

Q *My nephew broke out with chicken pox right after I visited his family. I'm twelve weeks pregnant. What can I do?*

A In all likelihood you are immune to chicken pox. First, ask your mother if she remembers you having had it as a child. If you had it, you have lifelong immunity. If you either do not know, or know for sure that you did not have chicken pox, you may get blood drawn to determine if you are immune. This should be done immediately. If the results show that you are susceptible, you may receive Varicella Zoster Hyperimmune Globulin (VZIG) within about ninety-six hours and hopefully avoid infection. Note that chicken pox poses significant risk of congenital abnormalities in the first trimester, and considerable risk if acquired right before delivery in terms of neonatal infection, but poses *very little* risk between about twelve and thirty weeks. (See Section 9: Medical Complications, Infections)

402

Q *Is there a varicella vaccine I can take before pregnancy if I know I've never had chicken pox?*

A Yes. Varicella vaccine (Varivax) became available in 1995. It may be safely taken three months before conception. The delay is due to theoretical risk, since the vaccine does contain live virus.

Acne Treatment

403

Q *I've been on Accutane for my acne. Do I need to stop it when I get pregnant?*

A Yes. In fact, you need to stop it before you get pregnant. Isotretinoin (Accutane) (Category X), as mentioned in the first part of Section 5, is one of the few known teratogens. It has been associated with a markedly increased risk of miscarriage and multiple fetal anomalies of different organ systems. These include abnormalities of the brain, skull, ears, eye, cleft lip and palate, congenital heart defects, absent thymus gland, and intrauterine death. The American Academy of Pediatrics does not consider Accutane compatible with breast-feeding.

Tretinoin (Retin-A) (Category C) has been shown to be teratogenic in animals but only orally. However, even at 320 times the normal dose it was not teratogenic topically. Certainly it would be wise to avoid this drug in the first trimester, but topical use beyond that is reasonable pending a discussion with your doctor. Topical Retin-A is completely metabolized in the skin.

The American Academy of Pediatrics has not determined whether it is safe to use while breast-feeding.

404

Q *My doctor has me on a new medicine for acne called Proscar. Is it safe?*

A No. It is absolutely not safe. Finasteride (Proscar) (Category X) is not indicated currently for the treatment of acne, although it is often used for this. The drug blocks the conversion of a precursor form of male hormone to a more potent one. It is known to cause birth defects in animals.

There is no known effect on the female fetus, but theoretically, exposure to finasteride during the critical developmental phase of the external genitalia from about ten to sixteen weeks could lead to ambiguous genitalia in the male newborn. (See Section 4: Fetal Development)

The American Academy of Pediatrics does not consider Proscar compatible with breast-feeding.

Antibiotics

405

Q *Are antibiotics safe in pregnancy?*

A In general, antibiotics are felt to be safe in pregnancy whether given orally, as a topical cream, or in intravenous form. This applies to all trimesters of pregnancy, with a few exceptions. (See table) In the absence of a specific allergy, all penicillins, cephalosporins, and erthromycins are safe. A partial listing of these would include:

Penicillins *(Category B)*	Oral: PenVeeK, Pentids, Unipen, Veetids, Amoxil, Ampicillin, Principen, Geocillin, Augmentin
	Injection: Bicillin, Geopen, Penicillin G, Timentin, Wycillin, Unasyn, Piperacillin, Ampicillin
Cephalosporins *(Category B)*	Oral: Ceclor, Anspor, Ceftin, Keflex, Keftabs, Ultracef, Cefzil
	Injection: Cefizox, Cefotan, Duricef, Ancef, Monocid, Cefoxitin, Rochephin, Kefzol, Mandol, Cefuroxime, Ceftazidime
Erythromycins *(Category B)*	Oral: Eryc, E.E.S., Erythromycin, Zithromax, Biaxin (Category C for lack of data), Dynabac, Ketek
	Injection: Erythromycin

406

Q *What about tetracycline? I was using it for my skin before I got pregnant.*

A Tetracyclines (Category D), including doxcycline (Vibramycin) and minocycline (Minocin), are often used to treat acne. They have traditionally been avoided due to their propensity to discolor teeth from about fourteen weeks on. There is no evidence of tetracyclines causing a problem prior to ten weeks. New data on this, released in 1997, may dispute the effect of doxycycline specifically on fetal teeth and bone. However, since reasonable substitutes almost always exist, all tetracyclines should be avoided until more data is obtained.

The American Academy of Pediatrics considers tetracyclines safe for breast-feeding.

407

Q *I have a yellowish discharge with a bad odor and my doctor says I have bacterial vaginosis (Gardnerella). He prescribed Metrogel, a cream form of metronidazole, but my friend's doctor told her that oral metronidazole (Flagyl) was dangerous in pregnancy. Who's right?*

A Metronidazole (Category B) is known orally as Flagyl and has recently become available as a cream for the skin or vagina known as Metrogel. Data on the safety of metronidazole has been conflicting for years. As of this writing it appears that there is no reliable data to suggest that metronidazole is unsafe in the second or third trimesters. It should be avoided in the first trimester. Likewise, a single large dose, as is used in the treatment of trichomonas, a vaginal protozoan that also causes vaginal itching and discharge, should be avoided, and prolonged low-dose therapy should be substituted instead.

The American Academy of Pediatrics advises caution with this drug while breast-feeding. If a single large dose of 2,000 milligrams is given, breast-feeding should be stopped for twenty-four hours after the dose.

Clindamycin (Cleocin) (Clindesse Cream) (Category B), used to treat bacterial vaginosis, has not been linked to any birth defects. It has not been implicated as a problem for the fetus in any trimester. The American Academy of Pediatrics considers clindamycin safe for breast-feeding.

Simple urinary tract infections (UTI), or bladder infections, can ascend more easily in pregnancy and become a serious kidney infection. What's more, kidney infection (pyelonephritis) has been associated with preterm labor. (See Section 9: Urinary Tract Disease)

Nitrofurantoin (Macrobid) (Category B), used to treat bladder infections, is felt to be safe in all trimesters. The American Academy of Pediatrics considers nitrofurantoin to be safe while breast-feeding.

Ciprofloxin (Cipro), which your doctor may have prescribed for bladder infections before you got pregnant, is one of the newer fluoroquinolones (Category C), as is norfloxacin (Floxin) and gatafloxicin (Tequin). This class of drugs has been associated with joint and extremity problems in animal studies, and fluoroquinolones should not be used in pregnancy. Talk to your doctor before you use any antibiotics you already have on hand.

Trimethoprim-Sulfamethoxazole (Category C) (Bactrim; Septra) is one of the most common antibiotics used for UTIs. While most studies show no association with birth defects, some caution is warranted. While sulfonamides seem to be fine in the first trimester, trimethoprim is a little worrisome because of several studies linking it to cardiovascular defects. Sulfa drugs, on the other hand, should be avoided in the late third trimester because of their ability to bind to bilirubin and potentially cause brain damage. (See Section 4: Digestive System—kernictirus)

In short, if the bacteria in question is only responsive to this class of drugs, then treat with it; otherwise seek substitutes, especially in the first and third trimesters.

Monuril (Category B) is a single-dose powder for UTI. It is felt to be safe in pregnancy simply because there is no teratogenicity in animals at any dosage. New in 1997, it is mixed into water and makes a drink similar to Kool-Aid, to be used as a one-time dose. Due to lack of experience as well as the availability of substitutes known to be safe, it would be reasonable to avoid using Monuril in the first ten weeks.

408

Q *I was hospitalized for pyelonephritis (kidney infection) at thirty weeks and they gave me gentamicin IV. A friend who is a doctor said that this could cause deafness in the baby. Is that true?*

A Some friend. You can ask your doctor, but if he chose gentamicin it was in all likelihood because the bacteria involved weren't sensitive to anything else. The aminoglycosides include streptomycin, kanamycin (Category D), and gentamicin, amikacin, and vancomycin (Category C). Streptomycin and kanamycin have been linked to ototoxicity, meaning damage to hearing and other eighth cranial nerve function. The other aminoglycosides have not been linked to any congenital defect, but are generally avoided in the first trimester because of their relationship to the other two known teratogens. Gentamicin and amikacin may be used for life-threatening infections such as pyelonephritis in pregnancy in any trimester if sensitivities indicate the necessity. Avoid the regimen of a single large daily dose, however, until more data is available.

A newer class of antibiotics, the monobactams such as aztreonam (Azactam), have been little studied in pregnant people, but unlike the aminoglycosides have no teratogenic effects in animal studies. They have very similar bacterial coverages to the aminoglycosides.

409

Q *My best friend was just operated on for a ruptured appendix and they gave her Primaxin at ten weeks. I'm a nurse and wondered if we could say that was safe?*

A Imipenem (Primaxin) is a newer drug of the carbapenam class; it is an injectable broad-spectrum antibiotic. There are no reports linking it to teratogenicity in humans, but there is little data available. It should be used only when sensitivities mandate it in a sick patient; otherwise anaerobic drugs with longer track records would be advisable, such as Cefoxitin.

410

Q *My husband and I both have tuberculosis. Are all the antibiotics prescribed for tuberculosis okay to use?*

A The antituberculous antibiotics include isoniazid (INH), rifampin, and ethambutol. None of these has been proved as the cause of birth defects with exposure in any trimester. INH has occasionally been implicated in various defects with first trimester exposure, but several large reviews found no association.[36]

In any event, the risks to the fetus of untreated tuberculosis far outweigh any potential concerns about the antibiotics.

Antifungals (Antimycotics)

411

Q *I'm only nine weeks pregnant, but I have a yeast infection and the OTC creams didn't work. Can my doctor prescribe something?*

A Just recently, many of the group of antifungals called imidazoles became available over the counter. These include Clotrimazole (Gyne-Lotrimin), Miconazole (Monistat), and butoconozole (Femstat and Gynazole-1) (Category B). All of these may be effective against vaginal infections caused by candida, torulopsis, and others. (See this section: Over-the-Counter Drugs)

Terconazole (Terazol) is a newer imidazole that treats some resistant strains of yeast but is available only by prescription. All of the imidazole antifungals are safe in pregnancy.

Ketoconazole (Nizoral) (Category C) is a slightly older oral antifungal. It has been used in human pregnancy with no adverse effects. In the Michigan Medicaid Recipient Study, 20 newborns were exposed in the first trimester with no increase in birth defects noted. It has been used to treat both Cushing's syndrome in pregnancy because it blocks both testosterone and cortisol synthesis, as well as systemic fungal infections in patients with HIV.

Fluconizole (Diflucan) (Category C) is a new oral agent for treatment of candida and other fungi. Diflucan has not been causally linked to birth defects. In rabbits, at doses sixty times normal, there was an increased abortion rate and thus the drug was classified as Category C.

It is probably prudent to avoid this medication in the first trimester. However, its use is reasonable and considered safe in the second and third trimesters for fungal infections that are resistant to the topical imidazoles.

412

Q *I've used Nystatin swish and swallow for thrush before. Is it safe?*

A Nystatin (Category B) is not known to be a teratogen. If possible, it would be wise to avoid all systemic antifungals in the first trimester.

413

Q *A friend of ours with AIDS had histoplasmosis. She got Ampotericin B but they called it "Amphoterrible." Is it really safe for her in pregnancy?*

Systemic infections with histoplasmosis, coccidioidomycosis, crypto coccosis, and systemic candidiasis sometimes respond to nothing else. Amphotericin B (Fungizone) (Category B) has not been linked to any adverse pregnancy outcome and may be used in all trimesters of pregnancy. It is sometimes called "Amphoterrible" because of its side effects, which include fever, headache, weight loss, nausea and vomiting, diarrhea, generalized muscle pain, and local phlebitis (clotting) at intravenous sites.

414

What about nail infections with fungus? I heard that the oral medicines for this are dangerous.

Griseofulvin (Gris-Peg; Fulvicin) (Category C) has been clearly linked to both miscarriage and birth defects in animals. Studies in humans are inconclusive. Since this drug is not used to treat life-threatening infections, it should be avoided in pregnancy.

Itraconozole (Sporonox) (Category C) has also been associated with embryotoxic and teratogenic effects in animals and therefore should be avoided in pregnancy despite the lack of human data. Tervinafine (Lamisil) oral and topical is probably safe and Category B.

Antivirals

415

My sister-in-law was just diagnosed with AIDS. Will she be able to take AZT now that she's ten weeks pregnant?

Zidovudine (AZT) (Category C) is an analog of thymidine, one of the basic building blocks of DNA, and is one of the first drugs to be successful in inhibiting the AIDS (HIV) virus. It has been clearly shown to reduce the levels of virus transmitted to the fetus from an infected mother, and therefore the rate of newborns with HIV. While there is some debatable evidence about a risk of fetal anemia when given in the first trimester, the outcome of fetal infection is thus far uniformly fatal. For that reason, Zidovudine is currently recommended for treatment of pregnant women known to be infected with the HIV virus.

416

What about use of the protease inhibitors in pregnancy?

Protease inhibitors Crixivan (Category C), Invirase (Category B), and Norvir (Category B) have all been used in human pregnancy to treat HIV-positive patients. There are no reports of human birth defects attributable to these drugs at this time, but there is little experience.

There is little information yet available about the outcome of fetuses whose mothers were treated with protease inhibitors in pregnancy. In rats and rabbits there appears to be no evidence of teratogenicity, but there are no adequately controlled trials in humans. There have been isolated reports of supranumary (extra) ribs in rats with Crixivan, but not with the other drugs. It is likely, however, because of their ability to render viral levels undetectable in some HIV-positive patients, that data on early exposure in pregnancy will rapidly accumulate even in the absence of controlled studies. AZT will dramatically reduce transmission to the fetus currently and is known to be safe.

417

Q *I've got herpes and I'm a neonatal ICU nurse. I've seen the devastation of herpes in newborns. Can I use Zovirax or Valtrex to prevent a recurrence in the third trimester?*

A Zovirax (acyclovir) and Valtrex (valcyclovir) (Category C) are both agents effective against the herpetiviridae family of viruses, including both herpes simplex (oral and genital herpes) and varicella (chicken pox). Valtrex is in fact metabolized into acyclovir, but achieves much higher blood levels. Famvir (famcyclovir) is felt to be equally safe in the second and third trimester as Valcyclover.

The Michigan Medicaid Recipient Study reviewed 478 newborns with first trimester exposure to acyclovir and found no evidence to support a risk to acyclovir.[37] New data from the University of Texas Southwestern in Dallas would seem to indicate that acyclovir may be used not just for life-threatening varicella pneumonia in pregnant women, but also for first-time herpes infections as well as suppression of late trimester recurrences, thereby lowering the number of C-sections performed.[38]

The American Academy of Pediatrics considers acyclovir to be compatible with breast-feeding despite the fact that the drug is concentrated in breast milk. (See Medical Complications, Infections)

418

Q *My doctor was using interferon A to treat my venereal warts (HPV). Can that continue during my pregnancy?*

A Interferon A (Intron A) (Category C) has not been shown to cause birth defects in humans, but there are no published reports of controlled studies in pregnant women to date. It has been used both locally and systemically by subcutaneous injection. It is effective against hairy cell leukemia and some viruses, but again, data is lacking on its safety.

More traditional means of treating venereal warts (condyloma), such as trichloroacetic acid (TCA), cryotherapy (freezing), or laser should be used in pregnancy.

Podophyllin as well as 5-fluorouracil are both topical compounds used to treat condyloma, or venereal warts, in nonpregnant women. They should not be used in pregnancy because of concerns about potential danger to the fetus.

Imiquimod (Aldara) (Category B) is a topical treatment for venereal warts that became available in 1997. It may work by stimulating your body's own alpha interferon to attack the HPV virus. While there are no studies in animals showing birth defects, there are no controlled studies in pregnant women. Currently, it is probably reasonable to confine pregnancy treatment to traditional surgical, freezing, or laser therapy when topical TCA fails.

419

Q *I work in a neonatal ICU and we've been treating a baby with respiratory syncytial virus (RSV) using Ribavirin aerosol. Is that safe for me in pregnancy?*

A Considering the minimum exposure passively, the risk is probably extremely small. Ribavirin is not recommended in pregnancy, however, due to its association with hydrocephalus and limb abnormalities in rats. It would be prudent to switch work assignments in order to avoid any exposure to the drug.

Other antiviral agents such as idoxuridine, trifluridine, and vidarabine were all developed as cancer chemotherapy originally. Because of their cytotoxic effects, they should all be avoided in pregnancy.[39]

420

Q *Everybody at work has the flu and I forgot to get vaccinated. Can I take amantadine to prevent it? I'm twenty-three weeks pregnant.*

A Amantadine (Category C) is used for Parkinson's disease as well as for flu prevention. It is a known teratogen in animals and there have been isolated reports of defects in human newborns. While the data is inadequate to draw conclusions, the current perception is that getting the flu would probably be safer than taking amantadine.

Antiparasitics

421

Q I've been diagnosed with trichomonas vaginalis and I itch like crazy. Is it okay to use Flagyl orally at thirteen weeks?

A Metronidazole (Flagyl) (Category B) has been mentioned elsewhere with respect to treatment of bacterial vaginosis. It is the only known effective agent for the vaginal/cervical parasitic infection, trichomoniasis. Several large studies have not found any association between metronidazole and birth defects, even with first trimester exposure.[40] However, because of a suggestion of cancer-causing tendencies in some animals, it should probably be avoided, at least at the one-time dose of 2,000 milligrams, in the first trimester. It is suspected that some problems may arise from the peak dosage levels. After twelve weeks, oral Flagyl or vaginal Metrogel may be used without restriction.

422

Q I've got pubic lice for the first time in my life and I'm twenty weeks pregnant. What should I do?

A You need to see your doctor and make sure of your diagnosis first. He or she may recommend gamma benzene hexachloride (Lindane), which may be used for both pubic lice (pediculosis pubis), head lice, and scabies (mites). Because this drug is absorbed through the skin and has been associated with bone marrow failure, neurotoxicity, and seizures, it would be wise to use a substitute if possible, certainly in the first trimester.

Pyrethrins with piperonyl butoxide (RID) (Category C) may be used for lice, but not for scabies. Despite its classification in Category C, it is preferred over Lindane in pregnancy because it is not systemically absorbed.

Crotamiton 10% Lotion (Eurax) may be used to treat scabies. Like pyrethrins, crotamiton is not systemically absorbed.

423

Q I'm sixteen weeks pregnant and we have a chance to go to Hong Kong and Singapore. Can I use malarial drugs to prevent infection?

A Chloroquine (Category C) is the antimalarial of choice for pregnant women. Malaria is endemic (present all the time) in many parts of Central and South America, India, Africa, and Asia. Primaquine, available for the same indication is less well studied and should not be used unless chloroquine-resistant malaria is encountered. Quinine (Category D), often used for chloroquine-resistant strains, should be avoided unless absolutely necessary. It has been associated with multiple defects in humans. Quinidine (Category C) would be a safer choice.

424

Q *I know to have my husband clean the kitty litter, or at least if I do it, not to breathe it in, to wash my hands afterward, and to avoid wiping my mouth with my hands. What if I get toxoplasmosis even with all these precautions?*

A (See also Section 9: Infections)
Toxoplasmosis may be treated if it is diagnosed by blood tests or by changes on your baby's ultrasound. Pyrimethamine (Category C) (also used for malaria) and sulfadiazine (Category B) may be prescribed together; sometimes spiramycin (Category C) (same family as erythromycins) may be given alone.

Because of the fetal teratogenicity of toxoplasmosis itself, it has been difficult to evaluate the safety of these drugs in pregnancy. On balance, the evidence is against using these medicines, since they have caused birth defects.

425

Q *My two year old has pinworm and the pediatrician says we should treat everyone in the house. I'm eight weeks pregnant. Can I be treated?*

A Yes, but pinworm (enterobiasis) is hardly a life-and-death disease.
Mebendazole (Vermox) (Category C) is the drug of choice for pinworm (threadworm), as well as more dangerous helminths such as trichuriasis (whipworm), ascariasis (roundworm), and uncinariasis (hookworm). Although mebendazole is teratogenic in rats, it is thought to have caused no human birth defects. In light of the fact that pinworm is not life-threatening, and that your husband and son may be treated, it is reasonable to wait until the end of the first trimester before you are treated.

Thiabendazole (Mintezole) (Category C) is used for the same indications as above, with the same lack of evidence for teratogenicity in humans.

Pyrantel pomoate (Antiminth) (Category C) is used for ascariasis (roundworm) and enterobiasis (pinworm). It has not been reported to have teratogenicity in rats. While there are no adequate human studies, if treatment must be given in the first trimester, this drug might be a more prudent choice than mebendazole.

Quinacrine (Atabrine) (Category C) has also been used to treat both malarial and worm infestations. This drug was shown to increase fetal mortality in animals, but without structural defects. Rare cases of questionable human defects have been reported with first trimester use. It should probably be avoided in favor of available alternatives.

Asthma

426

Q   *Can I still use my inhaler while I'm pregnant?*

A   Absolutely. In fact, asthma medicines are the easiest to discuss of all the medicines used for chronic diseases. You can use whatever you need. Inhalers are generally beta-adrenergic agonists, or agents that relax smooth muscles in the bronchi and small airways. They are also called sympathomimetic agents because they stimulate the sympathetic nervous system, and act as bronchodilators. Common ones include metaproterenol (Metaprel; Alupent), albuterol (Proventil; Ventolin), isopreterenol (Isuprel), and iso-etharine (Bronkometer). All are Category C drugs. None have been associated with birth defects, even after prolonged exposure in the first trimester. All, however, are capable in large doses of causing maternal and fetal tachycardia with accompanying drops in blood pressure. They also may increase maternal serum glucose. Used in the directed doses, however, they are entirely appropriate for asthma in pregnancy.

All of the beta-adrenergic agonists are known to slightly inhibit preterm labor and to decrease the incidence of neonatal respiratory distress syndrome.[41]

427

Q   *I'm taking Theodur. Will I be able to continue that in pregnancy?*

A   Yes. Aminophylline derivatives such as the theophyllines (Theodur) (Category C) are felt to be safe in pregnancy and are the chronic bronchodilators of choice. The Collaborative Perinatal Project reviewed 193 mother-child pairs with first trimester exposure and found no link to birth defects. Like the beta-adrenergic agonists, these drugs also tend to inhibit preterm labor and improve lung maturity.

They are classified as Category C because long-term effects of aminophyllines have not been studied after prolonged in utero exposure.

428

Q   *I was in the emergency room with an asthma attack when I was twenty-five weeks pregnant. Was that really adrenaline they gave me?*

In all likelihood it was. Epinephrine (adrenaline), ephedrine (both Category C), and terbutaline (Breathine) (Category B) are all common sympathomimetic amines. These agents, like others given in their class, cause bronchial smooth muscle relaxation. They are first-line choices for treatment along with the inhaled agents mentioned above. Additionally, terbutaline is now the most commonly used medicine to treat preterm labor.

429

My obstetrician says it's okay to use inhaled steroids, but I've heard steroids were dangerous. Should I use my steroid inhaler while pregnant?

Yes. Inhaled steroids have become almost an equal mainstay of therapy with the inhaled beta-agonist bronchodilators. Inhaled steroids include beclomethasone (Beclovent; Vanceril), fluticasone (Flonase), and dexamethasone (Decadron Respihaler). All are classified as Category C. None has been shown to cause birth defects even with first trimester exposure. The Michigan Medicaid Recipient Study looked at 595 first trimester exposures and found no linkage to adverse fetal outcome.

Dexamethasone is used orally ever increasingly in preterm labor to help advance lung maturity, with excellent success. Newer studies tend to show benefit for infants of both sexes and all races, contrary to earlier findings.

Fluticasone/salmeterol (Advair) diskus (Category C) may be used with caution, not as first line treatment.

Fluticasone (Flonase) (Category C) nasal inhalers for allergies may also be used safely in pregnancy.

430

I have a cromolyn sodium inhaler Can I still use it to prevent attacks?

Yes Cromolyn sodium (Intal; Nasalcrom) (Category B) helps suppress your immune system's mast cells and thereby prevent the release of certain chemicals that can cause bronchoconstriction. Two puffs taken up to four times per day may be used safely in pregnancy.

431

My doctor has me on a new drug called Accolate. Can I stay on it in pregnancy?

Zafirlukast (Accolate) (Category B) is not a known teratogen in animals at any dosage. It works by blocking leukotrienes, which are compounds that cause smooth-muscle constriction around airways. There are no reports of human teratogenicity, but no controlled trials in pregnant women.

There is every reason to believe that the benefits may well outweigh the risks if you respond well to the drug. It should not be used in breast-feeding, however, since it is extensively excreted in breast milk.

432

Q *I have some old Tussi-Organidin at home that I used for a bad cold. Can I use it to help break up the congestion in my chest? I'm afraid I'll get an asthma attack if I don't.*

A Don't touch that bottle! Tussi-Organidin (Category X) contains iodide and is known to be associated with fetal thyroid goiter, hypo-thyroidism, and even tracheal airway obstruction in the newborn. No iodide-containing preparations should be used in pregnancy, even though they are not teratogenic in themselves.

During pregnancy, for coughs, use the preferred antitussives guaifen-esin, dextromthorphans; for decongestion, use oxymetazoline and pseu-doephedrine; if you need an antihistamine, use chlorpheniramine and tripelennamine; if you need an anti-inflammatory agent, use cromolyn, prednisone, and beclomethasone.[42] (See this section: Headaches, Cold, and Flu.)

Anti-Inflamatories and Immunosuppressives

433

Q *Can I use oral corticosteroids?*

A Corticosteroids are potent anti-inflammatory medicines used for the treatment of asthma, allergies, bronchitis, skin disorders, and a large set of chronic collagen vascular (connective tissue) diseases. These diseases include systemic lupus erythematosus (SLE), rheumatoid arthritis, scleroderma, polyarteritis nodosa, Wegener's granulomatosis, temporal arteritis, and dermatomyositis. These related disorders are caused by autoantibodies. Many doctors feel that ulcerative colitis and Crohn's disease belong in this group as well. Essentially these diseases all involve errors of the human immune system, in which the body attacks any number of its own tissues. (See Section 9: Medical Complications)

All of these disease states have corticosteroids as the mainstay of their therapy. Prednisone (Category B) is by far the most common of these drugs. It is immediately converted to prednisolone in the body, and methyl prednisolone (Medrol) is another frequently used steroid. In the Michigan Medicaid Recipient Study, 501 first trimester exposures to these drugs were reviewed and the data did not support an association between the drugs and congenital defects. The summary of all information to date would suggest that these medicines pose an extremely small risk, if any, to the developing fetus.[43]

Dexamethasone (Decadron) (Category C) has also been used extensively in pregnancies. It is now used more frequently to promote lung maturity in premature labor, just as injectable Betamethasone has been used for years. There are no reports linking dexamethasone to birth defects in humans, and long-term follow-up of children who were exposed in utero has shown no adverse effects. It is classified as Category C because of toxic effects none of which have been seen in humans.[44]

Note that intravenous Cortisone (Category D), unlike the oral steroids mentioned above, has been associated with human defects in rare instances, and should rarely if ever be used in pregnancy.

434

Q *What other anti-arthritis drugs can be used in pregnancy?*

A Ibuprofen (Advil) and Indomethacin (Indocin) are both Category B until the 3rd trimester when they change to Category D due to their prolongation of labor, increased risk of abruption, bleeding post partum, and increased risk of fetal cardiac problems. Indocin may be used in the short term to inhibit preterm labor, but can be associated with a rapid reduction in amniotic fluid and must be monitored closely.

Disease Modifying Anti-rheumatic Drugs (DMARDS) used for arthritis and joint pains are categorized as biologic (Humira, Enbrel, Remicade and Kineret), as synthetic (Imuran, Sandimmune, Neoral, Gold compounds, Plaquenil, Arava, Methotrexate, penicillamine and Azulfidine) and as anti-inflammatories (prednisione and the non-steroidal NSAIDS such as aspirin and ibuprofen.)

All of these should be avoided in the first trimester if possible, but many are considered safe for the most part. The folate antagonist Methotrexate is contra-indicated in pregnancy and associated with miscarriage and multiple birth defects. Arava, or leflunomide is toxic in animals and is also contra-indicated and should not be used in pregnancy. Azulfadine, also a folate antagonist does not cause birth defects or miscarriage but the patient should supplement with folate if using this drug. Penicillamine is associated with connective tissue defects and should not be used in pregnancy at all. All of the NSAIDS can cause early miscarriage, closure of the ductus arteriosus, fetal renal toxicity, delayed labor and increased risk of abruptio placenta. Prednisone after 10 weeks is unlikely to cause significant problems, but continuous high dosage has been associated with growth restriction.[45]

Methotrexate, Arava, and Penicillamine are contraindicated in pregnancy. Azulfidine, if used, must include folate supplementation.[46]

435

Q *I have ulcerative colitis. Can I continue my Azulfidine?*

A Sulfasalazine (Azulfadine) (Category B, but D if used near term) is used primarily for treatment of ulcerative colitis and Crohn's disease.

As with other sulfa drugs, its primary risk is that it binds to bilirubin and causes its deposition in the newborn brain known as kernicterus. This risk, however, is only theoretical with sulfasalazine, since there are no reports of kernicterus even with its use right through delivery.

You should discuss its use with your doctor, but it is generally used without regard to trimester if needed to control a severe exacerbation of inflammatory bowel disease.

436

Q *I've had a kidney transplant. Can I stay on the drugs that I've been taking?*

A Yes. The benefits probably outweigh the risks in your circumstances, but discuss it with your doctor. Azathioprine (Immuran) (Category D) has been found to be teratogenic in rabbits. In humans, however, most have found the drug to be relatively safe.[47] Rarely, bone marrow suppression has been described in newborns.

Interestingly, azathioprine has been shown to markedly reduce the effectiveness of the IUD.

Cyclosporin (Category C) has not been shown to be an animal teratogen. In humans it has been used widely for heart and liver transplants as well as kidney transplants. There have been too few cases to draw definitive conclusions, but overall it would seem that the drug causes little risk to the fetus.[48]

Analgesics and Narcotics

437

Q *Can I use narcotic pain relievers safely? My oral surgeon wouldn't give me any after oral surgery because I was ten weeks pregnant.*

A Most data would suggest that use of hydrocodon would be reasonable in this circumstance. Narcotic pain relievers are all opiate derivatives, and are commonly used postoperatively. (See this section: Illicit Drugs, Heroin) They have not been linked to any human birth defects. They are, however, extremely effective postoperative pain medicines and, when used in prescription strength for short periods, pose no risk to the fetus in any trimester. Care must be taken, however, with many of the combination medicines that often contain aspirin, such as Percodan. Acetaminophen-containing combinations, such as Percocet, are preferable when possible (See this section: Over-the-Counter Drugs)

Codeine (Category C), hydrocodon (Vicodin) (Category B), meperidine (Demerol) (Category B), and morphine (Category B) are all classified as Category D if they are used in high doses and near term, (excluding intravenous and intramuscular narcotics in labor). It is probable that all could be used safely for brief periods during any trimester. Prolonged use should be avoided because of the risk of fetal addiction and subsequent withdrawal syndromes. Codeine is classified as Category C because several isolated defects have been found after first trimester exposure in multiple different studies, including the Collaborative Perinatal Projects review of 563 first trimester exposures.

Use of codeine should therefore be avoided in the first trimester.

The American Academy of Pediatrics considers all narcotics in prescription doses compatible with breast-feeding because of the small amounts excreted.

438

Q *Can I take Toradol in pregnancy?*

A Ketorolac (Toradol) (Category C) is an excellent nonsteroidal antiinflammatory drug (NSAID), particularly for postoperative pain relief. It is, however, an antiprostaglandin like all of the other NSAIDs, such as ibuprofen, and naprosyn, and may cause delayed and prolonged labor if used in the late third trimester. The manufacturer lists it as "contraindicated" in labor, because its uterine relaxant effect could increase postpartum bleeding.

Despite this, postoperative C-section patients are often administered a onetime dose of ketorolac if they are not otherwise at high risk for bleeding and are receiving poor pain relief from an epidural pump or a narcotic PCA (patient-controlled anesthesia) pump.

439

Q *What narcotics are commonly used in labor?*

A The first stage of labor may be as long as fifteen hours, and many people feel they need something more than emotional support. The narcotics morphine, meperidine (Demerol); butorphenol (Stadol), aphpadrodine, (Nisentil), and nalbuphine (Nubain) are the most commonly used in labor.

All are classified as Category B, but D when used late in pregnancy (excluding usage in labor). Butorphenol and nalbuphine have the added benefit of not being a respiratory depressant in the newborn.

These medicines have not been found to be teratogenic in animals, nor of course can there be an association with malformations when used for suppression of labor pain. Intramuscular delivery lasts longer, but could peak in the fetus about an hour after injection, and if this is near delivery, levels may be unacceptably high. Nisentil has fallen into disuse because of reported alterations of fetal heart rate and respiratory depression in the newborn.

440

Q *I've had awful headaches since about thirteen weeks. I'm seventeen weeks now. Can I take anything stronger than Tylenol?*

A Migraine or migrainelike headaches in the second trimester are usually vascular in nature and are related to expanding blood volumes. They usually resolve by about twenty weeks, but can be very severe.

Butalbital (Category C) is combined with acetaminophen and caffeine in Fioricet, and further with codeine in Fioricet #3. Butalbital is a short-acting barbiturate. Even with use in the first trimester there seems to be no risk of birth defects.[49]

It is a safe choice for severe pain after the first trimester even in combination with caffeine and acetaminophen. Its classification in Category C relates only to its class as a barbiturate and the confusion surrounding the potential for birth defects in drugs used to treat seizure disorders. Fiorinol contains aspirin and should probably be avoided.

Flextra DS is the same drug as Fioricet but without the caffeine. It is also felt to be safe in pregnancy after the first trimester.

441

Q *I use Imitrex for my migraines when I'm not pregnant. Can I use it in pregnancy?*

A No. Sumatriptan (Imitrex) (Category C) is used both by injection and orally for the treatment of vascular migraine and cluster-type headaches. While it has been found to be teratogenic in rabbits, there exists no evidence of teratogenicity in humans. However, Imitrex and other tryptans like it (such as MaxAlt, Relpax, and Frovea) should not be used in pregnancy because their mechanism of action involves blood vessel constriction, which could potentially jeopardize the fetus. Breast feeding mothers should discard milk for 12 hours following use.

Antihypertensives

442

Q *I have chronic hypertension and I plan to get pregnant soon. Can I stay on my captopril?*

A You need to stop your captopril and discuss an alternative with your doctor. Several drugs are considered completely safe in pregnancy, but many are not so clear, or are clearly contraindicated.

Angiotension-converting enzyme inhibitors (ACE Inhibitors) (Category D) such as captopril (Capoten) and enalapril (Vasotec; Vasoretic) should be avoided in pregnancy if at all possible. They have been associated with failure of the fetal skull to form properly, decreased amniotic fluid, and newborn kidney failure. ACE inhibitors decrease placental blood flow in animal studies and were often associated with death of the fetus. These drugs are contraindicated in pregnancy.

Olmesartan (Benicar), eprosartan (Teveten), and irbesartan (Avapro) are angiotensin receptor blockers and should be avoided as well if possible.

443

Q *Can I stay on my beta-blocker? I've been on Tenormin for years.*

A Discuss it with your doctor, who may wish to discuss other first trimester options, or let you continue it.

Atenolol (Tenormin) (Category C) is one of the most common of the selective beta-receptor blockers used for chronic hypertension alone or in combination with a diuretic. Other common ones are the original nonselective blocker (has other than cardiovascular effects) propranolol

(Inderal), as well as the cardioselective blockers nadolol (Corgard), timo-lol (Timoptic), metoprolol (Lopressor), and labetalol (Trandate), all of which are classified as Category C. Each has been associated in some reports with extremely small potential increased risk for birth defects with first trimester exposure. All of these associations were weak and subject to alternative explanations.

There are no adequate studies in the first trimester to say with certainty that all cardioselective beta-blockers are safe. Most of the data indicting any of these drugs relates to intrauterine growth restriction, and all this data is confounded by the fact that both chronic hypertension and preeclampsia may cause IUGR. Several British studies looked at atenelol and found it safe in pregnancy for chronic hypertension.[50]

With mild hypertension, it is not unreasonable to suspend treatment with these agents through twelve weeks and then reinstitute if necessary.

444

Q *Can I continue taking Calan?*

A In all probability, your doctor will let you continue with Calan, but it must be discussed in the context of your own circumstances. All of the calcium channel blockers are derived from verapamil (Calan; Isoptin) (Category C), nifedipine (Procardia, Adalat) (Category C) being the most prominent example. These drugs are commonly used to treat hypertension as well as supraventricular tachycardia (SVT) in pregnancy.

Verapamil has not been associated with birth defects after exposure in the first trimester, and nifedipine has only been weakly associated with one cardiac defect in a review of only thirty-seven patients. It is, however, tera-togenic in rats. Verapamil has been used intravenously to treat fetal tachy-cardia and orally to treat preterm labor. Both are reasonable options, due to the lack of viable alternatives. Nifedipine, however, may cause a severe drop in blood pressure if it is used intravenously; it should not be combined with magnesium sulfate in preeclamptic patients because there have been several reports of adverse effects.

445

Q *What about using diuretics?*

A Diuretics, like beta-blockers, have been used extensively in Europe to treat hypertension in pregnant women. In the United States their use is much less common.

Thiazides such as chlorothiazide (Dyazide, Maxzide, and others) (Category C) are the prototype for the entire class, which includes chlorthalidone, indapamide, metolazone, and quinethazone. In the Michigan Medicaid Recipient Study, 635 first trimester exposures were reviewed, with no association found to birth defects. Despite this, many consider diuretics contraindicated in pregnancy because of their tendency to decrease plasma volume and uterine perfusion. Most studies, in any event, have shown that their use did not improve outcome in hypertensive or preeclamptic patients. In addition, the thiazides have been associated in newborns with low platelets and consequent bleeding problems.

As a consequence, it is reasonable to advise avoiding diuretics of this class during pregnancy, except for treating acute cardiac conditions related to valvular disease or pulmonary edema (lung fluid).

There are no diuretics that are considered completely safe in pregnancy, at least not by all doctors. Loop diuretics such as ethacrynic acid and furosemide (Lasix) have not been studied well in pregnancy. Data is suggestive, but not conclusive, of some rare first trimester exposure associations with isolated defects. No adverse outcomes have been reported from limited second and third trimester use, but the same objections to use of any diuretic apply in that plasma volume, and thus uterine perfusion, may be decreased.

Spironolactone (Aldactone) (Category D) should not be used because it blocks the effects of male hormone and could feminize the genitalia of a male fetus.

Acetazolamide (Category C) is a carbonic anhydrase inhibitor. It has not been associated with birth defects in humans but has been associated with limb and vertebral spinal malformations in laboratory animals; therefore, it should be avoided in pregnancy. Despite this, the Collaborative Perinatal Project reviewed twelve cases of first trimester exposure with no defects noted.

446

Q *Which agents are considered safe to use for hypertension in pregnancy?*

A The list is short. Methyl dopa (Aldomet) (Category C) and clonidine (Catapres) (Category C) throughout gestation, hydralazine (Apresoline) (Category C) acutely and sodium nitroprusside IV (Nipride) (Category C) and Magnesum Sulfate IV ($MgSO_4$) (Category C) in emergencies.

Aldomet has been used for more than 30 years with no reports of adverse effects. Neither the Collaborative Perinatal Project nor the Michigan Medicaid Recipient Study found any association with birth defects.

Apresoline has likewise been used for many years, particularly as an injection to acutely control high blood pressure in severe preeclampsia. There have been no adverse effects reported.

Clonidine has been used more recently for treatment of chronic hypertension in pregnancy without ill effect, but data in the first trimester is very limited.

Nipride has been used for many years to treat life-threatening high blood pressure quickly by intravenous drip. Only its prolonged use poses a theoretical problem because one of the metabolites is cyanide, which can accumulate in the fetal liver.

$MgSO_4$ is the drug of choice for preeclampsia and superimposed preeclampsia. It is administered IV and has both anti-hypertensive and anti-seizure effects. (See Section 8: Preeclampsia)

A new class of anti-hypertensives called ARBs (angiotensin receptor blockers) such as Teveten, Avapro, and Benicar (Category C, but D in second and third trimesters) are effective, but have been associated with renal failure, hypotension, and even death in fetuses in the latter part of pregnancy. Once pregnancy is confirmed, these medicines should be replaced with safer options.

Anticoagulants

447

Q *I had a deep vein thrombosis (phlebitis) in my first pregnancy. What can I take to prevent it this time?*

A Heparin (Category C) is the preferred anticoagulant in pregnancy. It must be administered either subcutaneously by injection, usually twice per day, or intravenously if you are actually hospitalized for a blood clot during your current pregnancy. It is indicated for previous or current deep vein thrombosis, pulmonary embolus, and previous habitual abortion (repeated miscarriage) with positive lupus anticoagualant (LAC) and/or anticardiolipin (ACL).

Heparin is a large molecule that does not cross the placenta. There are no causative links between heparin and congenital defects. Risks include osteopenia (bone loss) and thrombocytopenia (low platelets) for the mother after prolonged use.

Low molecular weight heparin (Lovenox) may now be substituted in a once-per-day injection and the blood tests PT/PTT do *not* need to be followed as with traditional twice-per-day heparin therapy.[51]

448

Q *Can I take Coumadin? I've been on that ever since my pulmonary embolus four years ago.*

A Coumarin derivatives such as warfarin (Coumadin) (classified as Category D by some, as X by the manufacturer) is rarely used in pregnancy. While it has the advantage of oral administration, it is a small molecule and readily crosses the placenta. Fetal warfarin syndrome consists of a flattened nasal bridge, upper airway obstruction, low birth weight, blindness or optic atrophy, shortened fingers, dwarfing, developmental delay, seizures, scoliosis, deafness, congenital heart disease, and stillbirth. The critical exposure interval is at six to nine weeks of gestation.[52]

In short, warfarin should be avoided in pregnancy. It is, however, compatible with breast-feeding, according to the American Academy of Pediatrics.

449

Q *My doctor wants me to take minidose aspirin through my whole pregnancy because of my previous miscarriages. Can I do this safely?*

A Aspirin (ASA) (Category C) has completely different effects, depending on the dosage. At only 82 milligrams per day (one children's ASA) it may be used safely to help prevent preeclampsia in women who have a history of toxemia, chronic hypertension, or those who are prone to preeclampsia, such as women carrying twins. Newer data refutes mini-dose ASA's effectiveness as a preventative for preeclampsia.[53]

It is also indicated for women who are prone to habitual abortion (repeated miscarriage) and specifically those who are positive for the antiphospholipid syndrome with positive ACL and LAC. (See this section: Prescription Drugs, Heparin; see this section: Headache under Over-the-Counter Drugs)

Full-dose ASA (250 to 2,000 milligrams per day) should be avoided in the third trimester, because aspirin at this dose has been associated with newborn bleeding, delayed labor, prolonged labor, and maternal bleeding with or without placental abruption.

Anticonvulsants

450

Q *I've had a seizure disorder ever since I was a child. Can I continue to take Dilantin during pregnancy?*

Unfortunately, there is no simple answer. The safety of anticonvulsants used for the treatment of epilepsy is one of the most difficult issues to resolve in modern teratology. The majority of seizure disorders are treated with multiple drug combinations, thus confounding data uncovered to implicate a problem with one medication over another. On top of that, a seizure disorder by itself seems to be associated with a higher incidence of birth defects even when untreated. Women who have seizure disorders who are also on anticonvulsants seem to have about a two-to threefold increased risk of defects, thereby incurring a risk of about 6 to 9 percent.

Phenytoin (Dilantin) (Category D) has been associated with the Dilantin or fetal hydantoin syndrome, which is characterized by multiple abnormalities. These include craniofacial abnormalities such as a flattened nasal bridge, low hairline, short neck, wide-set eyes, cleft lip and palate, low-set ears, and ptosis (drooping) of eyelids. Other abnormalities include shortened fingers, absent nails, and congenital hip dislocation. Exposure in utero to Dilantin has also been associated with the later development of infant and childhood tumors. It should also be noted that Dilantin may lead to a folate-deficient state in the mother by inhibiting absorption from the intestines. Hemorrhagic disease in the newborn may also occur because of depressed production in the liver of vitamin K-dependent clotting factors.

Despite these findings, the total risk of any defect is in the range of 6 to 9 percent, and the risk of disaster to mother and fetus if seizures go untreated may be significantly higher. Therefore, your doctor may decide to continue hydantoin through pregnancy, despite its Category D classification.

The American Academy of Pediatrics considers Dilantin use to be compatible with breast-feeding.

451

Why would only about 7 percent of fetuses be affected by Dilantin and the other anticonvulsants?

No one knows for sure, but some people think there may be an inherited gene that causes some fetuses to have lower levels of an enzyme necessary for elimination of an epoxide metabolite of both hydantoin (Dilantin) and carbamazepine (Tegretol).

Probably carbamazepine (Tegretol) (Category D), which has been reported to have virtually the same problems associated with it as Dilantin, is no safer. Until about 1980, Tegretol was thought to be considerably safer, but more recent studies have shown this not to be the case.

The American Academy of Pediatrics considers Tegretol to be safe with breast-feeding due to low levels in breast milk.

452

Q *I use trimethadione (Tridione) for petit mal seizures. Should I continue this in pregnancy?*

A Trimethadione (Tridione) (Category D) has a long list of associated malformations. Rates are so high that most doctors agree that this drug should not be used in pregnancy, and another drug should be substituted for petit mal seizures.

Ethosuximide (Zarontin) (Category C) and methsuximide (Celontin) (Category C) should be used instead for petit mal seizures, because no linkage to birth defects has yet come to light.

453

Q *I was told Depakene was safer than the other anticonvulsants. Is that true?*

A Valproic acid (Depakene) (Category D) is certainly not safer than the other common anticonvulsants. Not unlike Tegretol, prior to 1981 the prevailing thinking was that Depakene was indeed much safer than other drugs, such as Dilantin. There have been a phenomenal ninety-two different types of malformation associated with valproic acid since then. It is strongly associated with neural tube defect if exposure occurs during the seventeenth to thirtieth day after fertilization; it is associated with defects of the heart, face, head and neck, skeleton and limbs, and skin and muscles, as well as defects of the bladder and kidneys.

The American Academy of Pediatrics considers Depakene compatible with breast-feeding because of its low concentration in breast milk.

454

Q *My doctor says we can control my seizures with phenobarbital alone and that this is safer than the other anticonvulsants. Is that so?*

A Phenobarbital (Category D) has been widely used as a sedative and anti-seizure medicine since shortly after 1900. Whether or not it is truly safer is difficult to conclude because it so frequently is used in combination with other drugs. That being said, it is true that there is no "syndrome" of typical defects known to be associated with phenobarbital.

The Collaborative Perinatal Project reviewed 1,415 first trimester exposures and found no reason to conclude that there was an increased risk in either major or minor categories of malformation.

It was, however, associated with hemorrhage in the newborn by depressing production of vitamin K-dependent clotting factors. It is, of course, also addictive and fetal withdrawal has been described.

Phenobarbital in pregnancy may be justified, however, if it is effective in preventing grand mal seizures. Discuss your individual case with your doctor.

Sedatives, Hypnotics, and Antianxiety Drugs

455

Q *Are any sedatives safe in pregnancy?*

A Many sedatives may be relatively safe after the first trimester. Hydroxyzine (Vistaril; Atarax) (Category C) is a sedative antihistamine belonging to the same category of drugs as meclizine (Antivert), and although teratogenic to animals in extremely high doses, human teratogenicity has never been proved. Because of rare, isolated birth defects associated with first trimester exposure in combination with other drugs, the manufacturer considers hydroxyzine to be contraindicated in the first trimester.

For use anytime after the first trimester, including during labor, there seems little reason to view hydroxyzine as anything other than safe.

Zolpidem (Ambien) is a non-benzodiazepine sedative hypnotic which may be safely used in the second and third trimesters.

456

Q *I've used Valium before as a muscle relaxant when my back goes into spasm. Can I take it in pregnancy?*

A Diazepam (Valium) (Category D) and some of the benzodiazepines, such as aprazolam (Xanax) (Category D), Klonopin (clonzaepam) (Category D), lorazepam (Ativan) (Category D), triazalam (Halcion) (Category X), estazolam (Prosom) (Category X), temazepam (Restoril) (Category X), and chlorazepate (Tranxene) (Category D) are used not only as muscle relaxants but more commonly as antianxiety medicines. They have been found to be teratogenic in rodents, in whom the defect of cleft lip has been noted. Earlier studies suggested that the frequency of this defect was increased in humans as well, but recent studies have refuted this.[54]

More recently, there has been agreement that the benzodiazepines are clearly associated with inguinal hernia, cardiac defects, and pyloric stenosis (narrowed small intestine). Used in labor, these drugs have been associated with respiratory depression, floppiness, and rapid loss of temperature in the newborn.

In summary, recent data does NOT support benzodiazepines causing any significant increased risk of birth defect, but does support association with "floppy infant syndrome" transiently after birth. Benzodiazepines used for anxiety should NOT be abruptly discontinued in pregnancy, even in the third trimester. [55]

Buspirone Hcl (Buspar) (Category B) is an effective antianxiety agent and has not been shown to be teratogenic in animals even at 30 times the normal dose. It is not chemically related to the benzodiazepines (valium group) nor to the barbiturates, nor is it considered a sedative.

There have been no reports of human malformations associated with buspirone, but the data is inadequate. Certainly if you become pregnant on buspirone but stop it at six weeks, there is almost no evidence to suggest that any damage might have been done. Continuing the medicine in pregnancy would depend on whether you and your doctor felt the benefits outweighed the unknown possible risks.

Chlordiazepoxide (Librium; Librax) (Category D) is probably safer than the other benzodiazepines, despite its classification as Category D. Neither the Collaborative Perinatal Project nor the Michigan Medicaid Recipient Study found reason to believe chlordiazepoxide was a teratogen. The fetus may experience symptoms of withdrawal, including tremulousness and irritability.

457

Q *Can my doctor give me phenobarbital over the short term as a sedative?*

A Phenobarbital (Category D) and derivatives secobarbital (Seconal), pentobarbital (Nembutal), and butalbital (Fioricet; Flextra) (Category C) have not been established as teratogens despite their rating. The rating has more to do with phenobarbital's traditional use as a combination agent in treating seizure disorders.

Fioricet is commonly used in the second trimester for headache. Seconal and Nembutal are frequently used to induce sleep in women having prodromal labor who are exhausted. (They are in labor with contractions for days, but have no cervical change.)

458

Q *I've used meprobamate in the past. Can I use it in pregnancy?*

A Meprobamate (Miltown; Equanil) (Category D) is little used as a sedative anymore. While several large reviews, such as the Collaborative Perinatal Project, found no association with defects, other studies have found a first trimester exposure risk as high as 12 percent.[56]

Meprobamate should certainly be avoided in the first trimester, since defects found included congenital heart disease, deafness, and deformed joints. With few indications, it would be best to avoid it completely in pregnancy.

Antidepressants

459

Q *My psychiatrist put me on Prozac and I'm doing really well, but now I want to get pregnant. What do I do?*

A Stay on it if your psychiatrist and obstetrician feel that it is critical for your well-being. If possible, discontinue the medicine from the time you find out you are pregnant until ten weeks of gestation.

Fluoxetine (Prozac) (Category C) is a serotonin reuptake inhibitor. This means that it alters the concentrations of a certain neurotransmitter at the nerve ending. At doses eleven times the human equivalent, fluoxetine has been shown not to be teratogenic in animals. While there are no well-controlled studies available in pregnant women,there are also no convincing reports of human birth defects felt to be causally related to fluoxetine.

Sertraline (Zoloft) (Category C), escitalopram (Lexapro) (Category C) venlafaxine (Effexor) (Category C), paroxetine (Paxil CR) (Category D), nefazodone (Serzone) (Category C), Fluvoxamine (Luvox) (Category C), desvenlafaxine (Pristiq) (Category C), and duloxetine (Cymbalta) are serotonin reuptake inhibitors (SSRIs; Effexor (Pristiq), and Cymbalta are actually SSNRIs) that have been shown not to be teratogenic in animals.

If possible these antidepressants might be discontinued from the time you know that you're pregnant to ten completed weeks. In 2004, the FDA added language warning of a *rare*, non life-threatening newborn withdrawal syndrome if SSRIs or SSNRIs are taken in the third trimester. You should discuss this additional information with your doctor and do *not* stop taking your medicines unless your physician is aware and agrees. I personally do *not* recommend stopping or tapering these medicines in the last trimester.[57]

A 2005 study by Alwan et al. found a tiny but statistically increased risk of omphalocoele and craniosynostosis with first trimester exposure to SSRIs, but primarily Paxil. The Swedish Medical Birth Registry[58] also found that Paxil exposure in the first trimester leads to a 1.78-fold increase in cardiovascular defects, most of which were ventricular or atrial septal defects and not life threatening. The overall malformation rate, however, was not increased at 4.8%. Still, most physicians would recommend not being on paroxetine in the 1st trimester. Do not simply stop an antidepressant at anytime without discussing it with your doctor beforehand.

460

Q *I had severe postpartum depression after my son was born two years ago. Is there something I can take to avoid it this time?*

A If postpartum depression (more serious than the "baby blues") was diagnosed and treated in your last pregnancy, there is something you can do. There is, of course, no way to predict if you will suffer postpartum depression again.

Make sure your obstetrician is aware of what you went through the last time. Together, you may simply decide to wait and see what happens but to treat aggressively at the first signs of depression, or go ahead and begin Prozac or another reuptake inhibitor a couple of weeks before your due date.

461

Q *I've been on my old tricyclic antidepressant, Elavil. Can I stay on it while I'm pregnant?*

A While no human studies suggest a risk, if possible these antidepressants might be discontinued from the time you know you're pregnant until ten completed weeks.

Amitryptiline (Elavil) (Category D) is a prototypical "tricyclic antidepressant," which is a clearly documented teratogen in animals. However, in the Michigan Medicaid Recipient Study, there were 467 first trimester exposures, with no evidence to support the contention that amitryptiline caused any birth defects.

Other tricyclic antidepressants include nortriptyline (Pamelor) (Category D), desipramine (Norpramin) (Category C), and doxepin (Sinequan) (Category C). While there have been isolated defects reported one at a time, the bulk of evidence suggests that these drugs are relatively safe in pregnancy.[59]

Bupropion (Wellbutrin) (Category B) has not been associated with any teratogenic effects in animals. It is a unique antidepressant not chemically related to the tricyclics, the serotonin reuptake inhibitors, or the monoamine oxidase inhibitors. There are no reports of birth defects in humans with exposure at any gestation, but the numbers are small. Zyban, the new pill advertised to help you stop smoking, is the identical drug, but is labeled to avoid use in pregnancy by the manufacturer.

462

Q *I have bipolar disorder and I take lithium. Will I be able to continue that in pregnancy?*

A Lithium carbonate (Category D) is a major tranquilizer used to treat bipolar or manic depressive disorder. Lithium is known to be a teratogen in both animals and people. Specifically, first trimester exposure has been associated with cardiac defects most frequently. In one registry, defect rates are reportedly as high as 11 to 12 percent of those exposed.[60] However, a prospective study in 1992 showed no evidence of a link to birth defects, with 148 exposures in the first trimester and 148 matched controls.

The use of lithium near term can lead to transient toxicity in the newborn, the most severe symptoms of which are floppiness, bradycardia, (slow heart rate), seizures, and shock.

In summary, the data is somewhat contradictory. Lithium should be avoided in pregnancy if possible, but particularly in the first trimester. If lithium is absolutely necessary, an effort should be made to skip the first trimester from six weeks to at least ten weeks, and to avoid the drug in the last two weeks of gestation as well.

Divelproex sodium (Depakote) (Category D), also used to treat bipolar disorder, is actually valproic acid, almost the identical formulation as Depakene. In short, it probably is no safer than lithium. (See this section: Anticonvulsants)

Lamotrigine (Lamictal) (Category C) is a newer drug used for controlling the depressed phase of bipolar disorder, and has little to no evidence of teratogenicty to date, but again, if possible, might be avoided from 6-10 weeks gestation.

Antinausea, Antiemetic, and Antidiarrheal Drugs

463

Q *Are there any prescription medicines I can use for my morning sickness?*

A Promethazine (Phenergan) (Category C) is an antiemetic antihistamine used for both severe morning sickness and with narcotics in labor. The Collaborative Perinatal Project reviewed 114 first trimester exposures and 746 total, with no evidence to support a causative relationship to any major or minor category of birth defects. Isolated defects have been reported rarely.

Promethazine is generally considered relatively safe at anytime in pregnancy. Avoiding it during the first ten weeks is probably wise, with over-the-counter medicines such as Unisom and Nestrex considered safer by many doctors.

Prochlorperazine (Compazine) (Category C) is a phenothiazine derivative used for nausea and vomiting. It has been found to be teratogenic in animals, but there is no clear evidence of birth defects in humans caused by Compazine. The Collaborative Perinatal Project reviewed 877 first trimester exposures and 2,023 total. No relationship was found to malformations, nor was there any effect on birth weight, mortality, or IQ followed out to four years of age.[61] Occasional extrapyramidal side effects (EPS) have been seen in pregnant women on Compazine with either torticolis or oculogyric crisis (neck muscle spasm, or eyes locked into the upward-looking position). While these side effects are frightening, they are transient and not dangerous. Treatment with Benadryl usually rapidly resolves the symptoms.

Chlorpromazine (Thorazine) (Category C) is another phenothiazine derivative used as a treatment for psychosis but also for nausea. The drug seems to be safe and effective for nausea throughout gestation, except during labor. In labor it has been associated with unpredictable drops in blood pressure.

Only one study, in France, showed a slightly increased risk of defects after first trimester exposure, and most other studies have shown the drug to be safe for intermittent antinausea indications.[62]

464

Q *I'm a nurse in an ICU and I've seen Zofran work for nausea postoperatively. Can pregnant women use Zofran?*

A Ondansetron (Zofran) (Category B) is a serotonin receptor antagonist used for nausea orally and by injection. It is extremely effective, relatively new, and at this writing, very expensive. It is indicated for severe nausea and vomiting induced by chemotherapy. There is no evidence to suggest that it is teratogenic in animals. While there are no reported birth defects after exposure in humans, the numbers are still small.

For severe hyperemesis gravidarum, in which treatment would otherwise require constant intravenous fluids and/or hospitalization, Zofran may certainly be considered.

465

Q *Imodium AD just isn't strong enough for my diarrhea. Can I have Lomita?*

A If possible, try to find the cause of the diarrhea before treatment. Even if not possible, diarrhea should have persisted for at least thirty-six hours before you and your doctor consider prescription treatment.

Diphenoxylate Hcl (Lomotil) (Category C) is a narcotic derivative medication for persistent diarrhea. It comes only in combination with atropine, a potent anticholinergic agent.

The Michigan Medicaid Recipient Study reviewed 179 newborns with first trimester exposure and did not find any association between Lomotil and birth defects.

466

Q *Can atropine and scopolamine be taken in pregnancy?*

A Atropine (Category C) is an anticholinergic agent. This means it works on certain nerve endings that control smooth muscles and some glands. It is available in both Lomotil and Donnatal and is used for diarrhea and irritable bowel syndrome. Donnatal also contains scopolamine and many inert ingredients.

The Collaborative Perinatal Project reviewed 401 first trimester exposures and 1,198 exposures overall and found no association between atropine and birth defects. For scopolamine, there were 309 first trimester exposures and 831 exposures overall, with no association between scopolamine and malformations.[63]

Scopolamine was used widely in the 1950s to induce twilight sleep for labor and delivery. It has fallen out of favor largely because of maternal tachycardia, fetal tachycardia, and other heart tracing changes, the potential for respiratory depression after birth, and the availability of better agents for pain relief in labor.

The American Academy of Pediatrics considers Donnatal and Lomotil to be compatible with breast-feeding.

467

Q *I've got irritable bowel syndrome and use Bentyl. Can I continue it when I'm pregnant?*

A Dicyclomine Hcl (Bentyl) (Category B) has been used by over 20 million pregnant women because it was the component of the antinausea medicine Bendectin that was removed in 1976 due to its ineffectiveness as an antiemetic. (See this section: Doxylamine) There appears to be no data to link dicyclomine with birth defects or other fetal problems despite exposure at any gestational age. A 1990 review stated the risk as "None."[64]

Hormonal Medicines

468

Q *I was still on the Pill when I found out I was pregnant. Is the birth control pill dangerous in pregnancy?*

A Oral contraceptives (Category X) all contain a form of synthetic progestin and a synthetic estrogen. Other than possible effects on development of sex organs, there is little evidence to link oral contraceptives (OCPs) to birth defects. The older acronym VACTERL (vertebral, anal, cardiac, tracheal, esophageal, renal, and limb) used to describe the types of birth defects that have been associated with sex hormone exposure should be discarded.

Only 0.07 percent of pregnancies exposed to OCPs may express any of these defects. Many investigators believe the actual risk to the fetus of birth defects other than those affecting the genitals is essentially nonexistent.[65]

All of the progestins have been associated with masculinization of the female fetus, but at an incidence of only 0.3 percent, or 3 in 1,000 exposures.

In short, if you become pregnant while on the Pill and stop it once you realize you are pregnant, at least before three months, your chances of a problem are extremely small.

The American Academy of Pediatrics considers combination oral contraceptives to be compatible with breast-feeding, but possibly a risk for decreased milk production. Progestin-only pills (Micronor; NorQD; Ovrette) have not been found to decrease milk production, and are safe and effective birth control while breast-feeding.

The new irritable bowel drug tegaserod (Zelnorm) (Category B) is felt to be safe after the first trimester.

469

Q *Can I continue to take Synthroid in my pregnancy?*

A Yes. Levothyroxine (Synthroid) (Category A) is not actually a medicine but a naturally occurring hormone produced both by the mother and the fetus. The degree to which the hormone crosses the placenta is controversial, but thought to be small. The Michigan Medicaid Recipient Study reviewed 554 first trimester exposures to levothyroxine (T4) and found no data to support an association between the drug and congenital defects.

470

Q *I was diagnosed with hyperthyroidism several months ago and I'm on PTU. Can I continue to take it in pregnancy?*

A Propylthiouracil (PTU) (Category D) may be used in pregnancy if you and your doctor think the benefits outweigh the risks. It is a very effective drug in that it prevents the production of levothyroxine (T4), but it also prevents the conversion of T4 to the more active T3.

If the drug is used through to term, it may transiently cause hypothyroidism in the newborn. It resolves on its own after several days, but in about 10 to 15 percent of the cases, the newborn may have a noticeable goiter (enlarged thyroid).

Note that despite its classification as Category D, it is considered the drug of choice for treatment of hyperthyroidism in pregnancy. Other drugs, such as carbimazole (Category D) and its metabolite methimazole, have been weakly associated with aplasia cutis (a scalp defect) and are thus felt to be potentially less safe.

Potassium iodide (Category D) is used as an expectorant, but when used to treat hyperthyroidism in the mother, it may inadvertently lead to goiter and hypothyroidism in the fetus at term. It should therefore be avoided in pregnancy.

471

Q *I have a pituitary adenoma and had to take Parlodel in order to keep my prolactin levels down and get pregnant. Is it safe to continue using Parlodel in pregnancy?*

A Since 1973, Bromocryptine (Parlodel) (Category C) has been used to treat infertility due to high prolactin levels whether from pituitary tumors or not. For the most part, bromocryptine has been stopped with the diagnosis of pregnancy. Large studies have failed to reveal any association between the drug and fetal malformations, despite isolated incidences of defects.

Parlodel is no longer indicated for the suppression of lactation. The Food and Drug Administration, in considering the high failure rate and the reported increased incidence of stroke, withdrew this indication in 1995.

Cabergoline (Dostinex) (Category C) was new in 1997. Like bromocryptine, it is a dopamine agonist (meaning it acts like the neurotransmitter dopamine), and it is used once to twice per week to treat prolactin-secreting tumors of the pituitary. While there are no associated fetal anomalies reported, it should also be stopped in pregnancy. Currently, it is not approved for lactation suppression in those who wish not to breast-feed.

472

Q *I've been diabetic since the age of eleven. Do I need to change my type of insulin when I get pregnant?*

A No, you don't. Insulin (Category B) is not a medicine, but a naturally occurring hormone. Infants of diabetic mothers are at about two to four times the increased risk for birth defects compared to infants of non-diabetic mothers.

Note that Humulin, or human insulin, does not cross the placenta, nor does it pass into breast milk. (See Section 9: Diabetes)

Anesthetics

473

Q *My dentist wanted to use a local anesthetic for a filling and I'm only nine weeks pregnant. Is that okay?*

A Local anesthetics ("caine" drugs) (Category C) are considered safe in pregnancy at any gestation when used in accordance with their labeling. These medicines are also used for labor epidurals and spinal anesthetics and have their own considerations in these circumstances. Drugs in this category include xylocaine (Lidocaine), mepivicaine (Carbocaine), bupivicaine (Marcaine), chloroprocaine (Nesacaine), tetracaine (Pontocaine), and ropivicaine (Naropin). (See Section 7: Normal Labor and Delivery, Pain Management)

474

Q *What about xylocaine viscous gel? I've always had some for aphthous ulcers (canker sores) in my mouth and for genital herpes. Can I use it?*

A Viscous xylocaine 2% may be safely used on mucosal membranes such as the mouth and vagina in dosages in accordance with its labeling. It is readily absorbed and theoretically could pose a problem if overdosed, but a little dab intermittently is not a significant risk.

475

Q *I'm having a wisdom tooth removed and my dentist says I'll need nitrous oxide in addition to a local anesthetic. Is nitrous oxide safe in pregnancy?*

A Nitrous oxide is a frequently used agent for dental anesthesia. Commonly called "laughing gas," it is also used in combination with other agents for general anesthesia during major surgery.

The Collaborative Perinatal Project found no evidence to suggest that nitrous oxide was a teratogen in humans even though some animal studies have shown birth defects in rodents.[66]

476

Q *Should women avoid general anesthesia during pregnancy, as I've heard?*

A It's all well and good to advise "avoiding" general anesthesia in pregnancy, but you'll have to figure out how to avoid appendicitis, gallbladder disease, car wrecks that cause ruptured spleens, broken limbs, etc.

There is little to no evidence indicting commonly used general anesthetics as causative of birth defects. Thiopental, a fast-acting barbiturate derivative used to put people to sleep, has not been associated with an increased risk of birth defects. Nor has halothane, an inhaled agent once used extensively to keep patients asleep during procedures. More recent derivatives of inhaled agents such as isoflurane and methoxyflurane have not been associated with an increased risk of malformations, but inadequate human studies exist to state this definitively.

A simple rule to keep in mind would be to delay elective surgery until after pregnancy. If emergency surgery is required, there is little evidence to suggest you should waste any recuperative energy worrying about the effect of the anesthetic.

477

Q *I understand that drugs may be used to immobilize a patient during surgery. Can it really be safe during pregnancy to take a drug derived from arrowhead poisons used in the Amazon?*

A Succinylcholine and curare are in fact related to poisons into which the tips of the arrows are dipped. These arrows immobilize prey after a non-lethal hit.

While they will immobilize you as well, (after you go to sleep) your body has enzymes that reverse the effect of these medicines by destroying them over time. The anesthesiologist can also add other drugs to hasten the reversal of their temporary paralyzing effect.

There is no data to support these medicines as human teratogens, although there are no widespread controlled trials to review. Before a procedure, you should always make sure the anesthesiologist knows you are pregnant, so that the safest, most minimal combinations of medicines available can be used.

Antipsychotic Drugs

478

Q *My sister has schizophrenia and is on Haldol all the time. Are drugs such as Haldol, used to treat serious mental illness, safe in pregnancy?*

There are several antipsychotic drugs. Haloperidol (Haldol) (Category C) is not felt to be teratogenic in any of the animal models in which it was tested. Extremely rare isolated cases of problems in humans have been reported, but no studies show a causal relationship between Haldol and congenital malformation. In 98 of 100 women exposed in the first trimester (two were lost to follow-up), no birth defects were found and there was no effect on fetal outcome.[67] Use in pregnancy depends on the obstetrician and psychiatrist determining together if the minimal risk is outweighed by the benefit.

The American Academy of Pediatrics does not recommend breast-feeding while on haloperidol.

Thiothixene (Navane) (Category C), used to treat psychosis, is a close chemical relative of another major tranquilizer, trifluoperazine (Stelazine). Neither has been shown to be teratogenic in animal studies. Very little data is available, but the Michigan Medicaid Recipient Study reviewed thirty-eight first trimester exposures and did not find an increased risk of birth defects. Continuance in pregnancy will depend on the obstetrician and psychiatrist determining together if the minimal risk is outweighed by the benefit.

Chlorpromazine (Thorazine) (Category C) is the prototypical phenothiazine from which other antinausea medicines have been derived (See this section: Prescription Drugs, Compazine and Phenergan). Thioridizene (Mellaril) is closely related. The phenothiazines in general have not been considered dangerous in pregnancy during any trimester. The Collaborative Perinatal Project reviewed 142 first trimester exposures, and 284 exposures at any time, with no relationship to malformations noted.[68] Rarely, extrapyramidal side effects (EPS) have been noted in newborns of mothers on Thorazine. These include tremors, increased muscle tone, and spasticity, but the vast majority of reports show no effect on the newborn.

For use as both an antiemetic and antipsychotic, the phenothiazines seem to be a group of drugs with very low potential for adverse fetal effects. Zyprexa (olanzapine) (Category C) is a newer antipsychotic in the thienobenzodiazepine class. Despite its class, no human adverse side-effects have been documented.

TOCOLYTIC (PRETERM LABOR DRUGS)

479

Q *What drugs have been used in preterm labor?*

A (See also Section 8: Preterm Labor)
Quite a few more than have ever been shown to actually work. Many drugs halt preterm contractions temporarily, but as to actually prolonging

gestation and preventing preterm delivery, very little has been shown to be any more effective than intravenous hydration and bed rest.

There is reason to believe as of 2006 that our current pharmacologic methods may be helpful in prolonging gestation on average from three to five days, perhaps long enough to get steroids such as Betamethasone or oral Dexamethazone on board to help mature the baby's lungs. Both are Category C. (See this section: Anti-inflammatory and Immuno-suppressive Drugs)

The list of tocolytics is long and includes beta-mimetics such as terbuta-line (Brethine) (Category B), ritodrine (Yutopar) (Category B), and fenoterol and salbutamol (Category C). Salts such as magnesium sulfate ($MgSO_4$) (Category B) are used extensively. Antiprostaglandins such as indocin and ibuprofen (both Category B, both D late in third trimester), and aspirin (Category C) have been used.

For many years pure ethanol alcohol (ETOH) (Category D) was used. Calcium channel blockers such as nifedipine (Category C) and verapamil (Calan SR) (Category C) have been used.

All of these drugs are discussed further in Section 8: Preterm Labor.

480

Q What's the bottom line on these tocolytic drugs?

A The bottom line is that large meta-analyses of treatment with any of these medicines has failed to show any but the smallest benefit in terms of actually extending gestational age.

Of the beta-mimetics, terbutaline used orally and subcutaneously has virtually supplanted the other types of beta-mimetic in the United States. Its use certainly seems safe when dosed appropriately. Although it stops some contractions, its ability to stop true preterm labor is in doubt.

Magnesium sulfate ($MgSO_4$) has gained increasing popularity in recent years as cost and complications eliminated ritodrine from com-mon usage. $MgSO_4$ may also be used safely when given in a very regi-mented intramuscular fashion, or more often with a computerized infusion pump. It would seem to be effective, or at least as effective as intravenous hydration and bed rest, at prolonging gestation an average of three to five days when true preterm labor with cervical change has been documented.

Calcium channel blockers are rarely used; animal data suggests they may decrease uteroplacental blood flow and thus decrease oxygen to the fetus. Indocin and the antiprostaglandins have been associated with decreased amniotic fluid. (See Section 8: Preterm labor)

COMPUTER DATABASES AND SOURCES OF REPRODUCTIVE RISK INFORMATION

Micromedex, Inc.

REPRORISK (REPROTEXT, REPROTOX, Shepard's Catalog of teratogenic agents and TERIS) Englewood, CO (800) 525-9083

National Library of Medicine, MEDLARS Service Desk

GRATEFUL MED (TOXLIN, TOXNET, MEDLINE) Bethesda, MD (800) 638-8480

Reproductive Toxicology Center

REPROTOX Columbia Hospital for Women Medical Center Washington, DC (202) 293-5137

Shepard's Catalog of Teratogenic Agents

University of Washington Seattle, WA (206) 543-3373

Teratogen Information System

TERIS and Shepard's Catalog Seattle, WA (206) 543-2465

WEBSITES

Drug Lists
  http://www.rxlist.com

Environmental Exposures and Risks
  http://www.marchofdimes.com/aboutus/681_9146.asp

FDA
  http://www.fda.gov

Fetal Alcohol Syndrome
  http://www.cdc.gov/ncbddd/fas/

Lead and Mercury Exposure
  http://www.balanceyournutrition.com/In_Focus_mercury_toxicity.htm

Smoking/Second Hand Smoke
  http://www.marchofdimes.com/professionals/14332_1171.asp
  http://www.expectantmothersguide.com/library/pittsburgh/smoking.htm
  http://www.fensende.com/Users/swnymph/refs/smoke.html
  http://www.medicalnewstoday.com/medicalnews.php?newsid=28119

Quit Smoking

Call 1-800-4-CANCER

http://www.cdc.gov/tobacco/how2quit.htm

http://www.ahrq.gov/consumer/helpsmok.htm

Substance Abuse

To Quit Drugs

Call 1-800-62-HELP or 1-800-COCAINE

http://www.nlm.nih.gov/medlineplus/pregnancyandsubstanceabuse.html

To Quit Drinking

Call 1-800-ALCOHOL

Teratology Drug Effects

http://www.otispregnancy.org/

http://teratology.org/

Toxins

http://www.earthyfamily.com/A-protect.htm

http://www.checnet.org/healtheHouse/education/
    quicklist-detail.asp?Main_ID=845

http://womenshealth.about.com/cs/azhealthtopics/a/envtoxrephealth.htm

http://www.who.int/topics/poisons/en/

SUGGESTED READING

Briggs, CG, RK Freeman, SJ Yaffe. 1994. *Drugs in Pregnancy and Lactation.* 4th Ed. Baltimore: Williams & Wilkins.

Friedman, JM., JE1994. *Teratogenic Effects of Drugs: A Resource for Clinicians* (TERIS). Baltimore: Johns Hopkins University Press.

Gilstrap, LC, BB Little. 1992. *Drugs and Pregnancy.* New York, Elsevier.

Rayburn, WH. FP Zuspan. 1992. *Drug Therapy in Obstetrics and Gynecology.* 3rd Ed. St. Louis: Mosby Year Book, Inc.

ORGANIZATIONS

Clearing house for Occupational Safety and Health Information, 4676 Columbia Parkway Cincinnati, OH 45226

OSHA, 200 Constitution Ave., Washington, DC, 20210

Section Six

Prepared Childbirth

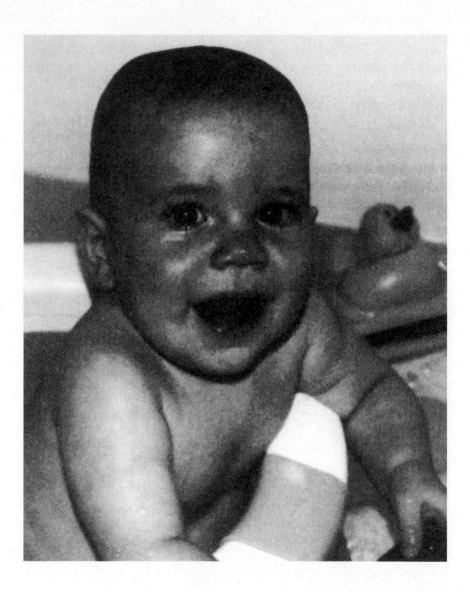

INTRODUCTION

What is prepared childbirth anyway? Prepared childbirth means simply the acquisition of knowledge about the birth process. This process includes pregnancy, labor and delivery, and care of the newborn. Preparation includes learning what to expect, when to expect it, what to do, and how to do it.

Holding this book in your hands is a significant part of prepared childbirth. Franklin D. Roosevelt is only one of several wise people who have noted that the only thing we have to fear is fear itself. Education dissipates fear. The only reason we feared the dark when we were four was because of the things we conjured up in our imagination to fill the void in our vision. When mom turned the lights on, presto change-o, the monsters were vaporized.

Prepared childbirth is an educational process by which you can enlighten yourself and vaporize your monsters.

The organization of this book is such that much of what would normally be categorized under "Prepared Childbirth" has been covered elsewhere. The facts you need or just may want to know about: What to do Before Pregnancy, Physiological Changes, Prenatal Care, Fetal Development, Drugs and Pregnancy, Obstetric Complications, and Medical Complications are found in the appropriate sections.

Consequently, this section deals primarily with childbirth classes, partner involvement, relaxation and breathing techniques, and emotional changes.

PREPARED CHILDBIRTH CLASSES

481

Q *Do I really need to go to a course where we sit through lectures?*

A Hey, even I sat through those classes with my wife! Admittedly, she introduced me as a shuttle craft pilot so that people would direct their questions to the teacher! If you haven't had a baby before, I think classes are an excellent idea. Your own doctor may offer classes in his or her office, or almost always the hospital in which you will give birth will provide a course. There may be a short course available for only two three-hour sessions, and/or a more in-depth study available for two to three hours per week over four to six weeks.

482

Q *Does my husband need to come too?*

A Responsibility for bringing up a child nowadays includes being present at his or her birth. If at all possible, I would encourage your husband to attend classes with you. Husbands can be a tremendous source of support and encouragement during labor, or they can be essentially worthless to everyone involved. His attending classes is one way to work toward the former!

Even though the baby isn't going to come out of his body in the literal sense, your partner may feel almost as though it is. In a loving relationship, the two of you really do become one in a sense. While your labor experience and his differ physically the two of you will surely share similar emotions. Certainly a working knowledge of what is going on allows him to be more helpful to you and to keep his own head together.

483

Q *When should I take childbirth classes?*

A Most doctors would like you to start around the beginning of the third trimester and finish up within three or four weeks of delivery. That way you've been pregnant long enough to experience some of the major changes in your body and can ask questions as needed, and you'll finish close enough to delivery not to forget everything you've learned. Ask your doctor when to sign up for the courses.

484

Q *But what if I do forget everything I've learned?*

A You won't. Besides, Labor and Delivery nurses will be there to remind you of what you learned, and they'll be with you through your whole labor.

485

Q *Does everyone take prepared childbirth classes?*

A No. But they probably should. Surveys have shown that most couples take classes with their first pregnancy. Many hospitals and health care providers make classes mandatory. For many years in our institution, documentation of class attendance was required for the father to be permitted in the Delivery Room. Now all deliveries take place in LDR (Labor, Delivery, Recovery) rooms and the classes are no longer mandatory, but we still strongly recommend them. Check with your obstetrician or midwife to make sure you fulfill the education requirements at your hospital or birthing center.

486

Q *Should we take the classes if we've already had a baby?*

A Most institutions will offer a "refresher course" that meets only once or twice rather than several times over many weeks. It is a good idea to consider attending. You may feel as if you don't need it, but the time is well spent just for the chance to focus on your spouse for a few hours with the other cares of your daily life briefly forgotten.

487

Q *What about sibling classes?*

A Sibling classes might well be available to you second and third timers and are a great way to involve your little one in the process. It's important that your children fully realize that you and Daddy are happy about this upcoming event and that the baby in Mommy's tummy is a good thing. All too soon your child will realize that the baby seems to be in competition for the love and affection previously reserved exclusively for him or her. Anything to make your older children feel part of the process is a good idea. Having the new baby give them a present right after delivery is a great idea. Putting your children's pictures on the inside of the bassinet so the baby can "see" his big brothers and/or sisters reassures them that they are still very important members of the family.

488

Q *In addition to sibling classes, how else can we prepare our three year old to deal with the new baby?*

A Sibling classes will be one of the places where you could learn other things to do. In addition to the ideas above, do anything that involves your child in the preparation process. This can include helping with changes to the nursery (his or her "old" room), going shopping with Mom, and going to the doctor with her to hear the baby's heartbeat.

Bring out the pictures of your first child's birth and first few weeks at home. Let your child see what he or she looked like as a newborn, *how much* attention was given to him or her, and how many pictures were taken.

Make sure your child knows over and over that no matter what changes, your love for him or her will never change.

Show your child ahead of time where Mom will have the baby, and where he or she will be during that time. A good present for your child is one of those "I'm a BIG Sister/Brother" T-shirts, which they can put on when they get the phone call telling them that their new sibling has arrived on the planet.

Be sure that the rest of your family and friends know how important it is to acknowledge your older children when they are present, before going on and on about the new baby.

489

Q *I've heard that older siblings tend to "regress" after the new baby comes home. Will I all of a sudden have two in diapers instead of the one I planned on?*

A Let's face it, this is flat-out competition for your time, and your first child is not likely to go down without a fight (sibling rivalry begins right here.) What you must do is help him or her realize that while the competition for time is unavoidable, this is not a competition for love and affection. Save special time each day for you, your husband, and your first child and make sure they know how important they are to you. It takes a little while for young children to realize that you can love more than one person. You might point out that he or she loves Mommy and Daddy at the same time, so you can love your older child and the new baby at the same time as well.

490

Q *What's a "doula"?*

A A doula is a woman trained to support you throughout your labor. She is specially trained in techniques to help you relax and to help you take command over your own sensations. Doulas are not trained in the skills of delivery itself, as are certified nurse midwives and obstetricians, but they certainly may be knowledgeable in that area. Some hospital systems have labor nurses who are also trained as doulas. In other systems, doulas may be hired on a case by case basis.

491

Q *I've heard of Lamaze, LeBoyer, and Bradley classes for prepared childbirth. What is special about each of them?*

A Birthing "methods" should work not only toward helping you as a couple relax and cope with the process, but also should help to strengthen your relationship with, and trust in, your provider.

Lamaze refers to a set of precepts, which, followed as guidance, are designed to help the patient and her partner have as enjoyable and relaxed an experience as possible, given that pain is known to be a part of childbirth. Specifically, Lamaze emphasizes techniques of breathing and relaxation to help you cope with labor.

LeBoyer refers to another set of precepts, not unlike Lamaze, but emphasizing the avoidance of the "trauma" of childbirth to the newborn. Specifically, it's most well-known characteristic is that of using warm bath-water to ease the baby into the world.

Bradley refers to a method that emphasizes inner "focus" with several methods of relaxation. It is used by those who feel strongly about avoiding pain medication in childbirth, almost in any circumstance. Unfortunately, some Bradley classes also teach (erroneously) that modern obstetric medicine as practiced by board certified obstetricians is overly "interventional." The reason that this is unfortunate is that this attitude often unwittingly sets up an adversarial and even confrontational relationship with the patient or more frequently her spouse, who has taken on the role of "protector" While everyone would like to believe that childbirth is "natural" and requires no intervention, one in a hundred women died in childbirth in 1900 and now one in ten thousand do. Sometimes intervention can be lifesaving, even if it's not exactly the way you planned it.

Be sure if you decide to take Bradley classes that you discuss it with your provider ahead of time. It can be an excellent approach as long as you and your obstetrician and midwife are working toward the same goal.

FEMALE REPRODUCTIVE ANATOMY AND TERMINOLOGY

492

Q *I'm embarrassed that I don't know much about my own anatomy in my genital area. What will I need to know?*

A Don't be embarrassed. Many men and women have woefully inadequate knowledge when it comes to the female reproductive tract. The following are some common questions about anatomy involved in the birth process. The answers will also define most of the terms you will need to know.

493

Q *What exactly is the uterus?*

A   The uterus, or womb, is actually a large muscular bag. Its walls are made of smooth, or involuntary, muscle, meaning you can't just squeeze this bag whenever you want to, but only when the conditions are right for your body to expel something inside it. When the uterus squeezes by tightening its muscular wall, it is called a contraction.

The lining of the uterus is not muscle, but specialized tissue called the endometrium. During pregnancy, this lining responds to hormonal changes and thickens into a very special tissue called the decidua, which allows the embryo to implant and the placenta to grow.

The very top of the uterus is called the fundus, and the bottom is the cervix. The cervix is specialized tissue as well. Normally it is firm and rubbery. It feels like the tip of your nose when you feel for it with a finger in the vagina. As later pregnancy approaches, the cervix begins to thin out, or efface. Some of this thinning may occur before labor, but by definition the effacement process must be completed during labor. Once the cervix has become paper-thin it can retract over the descending head of your baby.

494

Q   *What are the parts of the vagina called?*

A   When most people say "vagina" they really mean the vagina and the structures surrounding its outer opening, the vulva. The vagina is a muscular tube that extends from its outer opening between the urethra and the rectum up to its fusion with the outer sidewalls of the uterine cervix.

Most of us have realized since about age eight or nine that babies normally come out using the same route that "they" used to get in. Visualizing a swarm of microscopic sperm negotiating the vagina, the cervix, the endometrial lining of the uterus, and then the fallopian tubes stretches the imagination considerably less than imagining how something the size of a baby is going to retrace those steps. Your vagina stretches to accommodate nine months of baby growth.

The vestibule of the vaginal opening is made up of the clitoral hood and clitoris located below the pubic bone and specifically below the arch formed where the larger outer lips (labia majora) of the vulva fuse. The lesser inner lips (labia minora) of the vulva fuse just at the clitoris. The small opening immediately below the clitoris is the urethra, the opening to the channel that leads to the bladder. The remnants of the hymen then form the inner ring that borders the vaginal orifice (opening), also referred to as the introitus. The hymeneal ring, the labia minora, and the flattened labia majora all circle the opening of the vagina and fuse at the bottom of the opening, an area called the fourchette. Right below the fourchette is a small area called the perineum, where several muscles come together from the left and the right. Immediately behind the perineum is the anus.

All of these structures—the clitoris, urethra, vaginal orifice, and anus—are enclosed by specialized muscles of the pelvic floor. One in particular, the pubococcygeus muscle, originates in the pubic bone and wraps around the vagina; its fibers cross like a figure eight at the perineum, and then travel around the anus and insert on the coccyx. This is one of the muscles you strengthen with Kegel exercises. (See Section 2: Exercise in Pregnancy)

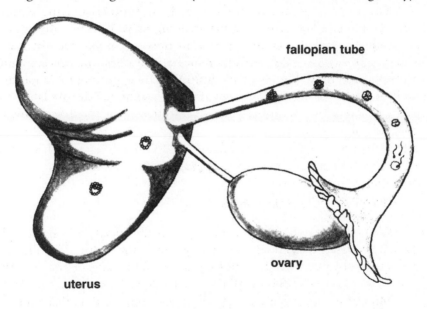

fallopian tube

ovary

uterus

495

Q *Where are the ovaries and what do they do in pregnancy?*

A The ovaries are normally located behind the uterus and very close together. One end of each ovary is attached to a corner of the uterus (cornu) by the utero-ovarian ligament. The other end is attached to the pelvic sidewall by the infundibulopelvic ligament (IP).

The ovaries make estrogen all the time, and progesterone during the second half of the cycle after you've ovulated every month. In pregnancy, the ovaries make both hormones, but the placenta takes over in the first trimester and quickly makes many hundreds of times as much hormone as the ovary made. The ovary that released the egg for fertilization forms a corpus luteum cyst that usually persists through about twelve to sixteen weeks, when it normally disappears. Occasionally, the cyst is a source of minor pain in the lower abdomen toward the end of the first trimester.

As pregnancy progresses, the ovaries move upward with the rising top of the uterus. Toward the end of the pregnancy, they have actually been dragged up out of the true pelvis.

496

Q *What is the amniotic sac?*

A The amniotic sac is, in lay terms, the bag of waters. (See Section 4: Fetal Development) It is actually made up of two layers, the inner amnion, and the outer chorion. Near term there is roughly a liter of amniotic fluid surrounding the baby. It is largely fetal urine at this point, but it is in constant flux across the membranes and decidua and is fully replaced every three to six hours.

About one-third of labors begin with the sudden rupture of this sac and fluid leaking out the vagina. Two-thirds of labors begin with uterine contractions, and rupture of the membranes follows either spontaneously (SROM) or when your provider ruptures them artificially (AROM). If the membranes rupture too early in pregnancy this is called preterm premature rupture of the membranes and may be associated with infection and/or preterm labor (PROM).

497

Q *What is the pelvic inlet, the pelvic outlet, and the birth canal?*

A The pelvic inlet is the roughly elliptical area formed by the narrowest part of the funnel that makes up the bony pelvis. Viewed from the left side while standing, a line perpendicular to this plane (a line along the path through which your baby must pass) would go from about two o'clock to eight o'clock.

To visualize the pelvic outlet, picture a woman lying on her back, knees bent and legs spread apart. Looking toward the vagina, as a gynecologist does, the pelvic outlet forms a diamond shape, with the longer axis running from top to bottom.

The pelvic outlet is the diamond-shaped area bordered by the A-shaped pubic rami in front, and the V-shaped area in back formed by the ligaments that run from your "butt bones" back to the tailbone. The pubic rami come down on either side of the vagina from the pubic bone, and end at your "butt bone," or ischial tuberosity, on either side. You can feel these bones by raising your hips one at a time while sitting and placing your hands under each buttock. If you picture the area as a baseball diamond, the rock-hard bone you feel forms first and third base as viewed from below in the position described. Second base is the pubic symphysis just above the clitoris, and home plate is the tip of the coccyx.

Don't worry if you find yourself confused by this description. The important part is that your fetus must negotiate this path through the pelvic inlet, and then take a bit of a turn to exit under the pubic bone through the pelvic outlet. The channel from the pelvic inlet to the pelvic outlet is called the birth canal.

498

Q *Is everyone's pelvis shaped the same, just bigger or smaller?*

A No, there are many different shapes. To make the shapes easy to remember, anatomists have classified them into four groups.[1]
These are:

Gynecoid pelvis	Normal, rounded shape to the inlet
Android pelvis	Heart-shaped with point in front
Anthropoid pelvis	Egg-shaped, front to back longer
Platypelloid	Egg-shaped, front to back shorter

Traditionally, android pelvic shapes tend to be associated with OP positions (see next question for explanation of term) and platypelloid with transverse positions, often with arrest and failure to descend leading to C-section. The outside appearance of your hips has nothing to do with the shape of the inlet.

499

Q *What does OP mean?*

A Certain positions in which your baby may enter the pelvis can make it harder to negotiate this path. For instance, if your baby comes down occiput posterior (OP), or oriented so that it would come out face or "sunny side up," it can make pushing the baby out considerably more difficult.

Occiput refers to the back of the head. Posterior means "back," and anterior means "front." Thus, the position of the head can be described with terms that state where the back of the head is oriented. So, occiput anterior (OA) means the baby is facing down, or face toward your tailbone, as it should normally at delivery. Occiput transverse (OT) means the baby is facing either the right or the left side of your pelvis, as it does normally when it is halfway down the birth canal. Position is determined by using the examining hand in the vagina to feel for the fontanels.

500

Q *What are the fontanels?*

A Fontanels are the baby's "soft" spots. There are two major ones formed by the intersection of the sutures. Sutures are the seams that form the borders between the flat bones in the skull. Sutures and fontanels are not firmly attached to each other for years. If they were, then your baby's head might not fit through the birth canal and the brain would have no room to grow after he or she was born.

The frontal fontanel is diamond-shaped. The fontanel on the back crown of the head is triangular and called the posterior, or occipital, fontanel. It is by feeling for these openings in the bone that the obstetrician, midwife, or labor nurse can determine the position of the baby's head in the birth canal.

501

Q *What does caput mean?*

A Caput means "swelling" on the top of the baby's head. Caput is the result of the descent of the head through the birth canal. As the head molds to the shape of the birth canal, water under the skin over the skull may get compressed into the leading area, resulting in swelling. Usually this is the result of the head pressing against the cervical opening before it is completely dilated. Molding actually refers to the changing shape of the bones as they are compressed by the canal. (See "sutures" above.)

Caput resolves over the first twenty-four hours or so of life and poses no danger other than that your baby might look like a "cone-head" for the newborn pictures.

502

Q *My doctor said my baby was vertex. What does that mean?*

A Presentation is the general term that refers to the way the baby would come out if labor were to begin at that moment. Vertex simply means head down. The word cephalic means the same thing. These are good terms meaning "on the launch pad."

Breech means the butt is coming down first. If the legs are up around the ears, it is called Frank breech. If the baby is sitting Indian-style, it is called complete breech. If one or both feet are hanging down, it is called a single or double footling breech, respectively.

If the baby is lying across the uterus during labor, it is called a transverse lie and the baby cannot be delivered vaginally. The only other undeliverable position is called mentum posterior and means "leading with the chin," specifically with the chin down toward the tailbone.

503

Q *If effacement is thinning, what does dilatation (dilation) mean?*

A The cervix may begin to thin out toward the end of pregnancy. With first babies, however, it often doesn't dilate, or open, any more than about the diameter of a fingertip before the onset of labor. With subsequent pregnancies, the cervix may in fact open several centimeters, with little to no effacement, weeks before labor begins.

In labor, the cervix completes its effacement and begins dilating more rapidly. Complete dilation is taken to be ten centimeters. This is roughly the diameter of a baby's head and also happens to be about how far the average individual can spread the tips of the index and third fingers. While the cervix actually dilates completely to a slightly different extent with every baby (that is, just large enough to fit over the head), we call it ten centimeters in everyone.

Once you have reached ten centimeters and are completely dilated, the second stage of labor begins and it's time to push.

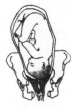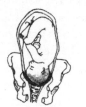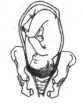

progressive enhancement

504

Q *What does the term "station" mean?*

A In the birth canal, station refers to the number of centimeters above or below the midplane of the pelvis at which one finds the presenting part.

The midplane of the pelvis is halfway down the birth canal and is referred to as "zero station." It is defined as the plane that passes perpendicular to the birth canal and through both the ischial spines. The spines are a bony protrusion that you can feel with your finger in the vagina, on either sidewall toward the back.

Each centimeter above the spines is given a number such that one centimeter up is called "-1 station," two centimeters is "-2 station," and so on. The same is true for distance below the spines, but the numbers are assigned plus signs. Thus "+3" means the baby's head is at the vaginal opening and delivery will be soon.

505

Q *My doctor said I wasn't engaged yet. What does that mean?*

A Engaged is the medical term for dropping, or lightening. Technically, your fetus is engaged when the bony part of the head is halfway down the birth canal. Realistically, it refers to the time during your final weeks of pregnancy when you suddenly have more room to breathe. When you feel the lower abdomen, the baby's head will no longer be easy to move from side to side. In a pelvic exam, your doctor will no longer be able to tap the head lightly and have it float away (ballotable). Instead, the head will be firmly wedged into the pelvic inlet.

506

Q *What are Braxton Hicks contractions?*

A Braxton Hicks contractions are usually painless, or close to painless, irregular tightenings of part or all of the uterine muscle. They begin as early as twenty-four to twenty-five weeks gestation and may continue with increasing frequency until just before labor. They make your belly feel like it is getting very hard for a minute or so and then softening. They may or may not be accompanied by back discomfort. By the late third trimester you may have twenty to thirty of these per day.

If before thirty-six weeks you think you may have had six to eight of these in an hour, you should drink fluids, lie down, and pay attention to any contractions over the next hour. If the contractions occur with the same frequency or more frequently you should call your doctor.

507

Q *What are the stages of labor?*

A You may feel like defining the stages of labor as panic, the long haul, and finished but they are a little better defined in medical terms. Labor means the regular, repetitive contraction of the uterus leading to the successive effacement and dilatation of the cervix.

The first stage occurs from the onset of these regular contractions to four to five centimeters of dilation. This stage may take many hours and averages about nine hours in a first labor.

The second stage occurs from four to five centimeters to complete dilation and is accompanied by descent of the presenting part to about halfway or more down the birth canal. Usually, dilation occurs more rapidly in this stage than the first. The cervix usually opens at least one to two centimeters per hour during this stage, so that the whole second stage is two and a half to five hours.

The third stage of labor is the expulsion of the placenta, or afterbirth.

Normally the placenta separates and uterine contractions force it out of the vagina between five and thirty minutes after delivery. If it separates partially and your bleeding increases markedly, the doctor may manually remove the placenta.

508

Q *What is an episiotomy?*

A An episiotomy is an incision made between the very back part of the vagina (fourchette) and the anus. The area between the vaginal opening and the anus is called the perineum and is where at least nine different muscle groups come together. It is more common with first deliveries and is usually performed only when this tissue starts to tear or if emergency delivery is required. (See Questions 550–555 in this section)

509

Q *What is an epidural anesthetic?*

A Epidural refers to the anatomic location in which a local anesthetic (for example, Xylocaine) may be placed through a plastic catheter in your low back. It is used for pain relief during both labor and delivery. Epidurals are usually placed after four to five centimeters of cervical dilation and, depending on the dosage and type of medication, may block more or less of your voluntary muscle activity as well as pain sensation. This may variably affect the progress of your labor, and the need for forceps, vacuum, or C-section. (See Question 766, Section Eight)

510

Q *Is a spinal block different from an epidural?*

A Spinal blocks are similar to epidurals only in that they both use local anesthetics and are placed via a needle in the low back. With a spinal block, anesthesia is time-limited and not given continuously through a catheter as with an epidural. Spinals are used primarily for anesthesia during delivery, not labor. (See Section 7: Normal Labor and Delivery, Pain Management)

THE FIRST STAGE OF LABOR

Relaxation Techniques

511

Q *I've heard friends talk about "active relaxation." What do they mean?*

A There are many times in life when the ability to separate ourselves emotionally from what is happening physically may be very helpful. We call this "tuning out' Prepared childbirth techniques, however, serve not to help you tune out, but to help you "tune in" to what's happening to your body, and thus help you take an active role in controlling the course of things.

Active relaxation then, involves many different techniques for consciously taking command of your body, and relaxing various muscles.[2] The goal is to make labor not something that happens "to you," but something that you direct with the help of your partner, nurses, doulas, and your midwife or obstetrician.

512

Q *When I sit in the dentist's chair, I try to think about sailing to help me relax. Is this the same sort of thing?*

A Not exactly. Thinking about something else is really a form of defensive "tuning out' As we mentioned above, prepared childbirth techniques involve "tuning in" and consciously controlling one's body. But you can use the same techniques you learn in Childbirth classes in all aspects of your life. Whether it's a visit to the dentist or the gynecologist, public speaking, test taking, a "discussion" with your spouse, a parent-teacher conference, a private "chat" with the boss, driving on the freeway, or sitting at a long red light, you can apply these methods and live more calmly and comfortably.

513

Q *How do you know exactly what muscles you need to relax?*

A First, you need to find out what isn't relaxed when you're tense. Some people feel as if they have to throw up, other people have to urinate, still others cough spasmodically. You may feel tension in your stomach or bladder, or in your shoulders, your forehead, the back of your head, your neck, your jaw, your chest, or your low back.

514

Q *Do people always know when they are tense and what makes them feel that way?*

A Tension can sometimes be close to free-floating anxiety. In other words, it's not always clear what makes a person feel tense. But everyone needs to be able to recognize tension as it expresses itself in his or her body.

Tension tightens muscles in different parts of the body for different people. You've probably noticed other signs as well. Some people tremble and shake, others get clammy skin and palms. Some people sweat profusely, others have dry mouth. Often the heart rate increases, even to the point of feeling the heart pounding in the chest. Some people develop itching, others just fidget—by cracking their knuckles, bouncing a crossed leg, or grinding their teeth. Some people bite their nails, others stutter under pressure.

515

Q *What will my partner be doing while I'm doing these relaxation techniques?*

A It is hoped that your partner will be part of the techniques. He will be trained to spot signs of your tension and pinpoint their manifestation in you. In other words, he'll know where you need to be touched the most, and he'll know what to say better than anyone else to keep you on track and goal-oriented.

516

Q *What are the active relaxation techniques?*

A There are four basic techniques commonly used. These include progressive relaxation, selective relaxation, touch relaxation, and visual imagery.[3]

517

Q *How does progressive relaxation work?*

A Progressive relaxation is designed to help you tune into your own body by concentrating on one muscle group at a time. You will learn to determine, through flexion and extension of each muscle, which ones have high baseline tone and are tense, and which ones are relaxed. Begin by locating specific muscle groups and consciously relax them until the entire body is relaxed.

- Practice by doing the following:
- Push your head against the pillow; hold briefly, then release.
- Arch your eyebrows; hold, then release.
- Clench your teeth tightly, then release.
- Open your mouth as wide as possible; hold, then release.
- First shrug, and then pull your shoulders downward; hold, then release.
- Bend one arm at the elbow and pull your wrist toward your face against the resistance created by placing the palm of your other hand against the wrist; release. (Be sure to release both arms simultaneously so as to avoid punching yourself in the nose.)
- Clench your fists; hold, then release; repeat several times.
- Extend your fingers to the maximum; hold, then release.
- Perform a pelvic tilt (See Section 2: Exercise in Pregnancy); hold, then release.
- Clench your buttocks together (as with Kegel exercises); hold, then release.
- Extend or stretch your feet and legs; hold, then release.
- Dorsiflex, or pull up, your feet; hold, then release.

Mentally review each muscle group that you can move, from head to toe. Contrast the difference in the way your muscles feel when they are tense and when they're relaxed.[4]

518

Q *How is progressive relaxation different from selective relaxation?*

A Selective relaxation seeks to isolate individual muscle groups and contract them while keeping all other muscles relaxed. The idea is to gain
control of your entire body, so that when the uterus contracts of its own
volition, you can consciously relax the rest of your body. For example, with
selective relaxation exercises you would:

- Contract the jaws, relax the rest of the body, and then relax the jaws.
- Contract the right arm at the same time as the left leg, relax the
  rest of the body, then relax the arm and leg.
- Progressive and selective relaxation are not actually used in labor, but
  serve as exercises to help you get in touch with your body and learn
  to focus.[5]

519

Q *How does touch relaxation work?*

A Touch relaxation involves stroking and rhythmic massaging by your partner's hands. This is best learned by example in class and perfected with
practice. You can be conditioned to relax certain muscle groups at your partner's touch. All of us in obstetrics have seen the beneficial, calming, pain-
reducing effect of a partner's touch. Massage of the low back in labor is a
particularly common relaxation technique.

Practice tightening, then relaxing the muscles of the forehead, jaw, arms,
shoulders, back, abdomen, and thighs at the gentle massaging touch of your
partner. After you have perfected this, try relaxing whatever muscle group
your partner touches without tightening these muscles first.[6]

520

Q *I've heard of using visual imagery for help in relaxing. How does that work?*

A Visual imagery can be used for relaxation just as it can for sexual excitation. You and your partner should either use the memory of a relaxing
place you have been together, or make one up. Talk about your imaginary trip
in detail. Specific descriptions of sights, sounds, colors, and smells help to
trigger the relaxing image.

521

Q *How are these techniques helpful in labor?*

A Once you have mastered all four of these relaxation techniques (and you will only do so by actually practicing on your own at home), you should be able to relax your body from its usual degree of tension almost instantly on your partner's command, or at his touch. As each contraction begins, you will then be able to relax every muscle in your body. This will not only save critical energy needed for the pushing phase, but it will allow you to better cope with each contraction.

Breathing Techniques

522

Q *I've heard about friends "hee hee hooing." Does that really help?*

A Breathing methods have long been advocated as a way to stay calm and deal with the pain of the first stage of labor. Many variations of paced breathing are used and different variations work for different people. Breathing strategies combined with visual imagery and the four relaxation techniques may be extremely effective if practiced prior to labor.

523

Q *My sister was taught to breathe rhythmically and more slowly than normal, but my best friend was panting. Is there a right and a wrong way?*

A Not so much right and wrong, but different for different women at different stages of labor. Some women use slow breathing (half the normal rate) throughout the early first stage, then feel the need to "pant" as the intensity of each contraction peaks closer to complete dilation. Your partner can help you stay on track with whatever you discover actually works best for you.

Usually it is best to count to a number you've picked ahead of time with each inhalation, whether you inhale through your mouth or nose. For example, with a slowed pace, your partner might count slowly to four either out loud or with his fingers where you can focus on them, and then count back down to zero with exhalation.

A variation of this is the "hee hee hoo" pattern. This is an effective-measure when pain gets intense and your partner really concentrates with you. You may focus on his fingers as he counts a number for each quick "hee" inhalation before the "hoo" slow exhalation. By varying the number of "hees" to each "hoo"—two hees, one hoo; three hees, one hoo; four hees, one hoo—then randomly, you are forced to focus your concentration on the pattern rather than the pain.

524

Q *How can I use visualization with breathing?*

A Visualization usually works best with slower-paced breathing early in labor. Any image that calms you and helps you focus on the completion of the process may be useful. Visualize climbing a mountain surrounded by spectacular scenery as you go up and up and finally over the peak in concert with the intensity of each contraction. Or picture waves rolling into the shore at the beach as you count slowly during inhalation and exhalation. Or visualize dancing slow to sensual music with your partner—whatever works best for you. Let your imagination be your guide.

Panic

525

Q *What if I just can't cope and start to panic?*

A Panic is not uncommon with a first laborer if she feels like her techniques aren't working or she can't remember the "right" thing to do. Either your labor nurse or your husband needs to take control forcefully when you start to "lose it" at the peak of contractions. This means your partner makes you look directly at him or her, establishes physical contact by grasping either your hands or, less frequently, your head, and insisting upon eye contact, instructs you to breathe with him or her and then demonstrates the pattern with the next contraction, and reassures you that everything really is okay. Your partner needs to remind you that each contraction brings you closer to the event you have anticipated for at least ten months.

The partner, nurse, doula, or doctor must take control briefly but firmly when either panic or perceived exhaustion sets in. The words "I can't" need to be extinguished from the patient's vocabulary. A situation can deteriorate needlessly when the support people are too timid.

526

Q *What if my support team still just can't get me to cope?*

A Rarely does a couple fail if both partners are dedicated to labor without medication (unmedicated delivery); have practiced and are comfortable with the relaxation, breathing, and visualization techniques described above; and have the assistance of dedicated knowledgeable support personnel. The women who end up with pain medication when that was not their intent did so because they entered the process with unrealistic expectations of themselves and also of labor.

Labor hurts. The techniques discussed do not make it not hurt, and should not be expected to do so.

527

Q *Is it a good idea to enlist my partner's support in helping me not to "cave in"?*

A No. Your partner is there to support you, not to fight with you or to inadvertently make you feel inadequate. For example, if your pain is worse than anticipated and you decide that you would like medicine to help with it, a reminder from your husband that you both had "agreed" to an unmedicated delivery will not be helpful. Your partner's role is to support your decision (except, of course, if it is dictated by panic). You don't need to be "reminded" that you planned an unmedicated delivery.

528

Q *Isn't a request for pain medication, whether intravenous or epidural, "caving in" or "throwing in the towel"?*

A Somehow the perception that taking advantage of what modern medicine has to offer indicates some sort of "failure" on the laboring woman's part has become pervasive in today's society. Nothing could be more inaccurate. Far from labeling you as a "failure," the recognition that you need additional support is a triumph of self-perception. The right medication, in the right dose, at just the right time, can salvage a wonderful experience from disaster.

529

Q *My neighbor hardly felt her contractions. She said it was no big deal and anybody ought to be able to do it "naturally."*

A Not all women are alike. Women perceive pain differently and it is not necessarily a question of being prepared. All physicians recognize that people are "hard-wired" differently. The fine peripheral nerve endings throughout the body are in neither the same concentration per square millimeter nor in the same location from person to person. I have had forty-year-old patients whose four children I've delivered and who trust me completely hit the roof when I do an office cervical biopsy. I've also had seventeen-year-old patients on their second visit who don't even feel the same procedure. This couldn't be if all women felt the same thing!

Some women do fine without pain medication, and others do not. Your ability to handle pain does not necessarily correlate with your degree of preparedness or dedication, and it is not a failure to ask for and receive medication when you feel as if you need it. Unless you are making the decision in a panic, your support personnel, including your husband, should be just that—supportive.

THE SECOND STAGE OF LABOR

530

Q *What is the second stage again?*

A The second stage of labor, begins when your cervix is dilated enough to allow passage of your baby's head, usually referred to as ten centimeters, and ends with the tip of the toes exiting the vagina.

531

Q *Can I use the same breathing techniques I learned for the first stage?*

A No. Whether you are unmedicated, lightly medicated, or medicated with an appropriately dosed epidural, you will feel an urge to "bear down" similar to that felt with the need for a bowel movement. Pushing or bearing down while holding your breath, often called Valsalva's maneuver, is virtually impossible to avoid. You may want to take a deep, cleansing breath as each contraction starts to build. This allows you to focus your energy and to relax all muscles but your abdominals.

The urge to push may come just because the baby's head has descended significantly, even if the cervix is not completely dilated. Usually your obstetrician, midwife, or labor nurse will be examining you and advising when it is best for you to start pushing. If for any reason you need to delay pushing when you have the urge, "panting" may be helpful for a short while.

Sometimes, especially with an epidural in place, it is wise to delay pushing for a while even after complete dilation. Occasionally, you may have no urge to push whatsoever, and it may be appropriate to simply allow the uterus to clamp down and continue moving the baby without your voluntary help, as some of your sensation returns.

532

Q *Do I need to be in a special position to push effectively?*

A Different pushing positions work better for different clinical situations and different people. For instance, if your baby's head is turned so that it does not have its face toward your tailbone, your labor nurse may recommend trying out several different positions.

Usually, pushing effectively involves concentrating all your energy in your abdominal muscles and relaxing your other muscles. That means avoiding "pushing with your legs" and avoiding "straining your face." Most often, curling your body into a "C" with your chin on your chest, your knees pulled up and out, and your back bowed rather than arched will be the most effective position.

533

Q *I've heard that squatting is a very good position. Can I do that with an epidural?*

A Squatting is an effective pushing position for many people. Whether or not you will be able to do this depends on your dosage and type of medication in your epidural, but also on the policies of both your doctor or midwife and those of the labor unit. I've had patients squat supported by their husband standing behind with his arms under her arms. Some LDR's are equipped with a squatting bar (similar to a roll bar on a Jeep) attached to the labor bed. With newer medicines in epidurals, squatting is often no problem.

534

Q *My sister was told to push on her side most of the time. Why?*

A There are several different possibilities. Sometimes the baby sits on its umbilical cord in certain positions and this can be detected by the fetal heart rate monitor or by the nurse listening to the heart during contractions. Sometimes a combination of medicine and pushing "on your back" can lower your blood pressure enough to affect the baby. Occasionally, pushing on your side may help an OP baby (a baby in the occiput posterior position) turn so that its face is toward the tailbone and it can better maneuver under the pubic bone.

535

Q *My friend said she couldn't tell which direction to push even though her epidural hadn't affected her leg mobility at all. What do you do then?*

A Dosing of the epidural may come into play here, but the most common immediate remedy is for the nurse, midwife, or doctor to put a gloved finger either firmly in the fourchette or on the perineum between the vagina and anus. You should try and push toward that point. A corollary to this is perineal massage, which either your nurse or doctor may do intermittently to help these tissues stretch out.

536

Q *If I push hard all at once won't I wear out?*

A Everybody can "wear out," and if the baby's doing well there's no rule against resting for a while. Think of pushing out the baby as similar to moving a tractor-trailer truck. The truck, like the baby, has inertia. You cannot move the truck by giving several short, quick pushes to the back of it. Slow, steady pushes, gradually increasing in intensity, are more likely to be effective. Once the truck starts to roll, it's easier to push. It's the same with delivering a baby. Your third push with each contraction should be your best. Typically, you may push to the count of ten, three to four times with each contraction.

537

Q *What else can help me push besides counting, following my urge, or feeling the touch on my perineum?*

A Some patients do better when they visualize the birth canal. Viewed from the side, the baby enters the pelvis at the inlet with its face turned to one side. As it descends, it slowly turns its face toward your tailbone and extends its neck so that its head pulls back and up under the pubic bone during delivery. Visualizing a path that curves down into your bottom and then up and out seems to help.

DECISIONS, DECISIONS, DECISIONS

Intravenous Access

538

Q *Will I have to have an IV?*

A Necessity of an intravenous line (IV) will depend somewhat on your doctor and the delivering institution. Many babies' and mothers' lives have been saved by immediate venous access. This does not mean that on arrival at the hospital or birthing center that you immediately need an IV. It also does not mean that your movement must be restricted to an IV pole with a bag.

Saline locks are small plastic catheters inserted in the vein and taped to your arm. They are no bigger than an inch or so long and pose no restrictions on movement whatsoever. If you should have a sudden problem, however, intravenous fluids and medicines can be given immediately.

539

Q *Why couldn't an IV be inserted only when and if I needed it?*

A It could. However, when things go wrong, they go wrong quickly. Many of the rare bad things that can go wrong in labor involve rapid blood loss. Blood loss collapses veins and in the heat of the moment precious seconds that may be critical to your baby's life or brain can be lost while someone is fumbling to insert an IV. A saline lock is no inconvenience once labor is diagnosed and should be used on all laboring patients if no IV is placed initially.

Facilities

540

Q *Should I look for a hospital with birthing rooms or LDRs?*

A In truth, you'd be hard-pressed to find a hospital without these facilities. There is general agreement that a more comfortable environment helps set everyone at ease. Once it was realized that bacteria live in the vagina all the time and that birth is about as sterile a procedure as planting geranium bulbs, birthing rooms that looked more like your own bedroom caught on rapidly. LDRs allow labor, birth, and recovery to occur in the very same room.

Anyone who has had to move to a delivery table with a "bowling ball" in her vagina will tell you that the experience was unpleasant.

Some facilities have you remain in the same room for your entire stay. Others, depending on volume of deliveries and room availability, often move you to a postpartum room once the original excitement has had an hour or two to dissipate and you realize that you're exhausted.

541

Q *Can a C-section be done in the LDR if need be?*

A All LDRs are equipped to do instrumented vaginal deliveries, including those using forceps or vacuum extractors. Some have the necessary attachments for anesthetic gases and the necessary lighting and room to function as an emergency operating room. However, most LDRs are simply close to an operating room standing ready for just such an event.

Preparation

542

Q *Some of my friends have had both shave preps and enemas. Are they both necessary?*

A A shave prep nowadays only involves shaving a small amount of pubic hair from the perineum between the vagina and rectum. Should you require an episiotomy or have a tear that needs to be sutured, it is virtually impossible to do with pubic hair constantly tied into the knots. Again, every women is different, and this is more of an issue for some than others. If you wish to avoid the itching of hair growing back in this area, trim the hair short yourself, or have your partner do it, as you near your due date.

Whether or not to have an enema is an item to discuss with your own caregiver. Although you don't need to have an enema, many women find it embarrassing to completely empty their colon as they push out their baby. If there is stool in the rectum, it will come out one way or the other because there simply isn't room for the head to pass through the birth canal without emptying the rectum.

You may either request an enema once it's clear that you're in labor, or if you feel like you're in early labor, administer a small Fleet enema at home before coming to the hospital.

543

Q *May I eat and drink in labor?*

A Women in labor are usually discouraged from eating solids. While it is true that people probably could eat in early labor without a problem, you never know when labor might progress rapidly or suddenly and necessitate general anesthesia. Pregnancy slows the emptying of the stomach. Even many hours after a small meal, the food may still be in the stomach. If you vomited during the induction of general anesthesia you could aspirate, causing lung damage or death.

Clear liquids may be permitted in labor and up to 2 hours before elective C-Section. These include water, fruit juices, Popsicles, carbonated beverages, tea, coffee, and sports drinks according to ACOG.[7]

Electronic Fetal Monitoring

544

Q *What is continuous electronic fetal monitoring?*

A There are two types of continuous electronic fetal monitoring (EFM)—external and internal. It is the fetal heart rate that is being monitored in both cases. With the external type, a flat, round ultrasound transducer is placed on your abdomen over the fetal heart and held in place with disposable elastic belts that go around your waist. The transducer is made of lightweight plastic and is about three inches in diameter. Often there is a second belt that holds a pressure transducer over the fundus of the uterus to detect when uterine contractions occur. Both are converted to an electronic signal, which appears on a tracing that is produced continuously by the machine.

The internal type, called fetal scalp electrode (FSE), is inserted through the vagina and cervix and affixed to the baby's scalp by a small curved wire that slips under the skin. A wire then tracks out of the vagina to a connection from the heart through the baby's body. This is more accurate than the averaging of rates done mathematically by an ultrasound external monitor.

Intrauterine pressure monitors (IUPC) also exist. An IUPC consists of another small catheter that is inserted through the cervix; the catheter runs past the baby's head and into the uterine cavity. An IUPC can actually measure the intrauterine pressure in millimeters of mercury generated by your uterine contractions, while an external pressure monitor only tells when the contraction occurs.

545

Q *When I get to labor and delivery, do I have to be on an electronic fetal monitor?*

A The answer should be no. While almost everyone would like to get a brief "strip," or record of the fetal heart rate in response to contractions over the first twenty minutes or so, you should be allowed to disconnect from the monitor and walk if everything is normal.

Electronic fetal monitoring became the nationwide standard of care in the late 1970s almost overnight. There was no credible evidence that instituting continuous monitoring would make labor and delivery safer. But because all doctors, midwives, and nurses know that obstetric disasters are often foreshadowed by slowing of the fetal heart rate, it seemed like a good idea.

Incentive for the use of such monitors was also provided by the nation's rising litigation crisis. Doctors erroneously thought that a record of fetal heartrate changes would help protect them from unfounded suits. Instead, they found that the monitoring strip usually provided ammunition for the plaintiff's attorneys in dealing with juries that lacked sufficient knowledge for appropriate interpretation.

A large recent study in Dallas at University of Texas Southwestern Medical School showed what had been long suspected all across the country. Continuous EFM did not diminish rates of fetal mortality and morbidity. In other words, use of EFM did not significantly statistically alter outcome. Even more distressingly, one thing EFM did do was raise the primary C-section rate for "fetal distress."[8]

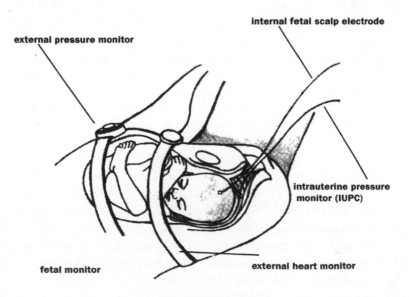

internal fetal scalp electrode

external pressure monitor

intrauterine pressure monitor (IUPC)

fetal monitor

external heart monitor

546

Q *If fetal monitoring doesn't change outcome, why are fetal monitors still used everywhere in the country?*

A EFM can be useful at times. In the Leveno study cited at the end of the last question, those patients who demonstrated heart rate decelerations by intermittent nursing auscultation were then put on fetal monitors. There are subtle findings better seen on EFM than heard audibly that may be critical to preserving your baby's health. The question is whether all laboring women need to be on monitors all the time. The answer would seem to be "no".

547

Q *What kind of conditions would require fetal monitoring for more than an initial evaluation?*

A EFM is indicated for several circumstances. In an otherwise healthy pregnancy, EFM may be recommended if there is meconium in the amniotic fluid, if you are more than ten days past your due date, if heart rate decelerations are either heard initially or are seen on an initial monitoring strip, or if you have received pain medication in the form of a narcotic or an epidural anesthetic.

If you are in labor with a condition that might adversely affect the baby's ability to tolerate the stress of labor (that is, the placenta's ability to function) a continuous EFM may be recommended. Such conditions include preeclampsia, chronic hypertension, growth restriction (IUGR), known decreased fluid before rupture (oligohydramnios), diabetes, vaginal bleeding of unclear source (possible abruption), or any of a number of other medical complications of pregnancy. You should be aware that studies indicate a wide variance in interpretation of EFM among health professionals. It has also been shown EFM can lead to higher rates of instrumented delivery and CS for perceived fetal distress, and that EFM changes are NOT at all predictive of cerebral palsy incidence.[9]

548

Q *Why would I need a fetal scalp electrode?*

A In some women, depending on how heavy they are, or how mobile the baby is, it may be very difficult to monitor the baby's heart rate. In situations where EFM is necessary and an external tracing is not possible, a fetal scalp electrode (FSE) may be recommended.

549

Q *Why would I need an IUPC?*

A An intrauterine pressure catheter is used either whenever you receive oxytocin (Pitocin) to start or increase the frequency and intensity of your contractions, or whenever you have failed to make any progress for more than two hours in the active phase (dilation of more than five centimeters). An external pressure monitor tells only when your contractions occur, not how strong they are. With an IUPC we can calculate Montevideo Units—the number of mmHg (millimeters of mercury) per contraction times the number of contractions in ten minutes—which provides a comparison of your labor to "normal" labor.

If you fail to progress after dilation of five centimeters, there are only three possible reasons: your contractions are inadequate, your baby is too big, or your baby is in a position that makes it difficult for the cervix to dilate or for the head to descend. At five to ten centimeters, the only variable that can be manipulated is the strength and/or frequency of contractions.

Episiotomy

550

Q *What exactly is an episiotomy and how do I know if I need one?*

A Episiotomy is the term for the incision sometimes made in the perineum, which is the tissue between the lower outlet of the vagina, the fourchette, and the anus. It is much more common with first deliveries than with subsequent ones, since in the former this tissue has never been significantly stretched.

551

Q *Will an episiotomy hurt?*

A If and when you need an episiotomy, it can be performed painlessly. If you have an adequate dose of an epidural anesthetic or a local anesthetic injected in the perineum, you should feel little pain, with the actual incision. Even when performed with no anesthetic, as long as it is done at the appropriate time (that is, when the tissue has stretched to the point where it has begun to tear on its own), you are unlikely to feel it as distinct from the discomfort of delivery itself. The compression of the tissue by the head decreases blood flow to the area, and in the same way that your arm becomes numb when you leave it over the back of a seat at the movies, transient numbness develops in the perineum as well.

Episiotomies are, of course, sore for several days after delivery. You will be given pain medication in the hospital, and your doctor will prescribe pain-killers to go home with as well. Don't be stoic after delivery. In this situation, narcotics are appropriate.

552

Q *Why do an episiotomy at all?*

A Good question. There are those who would argue against performing episiotomy under any circumstance; they may be the same people who have never struggled to sew the "exploded" bottom back together again. With extremely edematous (swollen) tissues, tears can be sudden and dramatic. If a ragged tear rips apart the nine different muscles that come together at the perineum (perineal body), the repair can be tedious and fraught with the danger of increased risk for infection, bleeding with hematoma formation, increased pain, increased pain with intercourse, and increased risk of incontinence to stool (loss of control over bowel movements).

553

Q *If I do perineal massage in the months before delivery, will it really help me avoid episiotomy?*

A No well-designed study suggests that perineal massage performed prior to labor has any benefit. Perineal massage involves kneading the tissue between the fourchette of the vagina and the anus. Analogous to nipple preparation, there is little evidence to justify it. Of course, if your husband does it, that could lead to sex and nipple stimulation, good for bringing on labor.

554

Q *Why is there such a controversy surrounding episiotomy?*

A There isn't. It just seems that way to the lay public. Obstetricians and certified nurse midwives almost always agree about when or if an episiotomy is indicated.

I do think there are times when episiotomies are performed where a little patience would have been more appropriate. Allowing the second stage to last a little longer, combined with perineal massage, will often obviate the need for an episiotomy, which, although it might have hastened delivery, served no other purpose.

555

Q *Why would a doctor perform an episiotomy if waiting longer would have made it unnecessary?*

A First, the advent of continuous electronic fetal monitoring has made doctors much more aware of heart rate decelerations during pushing. These decelerations may look ominous from a legal standpoint, but they usually pose little risk to the baby. However, they can influence the doctor's decision toward shortening the second stage with an early episiotomy. Statistically, a delivery performed in a birthing center, often by a midwife, is less likely to be continuously monitored; thus, the pressure of the fetal heart rate strip is not ever-present, even if decelerations are heard intermittently with a handheld Doppler device. Midwives might have the same episiotomy rate as doctors if they were under the same legal pressures and forced to use continuous monitoring by institutional standards of care.

Second, sometimes the unmedicated patient and her husband are literally begging for help in ending the second stage. This rationale should be rare. If couples are prepared with education and relaxation techniques, they will recognize the value of the sometimes longer second stage in shaping their baby's head and in thinning out the tissue of the perineum.

Third, some doctors perform episiotomies routinely after a certain time limit assigned to the pushing stage. This is unfortunate and I believe to be avoided.

Pharmacological Pain Management

556

Q *What medicines can I have in labor to help with the pain?*

A You may choose to have no medicines, medicines in your IV or as a shot in the hip, or either of these followed by an epidural when you are far enough along.

557

Q *Which medicines can I take safely in labor?*

A Narcotics such as meperidine (Demerol) and morphine, or the narcotic derivatives butorphenol (Stadol), alphaprodine (Nisentil), and nalbuphine (Nubain) may be given either intramuscularly (IM) or intravenously (IV). All of these are often given in combination with prochlorperazine (Phenergan) to counteract any nauseating effect of the narcotic. (See Section 5: Drugs in Pregnancy)

558

Q *At what point should I consider these medicines?*

A You don't have to consider them at all. However, if the breathing and relaxation techniques you have learned seem inadequate in terms of tolerating the pain, you might think about a little intravenous or intramuscular narcotic. If possible, do not make this decision in a state of panic. It is preferable that you use the techniques described above to regain control and then make your decision.

559

Q *Why would I want the shot if I could be medicated intravenously?*

A With intramuscular administration, the onset of action and side effects such as nausea are usually slower. Additionally, the pain relief lasts longer per dose, and is thus more even. However, the method of delivering the medication will be decided by your doctor, midwife, or nurse, in consultation with you.

Epidurals

560

Q *What exactly is an epidural?*

A (See Section 5: Drugs in Pregnancy)
Epidural refers to the anatomic place in the lower back into which local anesthetics are injected either intermittently or continuously. The result is temporary blockage of sensation and, to some extent, muscle function in the lower half of your body. You will be positioned either sitting on the side of the bed, curled over with your arms around a pillow, or lying on your side with your knees drawn up and your chin on your chest. As you bow your back like a Halloween cat, the skin over your

lumbar region is numbed and a needle is inserted there. This needle is advanced into a space just outside the one that contains cerebrospinal fluid (CSF). After a test dose is injected, a tiny plastic catheter is advanced through the needle and the needle is withdrawn. The entire procedure takes about five minutes.

561

Q *How is an epidural different from a spinal?*

A (See Section 7: Labor and Delivery)
Spinal anesthetics are similar to epidurals in that they are administered through a needle placed in the low back, either sitting or lying on your side, and the agent used is a local anesthetic or "caine" drug. Spinals, however, are used when rapid onset of numbing is needed for forceps deliveries or cesarean section. Unlike epidurals, the numbing only lasts a finite time, since no continuous catheter is put in place.

Spinals are considered a little more likely to give you problems such as low blood pressure, nausea, and vomiting. Spinal headaches, paradoxically, are less likely to occur than with an epidural. This is probably because the needle used for spinals has a much smaller diameter than the one used for epidurals. When an epidural needle inadvertently punctures the dura (filmlike lining) and enters the spinal fluid space, it leaves a bigger hole, causes a bigger leak, and is more likely to result in a headache. (See this section: Wet tap)

562

Q *How long does the pain relief last?*

A Most institutions offer continuous epidural anesthesia. In this circumstance, a computerized pump is used to continuously feed a small amount of the anesthetic solution into the epidural space. This pump may be set to give greater or lesser effect depending on the agent used and the height of the patient.

Epidurals may also simply be "capped." Then, medicine is intermittently pushed with a syringe into the catheter as a "bolus." With this method, the pain relief may wax and wane, at least to some extent.

When epidurals are used for C-section, they are often left in place for 48 hours to provide post operative pain relief. A pump is used to continuously fill the catheter, and to allow patient directed boluses, or narcotic, which provides pain relief without numbness.

563

Q *How do I know ahead of time whether to get an epidural?*

A You don't. It is unwise to make any absolute decision about what you are going to do in labor. Leaving the option open for regional anesthesia (epidural) does not undermine your ability to commit to an unmedicated delivery. The perception that acknowledging an epidural as a potential option leads to "failure" of the "natural" process is unfounded. It is exactly analogous to the belief that sex education in school leads to teenagers having sex. No data supports either contention.

564

Q *Is there a limited window of opportunity for an epidural?*

A Traditionally, epidural anesthetics have been instituted in the active phase of the first stage of labor, meaning when the woman is dilated five to ten centimeters. At one time, and in many places still, epidurals begun in the second (pushing) stage were considered contraindicated. With older anesthetics that caused significant motor (muscle) block, late institution of the epidural was felt to interfere with pushing. (See Question 766, Section Eight)

565

Q *Is it true that epidurals increase the forceps and C-section rates?*

A That is an extremely controversial issue, so much so that each camp is sure its perspective is the only one and simply views the opposing camp as wrong.

In general, studies in the obstetric literature have seemed to conclude that epidurals given too early in labor (before the woman is dilated four to five centimeters) and/or in too heavy a dose in the early first stage or in the second stage increase the rate of delivery with forceps or vacuum as well as the primary C-section rate. Studies reported in the anesthetic literature, however, seem to indicate the opposite. In short, most of these articles demonstrate that properly maintained epidural analgesia does not interfere with either stage of labor.

Both sides are coming together and starting to agree that agents with very little motor block, such as ropivicaine, combined with the use of the fast-acting narcotic fentanyl, are possible to use earlier in labor, and can also be used when the patient is completely dilated, as in the case of a very rapid labor in a woman who has had many previous deliveries. (See Question 766, Section Eight)

566

Q *What is a walking epidural?*

A Prior to the last decade, epidural placement required that the patient be confined to bed. More recently, narcotic-containing epidurals have been used very successfully for postoperative pain, whether C-section or otherwise. The last few years have seen the use of epidurals that contain only the narcotic fentanyl in labor as well. Laboring women have been permitted to walk around with the epidural catheter in place (the "walking epidural").

567

Q *Can I get a walking epidural too?*

A This is a good question to ask your doctor. Availability will depend on the anesthesiologists in your hospital, or possibly the obstetricians, if they are the ones to place the epidural in your system. Availability aside, your specific condition—for example, preeclampsia may be deemed inappropriate for a walking epidural.

568

Q *Does an epidural have any side effects?*

A In addition to the controversy over whether regional anesthesia can affect the cesarean section rate several undesired effects can occur. Probably the most common side effect noted is the epidural shakes. Frequently, people shake like a leaf shortly after epidural placement. While it may be due to a physiological change involving a sympathetic nervous block and dilated veins, others argue that the shakes are merely a manifestation of intravenous fluids that are colder than body temperature. In any event, the trembling is harmless, and usually resolves after a short period.

Epidurals may be difficult or impossible to place if you have severe curvature of the spine (scoliosis) or have had Herrington rods placed to correct this curvature.

Epidurals are contraindicated in women with some coagulation disorders (bleeding problems), severe preeclampsia, herpes outbreak on the low back, and known hypersensitivity or allergy to the "caine" drugs.

Hypotension (transient fall in blood pressure) may occur shortly after injection, depending on the dosage and the type of medicine. This is often avoided by giving at least a liter of IV fluid prior to placing the epidural.

The hypotension may be related to the epidural medicine blocking the nerves that control constriction of little arteries throughout the lower body. The drop in pressure can lead to decreased blood flow to the uterus and thus increase the risk of activating the defense mechanisms of fetal bradycardia or slowed heart rate. The vasoconstrictor ephedrine is also commonly used either preventively or in response to falling blood pressure with excellent success.

A wet tap occurs when the epidural needle was inadvertently advanced into the space containing cerebrospinal fluid, enabling some of the fluid to leak out. In about 50 percent of the cases, this can lead to a spinal headache whenever you sit up, which lasts for at least several days. It may be treated after the baby is born with a blood patch, which is blood drawn from your arm and then injected into the epidural catheter to form a clot over the hole and stop the leakage. Wet taps occur about 1 percent of the time.

Respiratory arrest (inability to breathe) may result if a large dose of medicine is accidentally injected into the spinal space. This is called a total spinal. Respiratory arrest is temporary, but it can be terrifying while others have to help you breathe. However, the possibility of respiratory arrest is so remote that some doctors, in practice for twenty years, have never seen it.

Even rarer are seizures, which can occur if a large amount of drug is inadvertently injected into a vein in the epidural space.

569

Q *Now I'm really confused. Should I get an epidural or not?*

A It is impossible to answer that question until you are in labor. Asking it beforehand demonstrates a misunderstanding of the process and the inherent variation from one woman to another. There is no doubt that the vast majority of women would successfully deliver babies without epidurals. They've done so for millennia.

Is it safe? Absolutely. Is it common? In our tertiary care facility with about five thousand deliveries per year, well over 80 percent of women choose epidural anesthesia. Rural areas with different personnel and facilities may have much lower rates. With Canada's socialized system, epidurals are becoming a rarity due to cost constraints by the government. They are also much more popular in some parts of the United States than in others.

But overall, they would appear to be safe, effective measures for pain relief of labor, delivery, and cesarean section. Few women voice regret at having made the decision to have an epidural.

Apgar Scores and Blood Gases

570

Q *What are the Apgar scores I always hear about?*

A Apgar scores were designed by Dr. Virginia Apgar in the 1950s and were intended to determine which babies needed the most support immediately after birth and at five minutes. Thus there are scores given at one minute of life and at five minutes. The categories for scores are heart rate, respiration (breathing effort), muscle tone, reflex irritability (response to stimulation), and color.

Zero, one, or two points are assigned in each of five categories, so a perfect score is ten. However, if a baby is normal, that does not necessarily mean it should get a ten. In fact, a one-minute score of ten is very rare and occasionally worrisome.

Initially, all newborns are blue to some extent. Well-oxygenated blood is shunted away from the skin to more vital organs such as the brain, heart, and kidneys. As a consequence, an initial Apgar score of eight is expected and a five-minute score of nine is frequent. Only if the five-minute score is below seven is there reason for concern about problems severe enough to require special support.

571

Q *Do low Apgar scores mean that my baby will have long-term problems?*

A In recent years we have learned that the Apgar scores have little to no value at predicting long-term health. This means that they have little prognostic usefulness. It turns out that even babies with very low Apgar scores may do well and babies with high Apgar scores may do poorly.

Contrary to what was originally thought, Apgars have almost no correlation with cerebral palsy. Over 90 percent of cases of cerebral palsy would seem to be related to some asphyxic (loss of oxygen) event weeks to months before birth. This means that labor is almost never the determining event for cerebral palsy.

Cerebral palsy is a congenital problem in which portions of the brain that control motor activity have been damaged. It is thought to be a result of decreased blood supply sometime during gestation.

572

Q *Are there other ways to determine how the baby tolerated labor besides the Apgar score?*

A Yes. Cord blood gases (CBGs) may be sampled. Before the placenta delivers, a double-clamped segment of the umbilical cord can be removed. Blood is then drawn from the umbilical artery that carries blood from the baby back to the placenta. This segment represents the state of the baby at the end of labor. Acid-base levels (pH), base deficit, and carbon dioxide level are measured. These values allow your doctor to know if your baby was especially stressed in labor.

Surprisingly, there is much less correlation than one would have thought between Apgar scores and CBGs. What is clear is that babies whose five-minute Apgars were over seven were not significantly stressed in labor. In general, the same would be true for babies with a pH reading of more than 7.10 and either a zero or small base deficit.

Circumcision

573

Q *What exactly is circumcision?*

A Circumcision is the surgical removal of the foreskin, which covers the head, or glans, of the penis. Without the procedure, the outer skin of the penis covers the head even with erection, but it is fully retractable.

574

Q *Why do some people advise against circumcision?*

A Circumcision for your newborn son is entirely elective. What does appear to be true is that the procedure is medically "unnecessary' The American Academy of Pediatrics has held since the early 1980s that the procedure shows no clear medical benefits for your son as an infant or as an adult.

Whether you should have your son circumcised for religious or social reasons is a different issue from the medical one. Although circumcision has been performed for nonmedical reasons for at least five thousand years, the vast majority of the three billion males in the world are uncircumcised.

575

Q *Who gets circumcised if it's not medically necessary and is not performed on the vast majority of the world's males?*

A Circumcision is a requirement of the Jewish faith and the Muslim faith. In addition, Americans, and particularly Caucasian Americans, tend to be circumcised.

576

Q *Are there any other reasons for having my son circumcised?*

A Yes. Little boys often compare their own penis with their father's. Differences in dimension, surrounding hair, and so on are unavoidable, but differences between father and son with respect to circumcision can be difficult to explain.

Many studies in the last century have led to conflicting conclusions about issues such as the incidence of sexually transmitted diseases with circumcised and uncircumcised males. Much of this data was confounded by socioeconomic class, with men of poorer family background having been less likely to be circumcised. Rates of circumcision increased dramatically once children began to be born in hospitals with increasing frequency around 1920.

It is true that personal hygiene is easier without a foreskin, the underside of which requires some effort to cleanse in the uncircumcised. But otherwise there appears to be little to no medical benefit to the procedure.

577

Q *We want our son circumcised. Is there more than one method of doing this?*

A The Gomco Clamp is the most common method used in the United States. The Plastibell is a close second. Both take about five minutes to perform and give essentially the same cosmetic result. Their only difference lies in how the tissue is occluded to prevent bleeding afterward. With the Plastibell, a small plastic ring tied around the corona (edge of the glans) should fall off in about one week. With the Gomco Clamp, the tissue has already been occluded with a metal clamp and a brief wait. Regardless of the method, circumcisions need to have Vaseline put on the cut edge for the first few days so they don't stick to the diaper.

Remember that all circumcisions look good on the first day, and not so good a day or two later. Don't panic. It is very rare that a circumcision leads to a medical problem.

578

Q *Who does the procedure?*

A In most places across the country, the obstetricians do the circumcisions. Pediatricians are second, family practitioners third, the Jewish mohel fourth, and the urologist last.

Whether or not an anesthetic should be used with your son's circumcision should be discussed with your doctor. Local anesthetics can have complications. A strong case can be made for using at least an anesthetic cream, but the vast majority of doctors do not do so. Older studies showed that crying times were actually longer with local anesthetic, after the procedure but not during it. This may be due to the "tingle" as the local wears off.

Newer studies, however, suggest that topical creams with lidocaine and prilocaine, such as EmLa Cream are safe and effective, with less agitation, lower heart and respiratory rate, and less crying demonstrated.[10]

Still, most doctors have done thousands of circumcisions without anesthetic and have seen the babies fall asleep after about 90 seconds once the clamp is on. The majority of obstetricians in 2006, nevertheless, choose to use some form of local anesthetic.

Bonding (See also Breast-Feeding)

579

Q *We'd like as much time as possible with our new baby as soon as she's born. Will we be able to hold her right away?*

A Every doctor and institution has different policies and procedures. However, in the absence of an immediate concern over your baby's health, you may have the baby in your arms as soon as the airway is suctioned out, the baby has been stimulated to inhale, and the umbilical cord is cut and clamped.

580

Q *We never want the baby to leave our sight. Will this be a problem?*

A Maybe. Almost every hospital has a receiving nursery where babies are warmed, suctioned if need be, cleaned off, and wrapped securely in blankets. In some institutions that normally doesn't occur until the baby is about an hour old. The first hour is spent with the parents in the LDR.

Many parents believe they are going to want twenty-four-hour room-ing-in, where the baby never leaves their room after the initial check-in. A very small percentage of mothers choose to do that once they have delivered. Labor is an exhausting experience, and as much fun as your newborn will be, most new mothers need to sleep. Often you will also have just taken narcotic pain relievers, which alter your judgment, reaction time, and ability to stay alert.

Nevertheless, some hospitals allow the option of twenty-four-hour rooming-in, and in many birthing centers this is the only option.

581

Q *We've heard that it is better to put the baby on the mother's chest immediately after delivery, without wrapping her up, so that she can find her own way to the breast when she's ready. Will we be able to do this?*

A Once again, these decisions will be dependent on your baby's health at birth and on the preferences with which you and your doctor are com-fortable. While it might well be true that some babies can instinctively find their way to the breast, it doesn't make it better to do this. There are many phenomena observed in nature that are not intrinsically *better.* One would be hard, pressed to find sociological or psychological evidence, rather than opin-ion, that any of the common bonding maneuvers is necessary for the growth and health of a normally adjusted young person.

582

Q *But isn't bonding with me essential in the first few moments of life?*

A No. We are not ducklings, and imprinting is not a human phenomenon. In fact, humans can be raised with no discernible deficit by people who are not their biological parents. Furthermore, there are many babies born who are premature or seriously ill who have virtually no early contact with their mother on an ongoing basis. There is data to show the tremendous ben-efits of human companionship, warmth, cuddling, cooing, facial expression, rocking, and so on even for the tiniest babies in the intensive care nursery—but not necessarily from the mother.

In summary, immediate contact with warm, loving, touching, sup-portive humans is important, and ideally that person should be you. But don't think for a minute that your baby or your relationship with your baby has been damaged if you are initially separated at birth for a medical reason. Love overcomes even less-than-ideal bonding, as shown by the success of infant adoption.

What to Bring

583

Q *I've been told to pack a bag. What will I really need?*

A Most of the things you will have thought of by yourself, so just check off the list below.

For Labor

- Stopwatch or watch with second hand
- Focal points; stuffed animal, and so on
- Slippers and robe
- Extra pillows
- Hard candies; lip balm
- Washcloths; mouthwash; toothpaste
- Contact lens case/eyeglasses
- Several sets of socks
- Roller or other tool for back massage
- Paper and pencil or pen
- Phone numbers of family members and friends
- Quarters for vending machines
- CDs or audiotapes (bring your own player if rooms are not equipped)
- Still cameras and/or video camera (instruct your poor husband on their proper use before labor begins!)
- Film for the camera

After Delivery

- Slippers and robe
- 2-3 nightgowns (breast-feeding fronts if preferred)
- 2-3 bras of at least one cup size larger than before pregnancy
- Nursing pads (if nursing)
- Clothes for going home (about what you wore at 20 weeks)
- Outfit and blanket for baby for going home
- Baby book to record fun facts, footprints, and so on
- Bedside travel clock
- Toiletries, hair and cosmetic items

- Something to keep you occupied (birth announcements, good book)
- Car seat (should be installed before the trip home—in backseat if the car is equipped with passenger air bags)

Postpartum
(See Section 10: After the Delivery)

NATIONAL ORGANIZATIONS WITH INFORMATION

Lamaze Childbirth Education ASPO/Lamaze
   1200 19th Street NW, Suite 300
   Washington, DC 20036-2401
   (800) 368-4404

ICEA (International Childbirth Education Association)
   PO Box 20048
   Minneapolis, MN 55420
   (612) 854-8660

Professional Labor Support DONA (Doulas of North America)
   1100 23rd Avenue East Seattle, WA 98112
   (206) 324-5440

SUGGESTED READING

ACOG *Guide to Planning for Pregnancy, Birth and Beyond*. American College of Ob/Gyn, 1995.
   ACOG Web Site: http://www.acog.com
   Main Switchboard 800-673-8444, (206) 638-5577
   Order Desk: 800-762-2264

Amis, Debby and Jeanne Green. 1996. *Prepared Childbirth the Family Way*. 5th Ed. Plano, TX: The Family Way Publications, Inc.
   To Order: (972) 403-0297

Eisenberg, A., H. Murkoff, S. Hathaway. 1991. *What to Expect When You're Expecting*. New York: Workman Publishers.

Iovine, Vicki. 1995. *The Girlfriend's Guide to Pregnancy*. New York: Pocket Books.

Jiminez, Sherry. 1983. *The Pregnant Woman's Comfort Guide*.

Parsons, Betty. 1987. *Preparing for Childbirth, Relaxing for Labor, Learning for Life*

Savage, Beverly. 1997. *Preparation for Birth: The Complete Guide to the Lamaze Method*.

WEBSITES

Prepared Childbirth

http://www.mjbovo.com/Pregnancy/LDPrep.htm

Diet

http://www.webmd.com/baby/tc/
        nutrition-and-weight-gain-during-pregnancy-topic-overview

http://www.healthcastle.com/pregnancy-diet.shtml

Due Date

www.americanpregnancy.org/duringpregnancy/pregcalc.html

Exercise in Pregnancy

www.childbirth.org/articles/pregnancy/safeexercise.html

Teens and Pregnancy

www.webmd.com and enter teen pregnancy in search engine

Section Seven

Normal Labor and Delivery

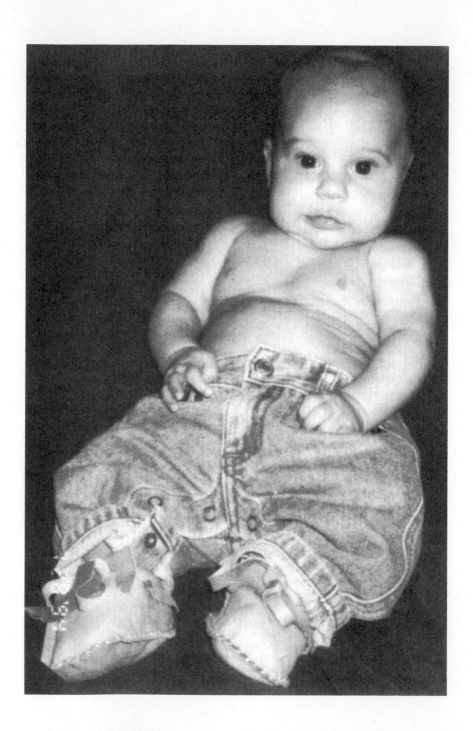

THE FINAL WEEKS

Pelvic Examinations

584

Q *When will the doctor start doing pelvic examinations?*

A You will recall that "term pregnancy" for singletons is defined as thirty-eight to forty-two completed menstrual weeks. Most doctors will do a digital pelvic exam using one or two fingers beginning at thirty-eight weeks to insure that the presenting part is the head, and to assess any cervical changes or descent of the presenting part. (See Section 8: Malpresentation)

585

Q *Will I have to get back in those stirrups again?*

A Usually not. Most of the time you'll be asked to lie on your back with your knees drawn up and out, and your feet resting together.

586

Q *After the pelvic exam, will the doctor be able to tell me when the baby is coming?*

A Unfortunately, your due "date" is really your due "month"! We should be telling you something along the lines of "Your baby's due sometime in the spring!" This would have tremendous psychological benefit over a specific "due date"! Cervical changes uncovered at the pelvic exam in the last few weeks may tell a little about how long your labor might be if it started that night, but tells little about when you are due.

Stripping Membranes

587

Q *What does stripping the membranes mean?*

A (See Section 8: Induction)
As you approach your due date, or if you have passed your due date, your doctor may perform a digital pelvic exam called "stripping the membranes"

hoping to stimulate labor. It is described in Section 8, and may or may not be effective.[1]

LABOR

588

Q *What is the definition of labor?*

A Labor is the occurrence of regular uterine contractions of increasing intensity that lead to the progressive effacement (thinning) and dilatation (opening) of the cervix.

589

Q *Aren't there different stages to labor?*

A A Labor is divided into three stages.

FIRST STAGE

Onset of labor to complete dilation Divided into latent (slow) phase (0-5 centimeters) and active (fast) phase (5-10 centimeters). Transition starts at about 8 centimeters and continues to complete dilation and the onset of pushing.

SECOND STAGE

Complete dilation to delivery of the baby

THIRD STAGE

Delivery of the baby to delivery of the placenta Rarely, some doctors name a Fourth Stage, when the uterus contracts to decrease blood loss after delivery of the placenta.

590

Q *I think I lost my "mucus plug." What does this mean?*

A Losing your mucus plug refers to passage of a glob of thick mucus often mixed with some bright red blood. This is painless and does not herald imminent delivery. This may or may not occur, and when it does, labor may be two days to a couple weeks away. Passing your mucus plug does not require any action from you or your doctor.

A mucus plug is not the same as a "bloody show." Bloody show implies a relatively larger amount of bright red blood mixed with some mucus, rather than mucus with a tiny amount of blood. Bloody show is a labor event, often becoming more apparent as the patient enters transition (dilation of eight to ten centimeters). The blood in bloody show is presumably from the more rapidly thinning and dilating cervix in the latter phases of the first stage of labor.

591

Q *How will I know for sure when I'm in labor?*

A Labor symptoms vary, so you won't necessarily know you are in labor until you know if your cervix is changing. Determining this by yourself at home tends to be somewhat acrobatic, so you may have to come to Labor and Delivery or your doctor's office to be checked.

You may suspect that you are in labor when you feel regular tightening of your tummy every four to five minutes for a period of at least forty-five minutes, and each tightening stays hard for forty-five seconds. (The little known "Thurstoni Rule of 4-5s") Start timing when the contraction begins, so that the interval goes from the beginning of one contraction to the beginning of the next. Usually these contractions will be strong enough that you clearly recognize them as different from what you've felt before, and they hurt enough to get your attention and make you stop what you're doing.

At this point, call your doctor, who will tell you whether or not to come to the hospital.

592

Q *My husband seems more nervous about my going into labor than I am. How can I calm him down?*

A There is nothing wrong with your husband being excited. If you attended childbirth classes several weeks before, be sure you continue to practice the techniques discussed under Prepared Childbirth. If you need to call the doctor because you think you might be in labor, have broken your bag of waters, or are bleeding, resist the temptation to have your husband handle the call. Doctors would much rather hear your voice than talk to an interpreter. Much as the labor nurse can tell a lot from your face, doctors can tell a lot from your voice.

593

Q *What if I go into labor and my husband is not nearby?*

A Part of preparing for childbirth includes planning for contingencies. You may wish to rent a pager for your husband if you don't have cellular phones. Remember that an average first labor will last about fourteen hours, so don't panic, you've got lots of time to reach him. It would be nice if babies just fell out the first time around, but it doesn't happen very often.

If your husband travels frequently for business reasons, ask him to avoid scheduling trips if possible from your thirty-eighth to your forty-second week. If that's not possible, find a good friend who will act as a backup. Consider hiring a doula. (See Section 6: Prepared Childbirth)

594

Q *My friend's daughter went into labor with her first baby and didn't even know it until she was dilated nine centimeters. Can that happen to me?*

A Only if you're the kind of person who wins the lottery on a regular basis! With first labors, painless dilation of the cervix at term is extremely rare. It is somewhat more common with women who have already had two or more children vaginally.

595

Q *I'm having my second baby. Might this labor be faster?*

A Most subsequent labors are faster than the previous one. If you had a twelve-hour labor (counting from when your first contractions were every four to five minutes), you might well have only a six-hour labor or less this time. Typically, the active phase, when you dilate from five to ten centimeters, and the second stage (pushing), are shorter than for first-time mothers.

596

Q *What is "precipitous labor"?*

A Precipitous labor is usually defined as a labor of less than three hours from start to finish. It is a reason for induction of labor with subsequent pregnancies. (See Section 8: Precipitous Labor)

Rupture of Membranes

597

Q *How can I tell if my water breaks?*

A Most often, there's not a lot of doubt about it. About one-third of women rupture their membranes before labor begins, and the rest do so in labor or the doctor does it for them. Usually there's a large gush as if you had just poured a glass of warm water in your underwear. Once your water has broken, it will continue to leak out until delivery.

Occasionally, if you have very little amniotic fluid or if the baby's head is already down in the birth canal (acting like a cork), your water may break with only a trickle. If you are uncertain, dry off your bottom with a towel and then sit on a clean dry towel for ten minutes. If your membranes have ruptured, you will usually be sitting on a wet spot. If you are still uncertain, call your doctor and go to the hospital or birthing center.

598

Q *What do I do if I think my water has broken?*

A Call your doctor anytime of the day or night if you either break your bag of waters, have painful regular contractions every four to five minutes for forty-five minutes, or bleed as heavily as you would in a menstrual period.

599

Q *I've heard it's bad if the fluid is green. Is that true?*

A Green amniotic fluid represents the passage of meconium from the baby's colon into the amniotic fluid. The vast majority of time this is simply the baby defecating and is not a sign of stress. Meconium, however, is not like bowel movements after birth. If the baby breaths it in at birth, it may be extremely caustic, leading to a serious reaction in the lungs. Meconium aspiration pneumonia can be fatal.

Consequently, you should be sure to let your doctor know that you saw green fluid. If this fluid is very thin, and stays the same throughout labor, your baby may simply need to have its airway suctioned out shortly after birth.

Thick meconium may represent a response to a decrease in the amount of oxygen reaching your baby either transiently or intermittently over a long period. Meconium in the fluid will be one of the reasons your provider may want you on the electronic fetal heart rate monitor continuously. (See Section 6: Prepared Childbirth)

600

Q *I was sure I ruptured with my last baby, but they tested me and said it was proba-bly just urine. I went into labor eighteen hours later and I still think I was right. Can you really lose control of your urine and not recognize it?*

A Losing control of your urine anytime after about twenty weeks is not uncommon. This usually accompanies coughing, laughing, sneezing, or jogging. Losing control and not recognizing it is harder to accept. While loss of urine has been used for years to explain gushes of vaginal fluid near term that test negative for amniotic fluid, there may be another explanation.

Recently several people have postulated that questionable rupture of membranes may actually be rupture of the chorionic membrane only, rather than the amniotic membrane. (See Section 4: Fetal Development; Section 6: Female Reproductive Anatomy and Terminology) The chorionic, or outer, membrane layer, contains only a very small amount of fluid as opposed to the large amount of intra-amniotic fluid. It is possible that when only the outer layer breaks, only a small amount of fluid comes out, and then does not continue to leak.

Doctors cannot predict when labor might begin after rupture of just the chorion.

ON ARRIVAL

601

Q *What will happen when I first arrive in Labor and Delivery?*

A Literally, the first thing that will happen is an experienced labor and delivery nurse will look at you and usually know to within a centimeter how dilated you are by your facial expression and breathing pattern. If it's appropriate, you'll usually sit down and be registered by a clerk and shown to a room a few moments later. You'll be shown where to change into a hospital gown, and then asked to empty your bladder and return to a bed.

Examination

602

Q *Will the doctor examine me then?*

A The doctor might examine you if he's already there, but usually a labor nurse will examine you and determine whether you are truly in labor or if you need to be observed over a couple hours to see if your contractions persist and your cervix changes.

603

Q *My mother had really fast labors with all five of us. Will my labor be as fast as hers?*

A Maternal history of rapid labors does have some bearing on you. While a maternal history of going into labor "early" or always carrying "late" does not have any relevance, a history of a first-degree relative (sister or mother) with a rapid first labor increases your chances of a rapid labor. Be sure to share this information with your doctor.

604

Q *Will I be sent home if I'm not in labor?*

A As long as your baby looks healthy on an initial monitoring strip, if your cervix fails to change over two hours, you might well be sent home. Don't let this embarrass you if it should happen. Women who have had three babies often can't tell for sure if they are truly in labor without being checked, observed, and rechecked!

605

Q *What will the nurse be looking for during the examination?*

A The pelvic exam has five components—Presentation, Station, Efface-ment, Position, and Dilation.

Presentation refers to which part of the baby is coming out first.

Station refers to the number of centimeters above or below the midplane of the pelvis (ischial spines) the presenting part is. (See Section 6: Female Reproductive Anatomy)

Effacement describes the thinness of the cervix compared to its original nonpregnant state, often expressed as a percentage.

Position denotes how far forward or backward the cervix is in its orientation as it protrudes into the vagina. Cervix "posterior" is hard to reach; cervix "anterior" is right beneath the pubic symphysis, and indicates a more advanced state than a posterior cervix.

Dilation describes how open the cervix is. Ten centimeters is considered completely dilated, big enough for the baby's head to pass.

606

Q *What if I come into Labor and Delivery with my bag of waters broken but not in labor?*

A About one-third of all labors begin this way. Some call this premature rupture of membranes (PROM), but the terminology is confusing. If this occurs prior to thirty-seven weeks, some doctors use the same term, or preterm premature rupture of membranes as a clarification. (See Section 8: Obstetric Complications)

At term, rupture of membranes is followed by the onset of labor within twelve hours in the majority of women. If rupture is questionable, your vaginal fluid will be tested with Nitrazine or pH paper. If the fluid is very basic (dark blue), this indicates that you have ruptured. If there is no color change, you may or may not have ruptured. Fluid can also be examined under the microscope for ferning. The ferning pattern would be present in amniotic fluid, but not present in normal vaginal secretions or urine.

What to do with you is more controversial still. Articles in the 1950s suggested drastic infectious consequences if you were not delivered by twenty-four hours after rupture. We now know that most of that infectious risk was brought on by people repeatedly putting their hands in your vagina and dragging bacteria up into the cervix. Consequently, most places in the United States will do nothing but observe and wait for labor to begin from six to twenty-four hours after documented rupture of the membranes.

607

Q *Don't I have to be induced right away if my bag is broken but I'm not in labor?*

A The balance of evidence through the mid-1990s suggests that waiting, without repeated pelvic exams, is the best thing to do if you are ruptured and not in labor. Whether your doctor waits six, twelve, eighteen, or

twenty-four hours will depend on what he or she believes in the medical
literature and what your individual circumstances are.

608

Q *What is prodromal labor?*

A Prodromal labor refers to the relatively rare circumstance in which you
have regular painful contractions for more than an hour, but no change
in your cervix to document the presence of labor. This can occasionally go on
for days. It is often caused by a very large baby or one in a position that makes
it difficult to "drop," or enter the pelvic inlet.

Often, in this circumstance the patient will be sleepless for thirty-six
hours or more and will be treated with either a narcotic or a phenobarbital
derivative such as Seconal or Nembutol in an effort to induce some much-
needed sleep. Frequently the patient will then awaken six to eight hours later
either in true labor or with contractions gone.

Monitoring

609

Q *Will I be placed on a monitor automatically?*

A (See full discussion of monitors in Section 6: Prepared Childbirth;
Electronic Fetal Monitoring)
Initially, probably so. It is prudent to monitor the baby's heart rate through at
least the first twenty minutes or so of contractions. If the baby appears healthy,
and your membranes are intact (the bag is unbroken) then you may be invited
to walk around while your labor intensifies. If your membranes are ruptured,
and your cervix is more than two to three centimeters but the baby's head has
not yet entered the pelvic inlet, some doctors, midwives, and nurses prefer
that you not walk for fear that your baby's umbilical cord might prolapse, or
come out into the vagina. This could compress the cord and be dangerous or
even lethal to the fetus. (See Section 8: Obstetric Complications)

610

Q *What is the difference between external and internal monitors?*

A (See Section 6: Prepared Childbirth; Electronic Fetal Monitoring for a
full discussion)

Fetal Heart Rate Decelerations

611

Q *What are they looking for on a fetal heart rate monitor?*

A Fetal heart rate is an indicator of many different things, including fetal temperature and, indirectly, stress. "Stress" may be caused by an intermittent decreased supply of oxygen. If this is occurring, it is a form of uteroplacental insufficiency, meaning that the placenta is not adequately supplying the baby.

Fetal heart rate interpretation is a subtle and complex task. It cannot be simplified to the absence or presence of decelerations.

612

Q *What are heart rate decelerations?*

A Fetal heart rate decelerations are exactly that, slowings of the fetal heart rate. The normal rate in labor may vary from around no to 170 beats per minute, but it may certainly go outside these ranges transiently without cause for alarm. The vast majority of the "decels" are physiological and not representative of any dangerous circumstance.

There are different types of decels. These decels are categorized by when they happen in relation to each contraction. If they occur at any time, they are called variable. If they occur before the start of the contraction they're called early, and if they occur after the start of the contraction and finish after the end of the contraction, they're referred to as late decels. They also have different characteristic shapes.

613

Q *Are some of these decels worse than others?*

A The physiology behind these heart rate changes is complex. In general, early and variable decels may accompany normal labor, even when they occur repetitively. Both may indicate intermittent umbilical cord compression or, particularly, head compression while pushing. These are usually not severe enough to be worrisome. Variable decels in response to head compression are a defensive reflex for the fetus. If you went to the newborn nursery and pushed on a baby's soft spot it would increase intracranial pressure. This triggers a reflex to slow the baby's heart rate defensively, lowering blood pressure. This is similar to what occurs in the pushing stage of labor. By the way, you'd get in big trouble if you actually went to the nursery and tried this!

614

Q *What about the third type, late decels?*

A Repetitive late decels are more likely to be a sign of significant stress to the baby, but it's not that simple. There are worrisome types of late decels and less worrisome types. Variability is thought to be even more important than actual rate.

615

Q *What is variability?*

A A healthy, well-oxygenated fetus will vary its heart rate by five to fifteen beats per minute almost constantly while awake. On the monitor this looks like a wiggly line. This is called beat-to-beat variability (BTBV) and is best assessed on an internal (fetal scalp electrode) monitor. There is also long-term variability, which is visible on an external monitor and reflects changes in rate over several minutes rather than from beat to beat.

A fetus is by definition not seriously compromised in terms of oxygenation if BTBV is present, no matter what the pattern of decels. Because there are entire books written on fetal heart rate interpretation, find out your doctor's opinion about your heart rate strip when he or she reviews it. Every situation has its own specific set of variables.

Decreased BTBV has causes other than decreased oxygen. Fetuses sleep in cycles of twenty to forty minutes and sleep will take the wiggliness out of the heart rate tracing. A similar effect occurs with administration of any of the narcotics mentioned earlier. Depending on agent and dosage, this effect may last from one to two hours.

Intrauterine Resuscitation

616

Q *If the doctor thinks there might be a problem, is a C-section mandatory?*

A Not necessarily. Intrauterine resuscitation means changing things for mother to improve the supply of oxygen to the fetus. Common maneuvers include increasing your IV rate, having you turn to your side, and administering oxygen by mask. Often these simple changes alone will be adequate to improve the FHR tracing.

617

Q *Other than a C-section, what else can the doctor do if my baby is having a lot of decels?*

A That depends on many factors. If you are in the second stage and the baby is at +2 station or better, your doctor may suggest delivery with forceps or a vacuum extractor. If you are still in the first stage and having repetitive decels of the variable sort, your doctor may recommend amnioinfusion.

618

Q *What is amnioinfusion?*

A Amnioinfusion involves using the intrauterine pressure catheter (IUPC) described above, and infusing saline (sterile salt water) into the uterine cavity around the baby. This fluid may increase the "cushion" around the baby so that umbilical cord compression is relieved. It may also serve to dilute meconium in the fluid and make it potentially less dangerous. It is a recent technique used extensively only since the mid1990s and may not be used in your institution.

619

Q *What happens if change of position, oxygen, increased intravenous fluid, and amnioinfusion fail to resolve the decels?*

A Your doctor will probably recommend delivery by whatever route he or she feels is fastest and safest at the time, be that forceps, vacuum, or cesarean section. (See Section 8: Obstetric Complications)

620

Q *Isn't it better if I'm up walking around in early labor?*

A Most providers would agree that ambulating in early labor is a good idea. Whether it actually hastens the latent phase is unclear, but at least it keeps your circulation moving, avoids stiffness, and alleviates boredom.

621

Q *Can I eat in labor?*

A Eating in labor is usually discouraged by most providers. The concern is that you might need immediate general anesthesia, and vomit can be aspirated (breathed in) and lead to a fatal aspiration pneumonia. Consequently, oral intake in labor is usually restricted to clear liquids, hard candies, and popsicles. (See Section 6: Prepared Childbirth)

FIRST STAGE

Progress: Dilation and Effacement

622

Q *After I've been checked, admitted, and determined to be in labor, when will I be checked again?*

A Rechecking the cervix is dependent to some extent on how far dilated and effaced you were on first examination. If your contractions remain at every two to four minutes and are of increasing intensity, you will be checked either when you feel that you need pain medicine, or when you have a significantly different sensation, such as pressure in the rectum.

623

Q *Do I have to dilate to make "progress"?*

A No. Especially with first labors, you may spend several hours in early labor without changing dilation. However, progress may be manifested by descent of the head, the cervix moving forward, or the cervix effacing. All of these things frequently occur with little or no dilation.

Pain Management
(See Section 5: Drugs in Pregnancy; Section 6: Prepared Childbirth)

624

Q *If I've been in labor for several hours, used my relaxation and breathing techniques, and still feel that I need pain medicine, what can I have?*

A (See Section 5: Drugs in Pregnancy; Section 6: Prepared Childbirth)
Pain may be managed in many ways in pregnancy. A large portion of Section 6 is devoted to questions in this area.

In the latent phase of labor, prior to dilation of five centimeters, pain medicine is usually restricted to the use of several different narcotics and their derivatives. Demerol, morphine, Stadol, and Nubain are the medicines commonly administered, often in combination with an antinausea phenothiazine sedative such as Phenergan.

All of these medicines may help you relax between contractions and regain control. Some women are concerned that narcotics make it easier to lose control, rather than help them regain it. Certainly everyone reacts differently. Often women who *must be* in control do poorly on narcotics. Narcotics tend to be disinhibiting in many women. However, for other women, they take the edge off just enough to avoid panic. (See Section 6: Panic)

625

Q *I've heard that narcotics cross the placenta. Couldn't that harm the baby?*

A Narcotics do indeed cross the placenta to the baby. If given in the proper doses at the correct times, however, there is virtually no risk to the baby. This is why they are used most commonly in the latent phase or early active phase of the first stage. (See Stages above)

Large doses of narcotic given close to delivery can lead to respiratory depression (slowed breathing) in the newborn. Usually stimulation is all the baby needs with occasional oxygen supplementation briefly. Rarely, the failure to breathe vigorously may be more severe. In that instance, the effect of the narcotic can be reversed in less than two minutes by giving a narcotic antagonist such as Narcan to the baby.

626

Q *Other than taking narcotics, what else can I do if my breathing and relaxation techniques seem inadequate?*

A These techniques are less likely to fail you if you have a professional doula in the room all the time, or if the labor nurses have been doula trained. (See Section 6: Prepared Childbirth) However, there are some other things that can be tried. Many women, especially those with back labors, benefit not only from massage to the low back, but also from a hot shower directed to the low back. In some centers, you may be able to take a warm bath as well. This is usually recommended when your bag of waters is intact and there is no reason for continuous monitoring.

Bring along music tapes or CDs to help you relax. These may be recordings with special significance to you and your partner, or simply the kind of music you enjoy the most. Be sure to check ahead of time if the labor room is equipped with CD or audiocassette players. If not, bring your own equipment.

Epidurals
(See Section 5: Drugs in Pregnancy; Section 6: Prepared Childbirth-Epidurals)

627

Q *When can I get an epidural if I want one?*

A When best to place an epidural, how to dose it, and what to dose it with, are all controversial areas in obstetrics and anesthesia. No one agrees on everything. In general, you may avoid a slowing of your labor which some doctors feel may occur with epidurals if you wait until the active phase of labor, when you are dilated four to five centimeters and the baby's head is down to zero station. If this is not your first labor, then these criteria may safely be relaxed somewhat. For instance, an epidural may be placed with the baby's head at -1 or -2 station and the cervix dilated only three to four centimeters with your second or third labor.

628

Q *What exactly is the controversy about?*

A (See also Section 8: Cesarean Section and Section 6: Epidurals)
One camp believes that regional anesthesia (local anesthetic used to block a large area of the body while awake) seriously interferes with the normal labor process. This interference can take the form of slowing or stopping the active phase, or, more commonly, interfering with descent during the second or pushing stage. This, they say and also show with the literature, increases the forceps, vacuum, and C-section rate.

The other camp thinks this is untrue. They have equally extensive literature to show that the labor epidural causes none of the above problems, and is merely an effective, safe, humane way to relieve a person's suffering.[2]

629

Q *How can the literature support both sides of the argument?*

A Easy. These studies are almost always comparing apples and oranges. Different "caine" drugs (Lidocaine, Marcaine, Ropivicaine, Nesacaine) can all have different effects. The effects differ even with the same drug from one provider to the next due to dosage and rate of administration if given continuously. Furthermore, they differ from one patient to the next due to rates of metabolism and also to exactly where the catheter is placed in the back.

630

Q *How can the catheter make a difference?*

A When an epidural is placed in labor, it is usually initially dosed through the epidural needle, and then a small plastic catheter is inserted. This catheter is advanced blindly, by feel, into the epidural space. The end that protrudes is then taped to your back and over your shoulder. Depending on the individual case, it is then attached to a computerized pump, which can deliver a very precise dose of the drug continuously.

If the catheter is either chinked in the space in your back, or advanced out an individual nerve root sheath, your pain relief will not be evenly distributed. Simply pulling back the catheter several centimeters may be all that's necessary to fix the problem.

631

Q *What is a "walking epidural"?*

A (See Section 6: Prepared Childbirth)
A walking epidural is just that, one which allows you to walk in labor. These are discussed in Section 6: Epidurals.

632

Q *What does the term "intrathecal" mean?*

A Epidural means "outside the dura." The dura refers to the layer of membrane that surrounds and encases the cerebrospinal fluid space. In labor, epidurals are placed significantly below the end of the spinal column itself and in the epidural space outside the area that contains cerebrospinal fluid.

Placing a needle into the "intrathecal" space is what we normally refer to as a spinal anesthetic. Spinals are quick to put in place, have a quick onset, and traditionally have caused complete numbness in the buttock, perineal, and under-thigh regions. This low spinal, used extensively before epidurals, was called a saddle block for obvious reasons.

In the late 1990s, regional labor analgesia has been achieved with intra-thecal narcotics such as sufentanil. A one-time injection mixed with a small amount of dilute bupivicaine gives about 130 minutes of "walking" pain relief. This is essentially a "walking spinal" and is used in some centers.

633

Q *When is a spinal used instead of an epidural?*

A (See Section 6: Prepared Childbirth)
Traditionally a spinal anesthetic has been used to establish a rapid-onset, dense block right before delivery. This is referred to as a saddle block because it numbs the areas that would roughly come in contact with a saddle.

It is also used with a larger dosage to establish anesthesia for C-section, when there is no time to wait for an epidural to "set up." Normally, it is not continuous (no catheter in your back), so therefore the block lasts for a limited time, about an hour.

634

Q *Will I have to have a catheter in my bladder if I have an epidural?*

A A foley catheter is not necessarily a requirement with an epidural, although one may be necessary in labor for several reasons. First, swelling of the external genitalia combined with descent of the baby's head and compression of the urethra may make urinating impossible for some women in the second stage. A more dense epidural that significantly alters sensation or one's ability to move may make voiding impossible or at least inconvenient even in the first stage.

In any event, a foley catheter is a soft rubber tube placed in the urethra (through which you urinate), with a small inflatable balloon which keeps it from falling out. It is then attached to a bag on the floor. The catheter can easily be removed at any time, and usually is removed with pushing or shortly before delivery in any event unless a cesarean is performed. With a cesarean, the catheter must be in place during the surgery to keep the bladder empty and out of the way, and is left in place for the first twelve to twenty-four hours after delivery.

635

Q *What kind of problems can one have with an epidural?*

A (See Section 6: Prepared Childbirth)
Epidural side effects are discussed extensively in Section 6: Epidurals.

636

Q *If I get an epidural after four to five centimeters, will I feel the contractions?*

A That depends on the dose and type of medicine. The goal would be
to relieve your pain, but still have you aware of when each tightening
occurs, and to do so without loss of leg mobility.

637

Q *What if the epidural doesn't work?*

A If an epidural catheter is in the right place, it will work. Some people may
get "hot spots," meaning areas that are less numb than others. Since the
medicine is distributed by gravity, this can often be corrected by positioning
the patient, by repositioning the catheter, or by removing it and replacing it at
a different interspace (space between the vertebrae).

Failure to Progress

638

Q *I know I will dilate more slowly in the latent phase than in the active phase, but what
if I'm not changing at all after some point and I am still less than four centimeters?*

A There is tremendous leeway given for slow progress in the latent phase.
The fundamental principle is patience. If the baby is tolerating contractions, you have no fever, and there is no sign of infection, then you simply
wait. If the contractions are becoming less intense after you've already made
progress and then stalled, there are several options.

The bag of waters can be ruptured if it is still intact. You can be
encouraged to walk if you've been lying down, or Pitocin augmentation
can be instituted.

639

Q *What is Pitocin augmentation?*

A Pitocin augmentation is the use of the synthetic hormone oxytocin,
administered intravenously by a controlled infusion pump, with the

intent of gradually strengthening the force of your contractions and bringing them to a frequency of at least every three minutes.

640

Q *What if I've made it past five centimeters but then stop dilating?*

A Failure to dilate further or descend further after five centimeters is called an active phase arrest. This means that your progress has stopped, or arrested. There are only a few reasons for this, and only one that we can do anything to change.

Your baby is too large to fit into your pelvic inlet. This is the least likely reason. It is called CPD, for cephalopelvic disproportion (or as mentioned earlier, I call it BNF, for "baby no fit")

Your baby is in a position where it cannot enter the inlet (for example, in occiput posterior face up position (See Section 6: Prepared Childbirth)

Your uterus isn't contracting well (Stupid Uterus Syndrome, or SUS as I like to call it)

Only the last reason can be actively corrected, by Pitocin administration. Babies can be manually rotated (head turned with the examiner's hand) or rotated with forceps, but not until the cervix is completely dilated and the head has descended in the second stage.

641

Q *Is an active phase arrest the only time Pitocin might be used in the active phase of labor?*

A No. Pitocin might be used if your progress has not halted, but is slower than normal. Usually, after you reach five centimeters, you will dilate about one to two centimeters per hour, often faster if it's not your first labor. If you progress less rapidly than this, it's called a slow slope active phase. This can be just because your uterus needs some help, or it can be a red flag that perhaps the baby is too big or in the wrong position.

642

Q *What is an IUPC?*

A (See Section 6: Prepared Childbirth)
IUPC stands for intrauterine pressure catheter. The external belt only tells us when you're contracting, not how hard. The IUPC actually measures the intensity of each contraction in mmHg (millimeters of mercury.)

This intensity times the number of contractions in ten minutes gives us the Montevideo Units (mU), which permits a comparison of the performance of your uterus to known standards generated over hundreds of thousands of labors.

If you reach more than 200 mU for over two hours and make no progress, it is extremely unlikely that you will progress any further and continuing labor might even be dangerous. This would constitute a reason for C-section. (See Section 8: Cesarean Section)

SECOND STAGE

Progress: Descent

643

Q *When does the second stage begin?*

A (See Section 6: Prepared Childbirth)
The Second Stage for more discussion) The second stage is the "pushing" stage and begins after your cervix is dilated ten centimeters as estimated on examination.

644

Q *What does descent mean?*

A After the cervix has dilated completely and retracted over the baby's head, the head will continue its movement down the birth canal. (See Section 6: Female Reproductive Anatomy) This movement is quantified with estimates of Station. Above the pelvic inlet (floating) is -3 or -4, halfway down the canal is 0, and crowning when delivery is imminent is +3.

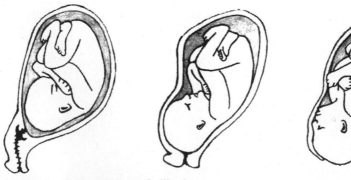

cervical effacement and dilation

The numbers refer to number of centimeters above (minus) or below (plus) the midplane of the pelvis defined as the line between the ischial spines. These are bony points that protrude from your pelvis into the lateral floor of the vagina.

645

Q *How long does it take to push the baby all the way out?*

A That varies tremendously. On average, you can expect to push about one-and-a-half to three hours with a first baby. Subsequent babies may take as little as one push over a two-minute period to just as long as your first labor. In general, pushing without an epidural may take a little less time than with an epidural.

The time it takes to push varies with epidural type and dosage as well as position of the baby. Pushing out a baby in the occiput posterior position may take a little longer, or the baby may even need to be rotated. (See Section 6: Prepared Childbirth)

Pushing may be approached in as many ways as there are people. In general, the idea is to concentrate your energies in your abdominal wall musculature. When partially reclining, you will pull your knees up and out, often with your husband and nurse supporting the underside of your feet. Pushing is accomplished with your chin on your chest and your body curled up like the letter "C After a cleansing breath as the contraction builds, you will inhale and hold your breath and then bear down similar to a bowel movement, usually for a count of ten. This is repeated three or four times with each contraction.

646

Q *Why do some women push for ten minutes and others for four hours?*

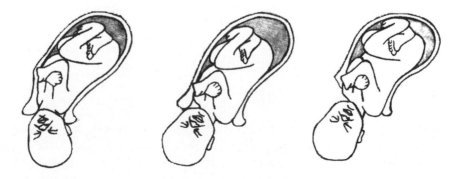

A Different-sized babies, different positions, different shapes to the pelvis, different amounts of numbness, and different degrees of stamina all contribute to this variance.

In general, deliveries subsequent to the first involve shorter second stages. The strong connective tissue that supports the uterus and bladder like a trampoline is stretched after the first vaginal delivery. This contributes to second babies feeling "lower" than first babies through the whole pregnancy, as well as making the second stage much easier.

Delivery

647

Q *What does "crowning" mean?*

A Crowning means that the "crown" of the baby's head is visible at the introitus! Once you can see the head start to stretch the perineum, and an area of the baby's head the size of a silver dollar is still visible between pushes, then you are crowning. Crowning implies that delivery is imminent, that is, it's usually only a few pushes away. It's time for your husband to find the camera and turn it on.

648

Q *Will I just deliver in bed?*

A Certainly women have done that for millennia, but nowadays we usually try to help "control" the delivery. This means breaking down the foot of a birthing bed so your provider can get close to you. With your feet positioned on pedals so that your legs are wide apart or, more frequently, with your lower legs in stirruplike supports, your doctor or midwife can comfortably help guide your baby's head down (below the level of the bed) and out from under the pubic arch.

649

Q *What is restitution?*

A Restitution means that after your baby's head is out, it will automatically turn to one side or the other, depending on which way the baby's chest is facing. After checking with a finger to make sure the cord is not around the neck, the head is gently guided toward the floor in order to help the anterior (front of your body) shoulder pass beneath the pubic bone. Once the shoulders are delivered, the rest of the body will try to "pop" out and along with it, often an ocean of amniotic fluid!

650

Q *What if the cord is around the neck?*

A A cord around the neck is called a nuchal cord and surprisingly happens with about a third of all deliveries. If the cord is felt with a finger to be nuchal, first an attempt is made to "reduce it," meaning to pass the loop over the already delivered head. If it is too tight, two clamps must be slipped by the head, placed carefully around the cord, with one jaw of each clamp between the neck and cord, closed, and the cord cut between. Otherwise, delivery will not be possible, or could rupture the cord. Rupture of the cord during delivery can cause catastrophic blood loss to the fetus, who has only about 280 cc of blood in all.

Some parents are concerned about the nuchal cord causing brain damage and even stillbirth by strangling the baby. Unfortunately, the misinformation about nuchal cords probably got started with compassionate doctors trying to explain otherwise unexplainable stillbirths. Babies don't breathe through their neck. They breathe through their umbilical cord. Thus, a cord wrapped around a leg, arm, or shoulder and chest is no different than one wrapped around the neck. Compression of the neck by the cord is rarely dangerous.

It is instead the compression of the cord, not the neck, that is potentially dangerous. Cords are very well protected by muscular vessels and a jelly-like substance called Wharton's jelly. It is tough to significantly compress a healthy cord.

651

Q *What is a shoulder dystocia?*

A Shoulder dystocia occurs when the shoulders are too wide to fit through the pelvic outlet. (See Section 6: Female Reproductive Anatomy). It is the obstetrician's worst nightmare, but can almost always be handled safely with a level head and a few maneuvers. (See Section 8: Shoulder Dystocia)

Episiotomy

652

Q *What is an episiotomy?*

A (See Section 6: Prepared Childbirth-Episiotomy)
Episiotomy is the term given to any number of types of incisions made, usually with scissors, into the skin between the back of the vaginal opening (fourchette) and the anus. This tissue is called the perineum. The purpose of the incision is to allow the vaginal opening to accommodate the size of the baby without tearing.

653

Q *Is it true that doctors do episiotomies and midwives don't?*

A No, it's not true. (See full discussion under Prepared Childbirth)

654

Q *Surely episiotomies must hurt a lot?*

A Episiotomies usually do not hurt severely when performed. Either an adequate epidural or saddle block is in place, local anesthetic is used as a pudendal block, or a local anesthetic is used just in the perineum. Even when there is no time for local anesthesia, the thinning of the perineal skin forces blood away from the area and there is a certain degree of numbing from this effect.

Episiotomies tend to hurt more afterward. The degree of pain will vary from one woman to the next, and is dependent on the type of episiotomy and repair performed.

655

Q *What are the types of episiotomy?*

A The midline episiotomy, as you would expect, involves a small incision straight toward the anus. A mediolateral episiotomy angles from the fourchette down and out at about thirty degrees off the midline, the intent being to avoid extension into the anus and rectum. A hockey stick episiotomy, also called a paramedian episiotomy, begins heading toward the rectum in the midline, but then swerves off to one side or the other just before the anal sphincter.

One type of episiotomy is not better than another. The type of episiotomy used is individualized to the particular patient and the particular delivery. Some women have long perineal bodies (distance from vagina to rectum) and others have very short perineums. Some women get tremendous swelling with pushing, making the tissue fragile and tearable like tissue paper, and others have no swelling and the tissue is more elastic. Some women have very large hemorrhoids and others have none.

Finally, your provider's training will dictate with which incisions he or she is most comfortable.

656

Q *Won't perineal massage prevent the need for an episiotomy?*

A Perineal massage performed during pushing may well help stretch out the skin as well as help you realize "where" to push. (See Section 6: Prepared Childbirth) It usually involves the thumb and first two fingers of the examiner, using one hand or both. Swelling (edema) is massaged out of the way, thinning the skin, and pressure is applied to the inside of the fourchette. This helps gradually stretch the tissue and may sometimes help avoid an episiotomy. Even with massage, about 70 to 80 percent of first-time laborers will need an episiotomy, or tear. A much smaller percentage may require episiotomy if they have already delivered vaginally in the past.

657

Q *Aren't we supposed to practice perineal massage at home before going into labor?*

A You may certainly practice, but there is no clear benefit until performing the massage in the second stage of labor. This is analogous to preparation of the nipples for breast-feeding. There is no good evidence that prelabor perineal massage prevents episiotomy.

658

Q *Is there a circumstance that almost always dictates use of an episiotomy?*

A Use of almost any type of forceps usually requires an episiotomy. The combined thickness of both forceps blades is necessarily added to the diameter of the head already coming through the introitus, and severe tears are more likely in the absence of an episiotomy.

659

Q *How is an episiotomy repaired?*

A Episiotomies are repaired with absorbable stitches. Often the incision must be closed in multiple layers. This is usually done with a continuous stitch, in and out, like hemming a skirt. These stitches do not need to be removed at a later time but disappear on their own after several weeks.

Your doctor may give you special instructions on how to care for an episiotomy after delivery, but a few constants exist. It is a good idea to place an ice pack on the perineum for the first eight to twelve hours after delivery. This will serve to decrease the swelling as well as relieve pain. Between twelve and twenty-four hours it is usual to switch to heat. Hot sitz baths followed by the dry heat of a perilamp placed between your legs in the bed, or the heat from a handheld hair dryer after the bath, is soothing and helps draw blood back to the area, promoting healing.

Rinsing the area with a squirt bottle after bowel movements is useful. Avoid constipation. If you have no bowel movement by about sixty hours after delivery, use milk of magnesia. If you have had trouble with constipation, consider using a stool softener such as Colace or Surfac twice a day from the time of delivery on. Remember, you can use flushable baby wipes on your own bottom instead of toilet paper. This might help with the hemorrhoids. (No reason to rub wood pulp on a tender area, is there?)

Forceps and Vacuum Extractors

660

Q *For what reason might my doctor feel forceps were necessary?*

A Forceps are used in three major circumstances—fetal distress, maternal exhaustion, and a time limit imposition. The type of forceps chosen will depend on the station, position, and molding of the baby's head.

661

Q *Is there more than one type of forcep?*

A Yes. Forceps are applied to either side of the fetal head, and then traction is applied on the handles that protrude from the vagina. Contrary to popular belief, the forceps don't squash the head, but work mostly by pulling on the angle of the jaw. The most common types of forceps include Tuckers, Tucker-McClain, Elliots, Liukhart, Liukhart-McClain, Liukhart-Tucker-McClains, Simpsons, Baby Elliots, Baby Simpsons, Keillands, Bartons, and Piper.

Each is for special circumstances, meaning position and station of the head, the degree of molding, and the amount of caput. The degree to which the head is canted front to back (asynclitism) is important as well.

662

Q *What's a vacuum extractor?*

A Vacuum extractors, like forceps, are instruments used to help get the baby delivered when you're either having trouble pushing it out, or it needs to be delivered in a hurry because it's in trouble (experiencing fetal distress). Unlike forceps, the instrument works by creating a vacuum over the crown of the head (suction), which allows traction to be applied.

663

Q *What's the advantage of using one over the other if both forceps and vacuum extractor are used to "pull" the baby out if I can't push it?*

A The advantages to a vacuum extractor are that it can be applied with little experience, is less likely to lacerate the inside walls of the vagina, requires no anesthesia, and does not increase the diameter of what needs to come through the vaginal opening.

The advantage of forceps is that more traction can be applied in circumstances where the vacuum extractor would just pop off, and they can be used for special tasks, such as rotating the head.

664

Q *What is the time limit on pushing?*

A The second stage of labor can be almost as variable as the first stage in terms of duration. Every mother and baby are different. However, problems tend to occur more frequently when pushing is allowed to exceed three hours without and four hours with an epidural.

665

Q *Maternal exhaustion sounds bad. When does that occur?*

A Maternal exhaustion means simply that you are no longer able to gather the energy necessary to continue pushing. The advice of your doctor and nurse are essential here. Sometimes you're right about the necessity to give up—the baby just isn't going to come out the vagina. Sometimes you just need a little help with forceps or vacuum extractor, and sometimes you just need a bit of forceful encouragement.

666

Q *How often do instrumented vaginal deliveries occur?*

A The incidence of forceps or vacuum deliveries varies geographically. It is influenced by the doctor's training, the use and kind of epidurals, and the ethnic heterogeneity of the population. In the United States, instrumented vaginal delivery occurs between about 6 to 20 percent of the time.

667

Q *I've heard that forceps are dangerous. I don't want to take a chance on my baby's skull being fractured, or the delivery affecting his intelligence. Shouldn't I just refuse to allow forceps?*

A In actuality, in experienced hands, the danger with forceps is more to the vaginal wall than to your baby's head. Forceps have been used since the mid-seventeenth century. Certainly in the hands of the novice, or in the hands of someone with poor judgment, any of the forceps listed above could be misapplied and potentially injure a baby. However, forceps can also save your baby's life. If, for example, your placenta pulls away from the uterine wall while pushing (abruption), and your baby needs immediate delivery, it may take ten to fifteen minutes to get the baby delivered by C-section in the best of circumstances. The ten minutes saved with forceps can be critical.

Large studies, including a 1991 review of 32,000 deliveries, all of which occurred at least seventeen years before, showed no difference in scores on intelligence tests among those delivered by forceps, vacuum extractor, or cesarean.[3]

Discuss these issues with your doctor ahead of time if you are particularly worried about this aspect of delivery. It may not even be an issue, because some obstetricians today prefer the vacuum extractor and rarely use forceps.

668

Q *What is different about outlet forceps and midforceps?*

A The exact definitions change from time to time, but both outlet and low II forceps mean that the baby is almost out. For forceps to be outlet, the sagittal or midline suture must go straight from front to back (AP, or anterior-posterior) and the baby's scalp must be visible between pushes. For low forceps, there may be a little turn to the baby's head so that the suture is off the midline by less than forty-five degrees, but the baby must still be +2 station or better.

Midforceps with or without rotation are used less frequently now that the cesarean has become so safe. This procedure involves attempting delivery with the head still at +1 station or above. It is much more likely to be associated with injury to the mother or baby than are low or outlet forceps. Over 90 percent of forceps deliveries performed today are done as low or outlet forceps and pose little or no danger.

669

Q *What are the dangers of the vacuum extractor?*

A The vacuum extractor was invented by Malmstrom in 1954. His device was a shallow metal cup attached to a chain for a handle. A rubber tube was affixed to a port on the dome so that a glass cylinder and pump could be used to generate the vacuum. Tremendous force could be applied, and it soon became clear that cephalohematoma was a potential complication. Cephalohematoma is bleeding under the scalp and, in rare cases, dangerous amounts of blood can be lost in this way.

Today's vacuum extractors are made of plastic. The cup is soft, not metal, and the amount of suction applied is controlled by a hand pump and gauge. Importantly, it is almost impossible to apply too much suction or traction because the cup simply pops off. This may lead to an increased caput, but cephalohematoma is extremely rare.

DELIVERY

670

Q *I want my mother and my husband in delivery with me . Is that a problem?*

This must be discussed with your provider. Different health professionals have different feelings about whom they are comfortable having in the delivery room. In general, your husband and one other person will always be allowed. Often, doctors and institutions will allow even more people to be present if you desire.

If you want to have your mother there, but not your husband's mother, make sure you handle the potential problem of hurt feelings honestly and tactfully long before your due date. Grandparents get extremely excited and concerned. Explain that you feel more comfortable with your own mother present. After all, it is you who have the risk and undertake the physical stress of the ordeal. Avoid the temptation to make an argument that there is more of a rationale for your mother's presence than your mother-in-law's. You don't have to justify your decisions about sharing your private moments with anyone.

Do not falsify your doctor's or the hospital's policies to justify your own arrangement of family members. If you tell them it's hospital policy to have only one other family member present when it is your desire, and not truly policy, then twenty people will stream out of the labor room next to yours and you'll have some " 'splainin' to do!"

671

Q *Can we have someone video the delivery?*

A Video cameras in the delivery area are usually permitted as long as a tripod is not used. Some institutions have prohibited video cameras because of the way tapes can be edited to portray a circumstance unfairly. This footage could potentially be used later in a civil suit.

Using a still camera is also a good way to capture the moment of birth. The flash will not hurt your baby's eyes.

672

Q *What will happen at the moment the baby comes out?*

A When everything goes well, those helping you will let you know as your final pushes are approaching. Many women prefer to use a large mirror so they can see the effect of each push.

The doctor or midwife will control the delivery of the head. This means they will use both hands to help ease the head out of the vagina. There are several maneuvers they can perform to try and keep you from tearing. They may instruct you to push less forcefully as the head comes out. Once the head is delivered you will stop pushing for a moment while the doctor checks for a cord around the neck and suctions out the baby's mouth and nose. Then your provider will ease out the shoulder under the pubic bone, and the rest of the baby usually pops out.

673

Q *When and how is the cord actually cut?*

A Usually, babies are held below the level of the table, head down, during suctioning of the mouth and nose and while stimulating the baby to cry. After excess blood has drained from the placenta into the baby, a plastic cord clamp is placed close to the baby, a metal clamp is placed on the side toward the placenta, and the cord severed between the two. Some obstetricians may allow your partner to cut the cord if the circumstances are appropriate and no emergency exists.

674

Q *When can I hold my baby?*

A In some institutions, you may hold your baby right away. In most hospitals the baby will first be stimulated to breathe on her own, but if no meconium is present and she gives a vigorous cry, you may have her immediately. A nurse will help you and your husband dry the baby, since newborns lose heat rapidly from evaporation. Then the baby may either remain on your chest skin to skin, or wrapped in a blanket as the situation demands.

Often, with babies who seem to be "gurgling" on lots of amniotic fluid, a few minutes with head down on the slanted radiant warmer combined with suctioning will help the baby become pink.

675

Q *Will my baby be pink right away?*

A Usually not. Babies have a lot going on in the first few minutes of life. (See Section 4: Fetal Development) The connection between the two upper chambers of the heart (foramen ovale) is closing. The connection between the pulmonary artery and the aorta (ductus arteriosis) is closing. The lungs are being expanded with air. The heart is pumping against massively increased pressures after the cord is clamped.

While all this is happening, the healthy baby shunts oxygenated blood away from the skin and into the heart, kidneys, lungs, and brain. This often leaves the skin with a bluish tint that is perfectly normal. After about four or five minutes of vigorous crying, the newborn will begin to send oxygenated blood to less essential areas such as the skin. Hands and feet may stay blue, however, for hours.

676

Q *What is that cheesy material I saw all over my sister's baby?*

A Vernix caseosa looks like cold cream and probably protects the baby's skin even better. (See Section 4: Fetal Development) It is actually desquamated (shedding) skin cells, but it serves to protect the fetus's skin in the latter weeks of pregnancy. Usually it is mostly gone by forty to forty-one weeks. This is a fairly reliable sign of gestational age, such that if a lot of vernix is present at delivery it is more likely that the baby is at less than thirty-nine weeks of gestation (or thirty-seven weeks from conception).

677

Q *How long will the baby stay with us?*

A (See Section 6: Prepared Childbirth)
Every institution has its own policies and procedures. In most, you will not be separated from the baby for at least an hour after delivery if it's healthy in all respects. In some hospitals, after an hour in which you may have breast-fed initially, and shown the baby to the proud grandparents, the newborn and your husband will head to the nursery to be checked in.

678

Q *Why might the baby not be allowed to stay with us?*

A If after five minutes your baby still appears blue, is working hard to breathe (nasal flaring, or chest or rib retraction), has suspected meconium aspiration, weighs more than nine pounds (could drop sugar levels rapidly), remains limp with poor muscle tone, or is suspected of infection, your baby might be taken to the nursery shortly after birth.

THIRD STAGE

679

Q *What is the third stage of labor?*

The third stage of labor is that time period between delivery of the baby and delivery of the placenta. Gentle traction on the umbilical cord may be applied by your doctor not to remove the placenta by force, but to help the placenta through the cervix and out the vagina after it separates. It usually takes about five to twenty minutes for the placenta to separate, and this is immediately preceded by an often sizable gush of red blood.

After the placenta has delivered, the doctor or midwife will often massage your uterus with one hand on your abdomen for several moments. Remember that bleeding from the uterus is controlled entirely by uterine contraction. You will receive oxytocin in your IV to help contract your uterus as well.

680

Q *I shook like a leaf after my last baby was delivered. Why does that happen?*

A Postpartum shaking is an extremely common phenomenon. It often occurs shortly after delivery and may be related to the rush of adrenal steroids and epinephrine released at the time of birth. After all, it is physiologically probably the most demanding thing your body has ever endured.

A similar phenomenon occurs after epidural placement or dosing, and seems to be equally harmless.

681

Q *What happens if the placenta doesn't come out?*

A Retained placenta with a normal term pregnancy is unusual. It is a much more frequent occurrence with deliveries under thirty-four weeks. If it occurs after vaginal delivery, the doctor will perform a manual removal of the placenta. In this procedure the entire hand is placed up through the open cervix and a plane of separation between the uterus and the placenta is developed with fingertips. The placenta is then peeled off of the wall with the gloved hand. This procedure is well tolerated with an epidural in place and not as well tolerated without.

Manual removal is more likely to occur if the placenta separates partially. This allows excessive bleeding from the placental bed, which is now exposed because the rest of the placenta keeps the uterus from contracting around it. The placenta must be completely removed in order to stop the bleeding.

682

Q *How is my bleeding stopped if the uterus won't contract after delivery?*

A (See also Section 8: Obstetric Hemorrhage)

Uterine atony (lack of muscle "tone") is more likely with a piece of retained placenta, very long labors, very short labors, large babies, and preeclampsia. If bimanual massage with the doctor's fist against the lower uterine segment (in the vagina) and the other hand on your abdomen massaging the fundus fails to stop the bleeding, then various medicines are used, including oxytocin, methergine, and prostaglandin (Hemabate). If these methods fail, other surgical options remain as discussed in Section 8.

Admissions Nursery

683

Q *What happens in the admission nursery?*

A Admissions nurseries vary from place to place, but many of the routines will be similar. At some institutions, the following things occur:

1. Vitamin K is administered intramuscularly (to prevent bleeding in the brain).

2. Blood pressure is taken in all four extremities.

3. A heel stick done for AccuCheck (blood sugar level).

4. Modified Ballard or Dubowitz testing is performed on all babies (assesses development and thus gestational age).

5. Antibiotic ointment (erythromycin) is placed in the eyes to prevent blindness from sexually transmitted diseases (mandated by state law).

6. Vital signs (temperature, pulse, blood pressure) are taken every thirty minutes over a two-hour period.

7. Admissions bath performed after one hour if temperature is higher than 98.4 degrees Fahrenheit and the respiratory rate is less than 66.

8. If the baby is stable, with no heart murmur, a normal three-vessel cord, then triple dye is placed on the cord (avoids infection at site).

9. The baby is offered sips of water after the bath and given some formula if bottle-feeding.

10. The baby's pediatrician is notified that assessment is done and made aware if the mother was Group B Strep +, had a fever, or had prolonged rupture of membranes.

684

Q *I saw the nurses "dropping" my best friend's baby into the bassinet and then laughing. Are these nurses crazy?*

A Part of the newborn evaluation outlined above includes assessment of the Morrow reflex. This reflex involves grasping the newborn by the arms while he or she is on her back and gently lifting off the mat. Being careful to keep the head in contact with the mat at all times, the baby is then released. The sudden movement causes the baby to make a clapping motion. The same startle reflex can be elicited with a sharp hand-clap over the baby. This Morrow reflex is a sign of a healthy, neurologically intact newborn.

You may also see the nurses scrape the bottom of the baby's feet. This is to elicit another reflex called the Babinski. Healthy infants will curl their toes upward, unlike adults, who should curl their toes downward.

The rooting reflex is assessed by stroking the cheek. The baby should turn its head to that side as if looking for the breast. The suck is evaluated with the little finger of the examiner pressed against the roof of the baby's mouth. An automatic sucking will occur and the palate may be assessed at the same time.

685

Q *If my baby's on oxygen supplementation, will I be able to nurse him?*

A Brief periods of suckling might be permissible, but this will vary with the circumstance. Babies are obligate nasal breathers, meaning that unless they are crying, they cannot breathe through their mouths. Breast-feeding is hard work and the breast may partially obstruct the nasal openings, making breast-feeding unacceptable while your baby is having breathing difficulties and on oxygen.

686

Q *I specifically told the nursery not to give the baby sugar water, and they did it anyway. Why would they do this?*

A Sugar water can be lifesaving, especially for large babies with low heel stick sugars. Low sugars (hypoglycemia) can lead to seizures and brain damage if untreated. So keep these issues in perspective. There is no evidence that sugar water will discourage your baby from breast-feeding. Once your baby is stable and hungry, he or she will eat what you offer, whether breast, formula, or sugar water.

687

Q *Why do newborns get shots?*

A The most common newborn injection is vitamin K, which is known to help avoid bleeding internally by helping the baby's liver make blood clotting factors. Some babies require hepatitis immune globulin and hepatitis vaccine if their mothers have positive blood test screens for hepatitis. Other injections would depend on the specific indications at the time.

SUGGESTED READING

ACOG Patient Education Pamphlets. *You and Your Baby: Prenatal Care, Labor & Delivery, and Postpartum Care.*

American College of Ob/Gyn, 1995
   Main Switchboard 800-673-8444, (206) 638-5577
   Order Desk: 800-762-2264 ACOG
   Website: http://www.acog.com

Eisenberg, A. Murkhoff, and H. Hathaway, 1991. *What to Expect When You're Expecting.* New York: Workman Publishing.

Focus on Labor and Delivery. (Video) 115 min. 1990. Four expectant couples attend classes. Order #HX46604

Special Delivery. (Video) 42 min. 1988. Several couples before, during and after birth, some with MD, some with midwife. Order #HX 46636
   To Order Call: 1-800-299-3366 ext. 287 Childbirth Graphics, Div of WRS Group Inc.

WEBSITES

Anesthesia in Labor
   http://www.aana.com/laboranddelivery.aspx

Labor and Delivery
   http://www.babycenter.com/pregnancy/childbirth/index
   http://www.nlm.nih.gov/medlineplus/childbirth.html

Section Eight

Obstetric Complications

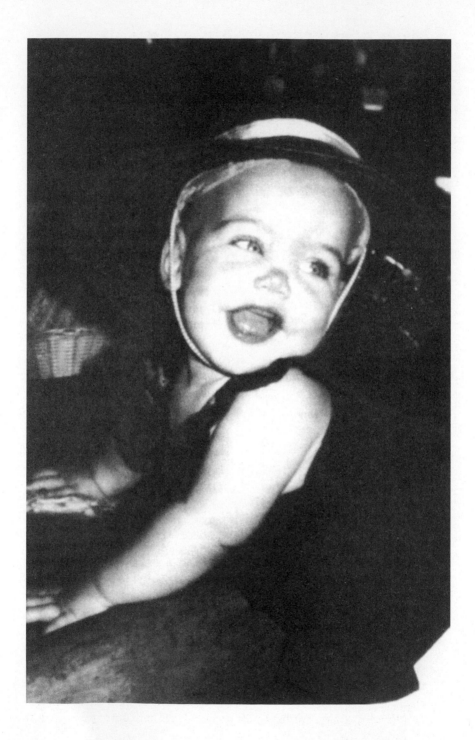

MOLAR PREGNANCY

(See Section 2: Miscarriage and Ectopic Pregnancy) Molar Pregnancy

688

Q *What is a "molar pregnancy"?*

A Molar Pregnancy is one of several types of gestational trophoblastic disease (GTD). It is seen in about one in a thousand pregnancies in the United States, but in as many as one in a hundred in some parts of Asia. In a molar pregnancy the uterus contains an abnormally growing placenta, but no fetus. Rarely this abnormal growth of the placenta can develop into an aggressive cancer called choriocarcinoma. All GTDs produce the human pregnancy hormone (HCG) and thus the disease's activity may be tracked with serial blood tests to follow the level of this hormone.

An excessive proliferation of the trophoblastic cells (see above) as well as swollen (hydropic) villi under the microscope, make the diagnosis of a hydatidiform mole. Most are genetically 46XX, with both X's coming from the father. Moles have a characteristic ultrasound appearance.

Gestational trophoblastic disease is divided into hydatidiform mole (either "complete" or "partial" sometimes with a fetus) and gestational trophoblastic tumors (invasive mole, choriocarcinoma, and placental site tumor).[1]

689

Q *What symptoms would make me suspect a molar pregnancy?*

A Most molar pregnancies are picked up on first trimester vaginal ultrasound nowadays. In the absence of ultrasound, persistent bleeding, failure to feel movement, an overly enlarged uterus, and an unusually high HCG level more than too days after the last menses all give clues to the diagnosis. Molar pregnancy may also be associated with severe hyperemesis (morning sickness).

About 20 percent of complete molar pregnancies go on to become gestational trophoblastic tumors even after evacuation by suction D & C. The diagnosis is made because HCG levels fail to fall to normal (lower than five). About 17 to 18 percent of the original moles become invasive moles, and about 2 percent become the malignant choriocarcinoma. All may be cured with methotrexate alone or in combination with other chemotherapy if diagnosed early enough.

If you have what you believe to be a complete spontaneous miscarriage on your own, but do not have any of the tissue that was passed to bring in so that a pathologist can examine it, you must have serial HCG levels drawn until they reach zero.

If you have had a molar pregnancy, you should use effective birth control for one year after HCG levels fall to zero; recently, six months has been considered acceptable.

ECTOPIC PREGNANCY AND MISCARRIAGE

(See Section 2 for full discussion)

THIRD TRIMESTER BLEEDING

690

Q *What do I do if I start bleeding later in pregnancy?*

A Call your doctor as soon as possible. Third trimester bleeding may be innocuous and nothing to worry about if, for instance, it is coming from a vessel in the cervix, but it might also be a sign of placenta previa or even placental abruption. (See Questions 691–696 in this section)

PLACENTA PREVIA

691

Q *What is placenta previa?*

A Placenta previa is simply the placenta "coming before," as the name implies. If the placenta implants so low in the uterus that it blocks the opening to the cervix, the baby either cannot deliver vaginally, or will do so with the potential for life-threatening loss of the mother's blood and/or fetal death by asphyxia as the placenta separates prior to delivery.

When the placenta is actually implanted across the opening of the cervix it is called a complete previa or total previa. If it either partially covers or nears the cervix, it is referred to as a partial previa or marginal previa, respectively. At term, slightly less than 1 percent of pregnancies actually have significant previas. Its incidence in first pregnancies is only one in fifteen hundred, but it is as high as one in twenty after a third delivery.

692

Q *How can previa occur in fewer than 1 percent of pregnancies when I know three women right now who were all told they had previas on their second trimester ultrasounds?*

A Placenta previa is "diagnosed" frequently at second trimester ultrasound; however, the lower uterine segment stretches more than the upper over the ensuing months and virtually all previas resolve, or seem to move away from the cervix. Of course, the placenta is implanted and can't move anywhere, but because of the way the uterus stretches, the distance from the placental edge to the cervix always increases, not vice versa. So the incidence of as high as 45 percent around sixteen to twenty weeks, of either low-lying placenta or placenta previa turns out to be extremely low at delivery. Usually the diagnosis in the second trimester will lead to a repeat sonogram around twenty-eight to thirty weeks to confirm that the previa has resolved.[2]

693

Q *Do I have to do anything different if I have a previa?*

A If a previa is still present in the early third trimester, sexual activity of any kind could lead to a catastrophic bleeding episode. This means any sexual activity that could cause orgasm must be avoided, not only intercourse, since the uterine contraction that accompanies orgasm may initiate the bleeding.

If the previa is still present by thirty-six weeks, a cesarean will be universally recommended when the time comes. If you have a bleeding episode with a known previa, you will be hospitalized. You are likely to have multiple episodes prior to delivery. Fifty percent of total previas and about 20 percent of marginals/partials bleed before thirty weeks.

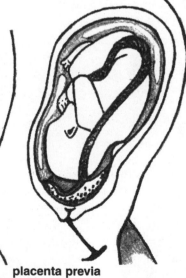

placenta previa

Timing of delivery will depend largely on gestational age and the severity of the bleeding. An attempt to assess lung maturity with amniocentesis is often made at thirty-six weeks, and if the lungs are mature, a cesarean can be performed electively. Elective C-section results in only 3 percent of the fetuses being anemic as opposed to emergency deliveries, where 28 percent of the fetuses are affected.[3]

As you can see, previa not only increases your risk of blood loss and surgery, but significantly increases the chances that you will be forced to deliver prematurely.

If you have already had a previa, your chances of having one again are about 8 to 10 percent. History of prior placenta previa or multiple C-sections are the strongest determinants of it occurring again.

Placenta accreta

694

Q *What is a placenta accreta?*

A Placenta accreta is a rare condition in which the placenta burrows not just into the lining of the uterus (the decidua), but actually into or even through the muscular uterine wall. In this circumstance, the placenta will not detach itself normally after delivery. When it burrows through the wall completely, called "percreta," maternal death is inevitable unless an emergency abdominal hysterectomy is performed.

Placenta accreta occurs with as many as 15 percent of placenta previas due to the thinner uterine lining in the lower uterine segment.

Vasa previa

695

Q *Is vasa previa different from placenta previa?*

A Vasa previa means "blood vessels coming first' In other words, it's not the placenta overlying the cervix as with placenta previa, but blood vessels in the membranes that carry fetal blood. This occurs only when the umbilical cord fails to insert in the body of the placenta, but instead attaches to the amniotic membranes some distance from the body of the placental disc. It occurs in about one in three thousand deliveries. With spontaneous or artificial rupture of these membranes, fetal death occurs about 75 percent of the time. Unfortunately, it is rarely diagnosed ahead of time, in which case an elective C-section could be performed, saving the fetus's life.

PLACENTAL ABRUPTION

696

Q *What is a placental abruption?*

A Placental abruption means the "abrupt" separation of the placenta from the uterine wall. It occurs in about 0.75 percent of pregnancies. The placental disc normally does not pull away from the wall of the uterus until sometime shortly after delivery. When it pulls away from the wall any time before delivery, whether in labor or prior to labor, there may be lethal consequences for the fetus and severe blood loss for the mother. Abruption severe enough to kill the fetus occurs in about one in four hundred deliveries, and the severe clotting disorder, DIC, occurs in about 30 percent of these cases. (See Section 9: Clotting Disorders)

Several factors increase the risk of abruption, including cigarette smoking, cocaine use, high blood pressure, trauma to the abdomen as in automobile accidents, uterine fibroids or uterine anomaly such as a septum, multiple repeat cesareans, and a very short umbilical cord. Parity (number of pregnancies) also increases risk, with incidence of less than 1 percent in the first pregnancy and more than 2.5 percent after three or more pregnancies.[4]

Abruptions present with vaginal bleeding 80 percent of the time, and usually in the third trimester. About 66 percent of women have pain in the abdomen, low back, or uterus. Uterine contractions, which classically are difficult to distinguish one from the other, or simply one continuous, unrelenting contraction, occur about 33 percent of the time. This type of contraction is called a tetanic contraction. At diagnosis, fetal monitoring shows a fetal distress rate of 60 percent, with 15 percent of fetuses having already died. In about 20 percent of the cases, the symptom is simply preterm labor until bleeding occurs or evidence of fetal distress develops.[5]

Treatment most of the time involves rapid delivery. Almost always this is by C-section. Vaginal delivery is sometimes appropriate when the fetus is determined on admission to have already died. With a very premature infant and/or a very small abruption, as evidenced by little bleeding and ultrasound evaluation of the clot behind the placenta, management may, rarely, be observation alone.

If you had a placental abruption with your last pregnancy, the risk of recurrence is quite high—perhaps as high as 1 in 8, or about 12 percent.[6]

PULMONARY EMBOLUS

(See Section 9: Medical Complications)

PREECLAMPSIA
(PREGNANCY-INDUCED HYPERTENSION)

697

Q *Are toxemia and preeclampsia the same thing?*

A Yes. Preeclampsia, which literally means "before seizure," is a pregnancy condition characterized by high blood pressure, edema (swelling), and/or protein spilling in the urine after the 10th week of gestation. It occurs in anywhere from 7 percent to 20 percent of cases, depending on definitions used for hypertension. In general, a blood pressure reading of over 140/90, and particularly a diastolic reading of more than 90 mmHg, combined with proteinuria, constitutes preeclampsia. Swelling is such a common occurrence with normal pregnancy that many experts feel it really has no place in the definition of preeclampsia.

Toxemia is a term developed early in this century based on a fundamental misunderstanding of the process. It was once thought that hypertension in pregnancy was due to circulating poisons, or "toxins," and thus the name. The term has been abandoned, as it should be.

Factors that clearly increase risk of preeclampsia include first pregnancy, twins, chronic hypertension, diabetes, family history, and advanced maternal age (over thirty-five) regardless of parity (number of previous pregnancies) and teen pregnancies. More controversial is the belief that poverty and being African American carry increased risk.

698

Q *What are the symptoms of preeclampsia?*

A One of the reasons for regular prenatal care is that preeclampsia, like diabetes in pregnancy, may have no symptoms at all early on. Preeclampsia is considered a vasospastic disease (blood vessel constriction) caused by the placenta; if you're going to get it, you've had it from the beginning of your pregnancy. Later on, preeclampsia of increasing severity is frequently associated with rapid weight gain over a short period, accompanied by increased swelling of not just your ankles, but particularly of your hands and face.

Severe preeclampsia may be suspected with a combination of symptoms involving the brain, eyesight, and abdominal pain. These include an intense headache, dizziness, and/or confusion; double or blurred vision;

scotomata (seeing stars); and very severe right upper quadrant belly pain just below the right breast. The symptoms may occur all together, or they may independently herald the onset of severe preeclampsia. Since placental abruption is also associated with preeclampsia, third trimester vaginal bleeding and abdominal pain over the uterus may also be symptoms of severe disease.

699

Q *What causes preeclampsia?*

A The cause is unknown. Some factor related to the placenta causes relative vasospasm (blood vessel constriction), which leads to increased blood pressure and transient damage to the kidneys that results in the spillage of protein.

For seventy-five years, experts have postulated different mechanisms with no uniform agreement. Recently it has been thought that some placental factor causes an alteration in the prostaglandin synthesis pathway such that a blood-vessel-dilating compound called prostacyclin is made in lesser amounts and a similar compound with opposite effects called thromboxane is made in greater amounts.[7]

Think of it like this. Your vascular system is a garden hose with the end clamped off. If you force more and more water into the hose, but the hose cannot dilate, the pressure inside increases. If the pressure inside gets high enough, the hose will start to leak. The pregnant woman's body normally retains water to expand blood volume in pregnancy. If her vessels don't dilate adequately, her blood pressure goes up. If the process continues, her "hoses" leak and she gets swollen, or edematous. When the kidneys have a relatively decreased blood supply because the renal arteries are constricted, they inappropriately retain more salt and water to correct what they perceive as an underfilled vascular space. A vicious cycle is then set in motion, and it can only end with delivery and removal of the placental products causing the problem.

700

Q *How is preeclampsia treated?*

A The only "cure" for preeclampsia is delivery. If you are diagnosed at a gestation where the risk to your fetus is estimated to be too great to recommend delivery, then that risk is balanced against the risk to your own health. Your doctor may well recommend bed rest on your side, either at home with home monitoring, or if severe enough, in the hospital. Hospitalization for severe disease may lead to the use of medicines such as hydrazoline (Apresoline) for your blood pressure and intravenous magnesium sulfate, both for your blood pressure and to prevent seizures.

Bed rest helps because it gets your enlarged abdomen off the major blood vessels that return blood to your heart, as well as the ones that supply blood to your kidneys and uterus. So, bed rest on your side—left a little better than right—improves cardiac output, improves blood supply to your kidneys, and improves oxygen and nutrition to your baby. Your kidneys are confused; they think they have to retain much more salt and water. If you supply them with more blood, they relax a little. The result is that you urinate more and, in a very short time, may improve your blood pressure and lose many pounds of edema fluid.

The danger of preeclampsia to your baby is that it leads to decreased blood supply to the uterus and also leads to blood vessel spasm in the placenta. In short, the placenta isn't as healthy as it should be and this can lead to growth-restricted babies and babies who tolerate the stresses of labor poorly. It is also associated with an increased risk of placental abruption (which is often lethal to the fetus), increased risk of premature delivery, and increased risk of maternal seizures and blood-clotting abnormalities such as diffuse intravascular coagulation (DIC). Seizures and DIC, although they are maternal problems, can prove to be extremely dangerous for your baby indirectly.

Preeclampsia means "preseizure." A small percentage of women with preeclampsia will go on to develop generalized tonic-clonic seizures and thus become labeled eclamptic. Seizures are dangerous due not only to the fact that they are a sign of cerebral edema (brain swelling), which can be fatal, but also because seizures are a hallmark of severe disease. Eclampsia is increasingly likely as term approaches, and seizures occur either before, during, or after delivery, with 97 percent developing before twenty-four hours after delivery.

But preeclampsia may also lead to blood-clotting problems such as DIC, as well as thrombocytopenia (low platelets). When these occur together with severe effects on your liver, it is called HELLP syndrome (H-Hypertension, EL-Elevated Liver Enzymes, LP-Low Platelets). Preeclampsia may adversely affect not only the liver, but also the kidneys, brain, heart, and lungs.

Preeclampsia can kill you. However, appropriately managed with magnesium sulfate, hydralazine, and timely delivery, the death rate approaches zero. Death is usually due to the very rare event of liver capsule rupture and bleeding internally, to hemorrhage associated with abruption of the placenta, or to untreated eclampsia.[8]

701

Q *What is DIC?*

A Diffuse intravascular coagulation (DIC) is a process more than a disease in that it usually is a complication of other diseases. These diseases include septic shock (overwhelming infection), preeclampsia, and placental abruption. The "LP" part of HELLP syndrome refers to low platelet levels that are often a part of impending DIC.

In DIC, also called consumptive coagulopathy, the underlying disease leads to the exhaustion, or consumption, of all of the body's clotting factors. Clotting factors are proteins made by the liver. With no clotting factors available and a concurrent lack of platelets, the patient may have life-threatening bleeding into a body cavity such as the lungs, or blood loss from any other traumatic insult to the body. These patients continue to bleed even from needle sticks.

DIC may be treated in a number of ways, including first whole blood transfusion, fresh frozen plasma, and, rarely, platelet transfusion.

702

Q *Can I do something to prevent preeclampsia if I'm at increased risk due to twins, previous preeclampsia, or chronic hypertension?*

A Possibly. Minidose aspirin (ASA) has been advocated by many since the late 1980s as a mechanism to prevent preeclampsia. You should discuss its use with your doctor if you have any of the factors that put you at high risk for preeclampsia such as hypertension, twins, or previous history of preeclampsia. Experts are not agreed on its effectiveness.

Minidose ASA alters the prostaglandin synthesis pathways and decreases the production of the type of prostaglandin that tends to dilate vessels to a lesser degree than it decreases the type that tends to constrict them (relative dilation).[9] Although some experts think that there is a beneficial effect to taking an 82-milligram children's chewable ASA every day, instituted at the beginning of pregnancy in women at high risk of preeclampsia, almost everyone agrees that it is ineffective once symptoms and signs of preeclampsia have begun.[10] At least one study also showed a slightly increased risk of placental abruption with minidose ASA, but recent studies have not confirmed this and have reaffirmed the reduction-in the rate of preeclampsia in women receiving a baby aspirin per day.[11]

IUGR AND OLIGOHYDRAMNIOS

703

Q *My doctor sent me for an ultrasound because the baby seemed to measure too small for its gestational age. We saw the report and it kept referring to "retardation" and now we're terrified. What's going on?*

A The term Intrauterine Growth Retardation (IUGR) is a misnomer. Recently a better term has been applied, with "retardation" replaced by "restriction." (See Section 3: Prenatal Care, Tests of Fetal Well-Being) It simply means that the placenta is not functioning as well as it might in supplying oxygen and nutrients to the baby, resulting in the fetus's growth rate being slowed or restricted. Thus, IUGR may be thought of as due to placental insufficiency. Estimated fetal weight is less than 10 percent of expected for the gestational age.

With IUGR, the placenta appears to provide inadequate nutrition to the fetus with resultant slowed growth. However, the fetal circulation is designed to favor, or spare, the head, heart, and kidneys. If head growth is disproportionately greater than body growth, it may indicate asymmetric IUGR. Asymmetric IUGR is self-explanatory with head-sparing. Placental insufficiency is by far the most common cause of IUGR. A much less frequent condition is symmetric IUGR, which is associated with infections such as congenital syphilis, cytomegalovirus, and hepatitis, or with genetic abnormalities.

704

Q *What can cause placental insufficiency?*

A Hypertension and preeclampsia are the most common easily identifiable causes. Other causes include chronic renal disease, chronic hypoxia (congenital heart disease or life at high altitude), sickle-cell anemia or other inherited anemias, abnormalities of the placenta and/or cord (see Section 4: Fetal Development), and the presence of two or more fetuses.[12]

705

Q *How would I know if my baby was growth-restricted, or had IUGR?*

A You probably wouldn't know without regular prenatal visits at which your fundal (uterine) height is measured. Fundal height, combined with the best data possible to determine true gestational age, are the two factors that most often lead to the diagnosis. Occasionally, decreased fetal movement could tip you off. But the diagnosis is made nowadays by serial ultrasound ordered because of a high index of suspicion. Definitive diagnosis can never be made until birth. Small for Gestational Age (SGA) is a term which includes IUGR basics, but also those which are just "constitutionally" small, meaning mom and dad are small also.

706

Q *What does the doctor mean when he says I have decreased fluid?*

A Oligohydramnios means decreased amniotic fluid. Toward the third trimester, the amniotic fluid is largely fetal urine. If placental insufficiency exists, the fetus's kidney output may fall, resulting in decreased fluid. Oligohydramnios may also be associated with genetic abnormality, indomethacin therapy for preterm labor, occult (unrecognized) preterm PROM, and post-term pregnancies. Potter's syndrome (renal agenesis or lack of kidney formation) leads to the almost complete absence of amniotic fluid.

Severe oligohydramnios may be dangerous not only because it implies reduced placental function, but also because umbilical cord compression is more likely. This could lead to intermittent decreased oxygen supply or, in rare cases, even to fetal death.

707

Q *What are the common causes of IUGR?*

A Asymmetric IUGR, the more common type, which is caused by placental insufficiency, is associated with a number of medical complications of pregnancy. By far the most frequent are those associated with high blood pressure. These include chronic hypertension, pregnancy-induced hypertension, preeclampsia, and superimposed preeclampsia. IUGR may also be associated with chronic diseases such as systemic lupus (SLE), ulcerative colitis, Crohn's disease, and maternal renal disease such as glomerulonephritis.

Bed rest and adequate hydration, combined with continued treatment of any underlying disease, is the best that can be done. When the risks of intrauterine life outweigh those of potential prematurity, delivery should be accomplished. This may be by induction or by planned C-section, depending on the baby's position and severity of IUGR and/or prematurity.

RH DISEASE (ISOIMMUNIZATION)

(See also Section 3: Rhogam)

708

Q *I'm Rh negative. Does that mean I have Rh disease?*

A No. Rh factor refers to a certain glycoprotein that is found on the red blood cells of most people. When this factor is present, people are said to be Rh positive; when it is absent, Rh negative . If you happen to be Rh-negative but some Rh positive cells get into your blood either from transfusion or by delivering a baby, your immune system will learn to recognize those positive cells as the enemy! It will then attack the enemy cells with IgG antibodies in the future. Once your immune system has memorized the positive cells as foreign invaders, you are said to be Rh-isoimmunized, or sensitized.

709

Q *How is that a disease?*

A Once your immune system is trained, it will send out IgG antibodies to attack any red cells with Rh-positive factor. The problem stems from the fact that these IgG antibodies cross the placenta. So, if you are Rh negative with a first pregnancy, your fetus is at no risk. If you get sensitized with the birth of an Rh-positive child, all of your subsequent pregnancies are in jeopardy.

The actual disease causes fetal anemia with resultant heart failure. Heart failure in utero causes hydrops fetalis, also known as erythroblastosis fetalis, with edema (swelling) of the fetal extremities, scalp, and buildup of fluid in the baby's abdomen (ascites).

Hydrops was once uniformly fatal, but now may be treated in utero with transfusions into the baby's abdomen, where the transfusion is absorbed, or directly into the umbilical cord. If you are far enough along, usually greater than thirty-four weeks, delivery is recommended, with possible exchange transfusion of the baby shortly after birth.

710

Q *Can I avoid getting Rh disease?*

A Yes. Rhogam is a medicine given at about twenty-eight weeks and also shortly after the birth of an Rh-positive baby. The Rhogam destroys any cells from your baby that may have leaked into your bloodstream before your immune system can learn about Rh-positive cells being the enemy. This occurs less than 5 percent of the time before delivery. Ninety-five percent of sensitization occurs when the baby's blood comes in contact with yours at birth. Administration of Rhogam has virtually eliminated the problem of Rh disease in the population of women who seek prenatal care.

GESTATIONAL DIABETES (GDM)

(See also Section 9: Medical Complications-Diabetes)

711

Q *My friend had gestational diabetes and had a ten-and-a-half-pound baby. Is that common?*

A Macrosomia, or big babies, is one of the potential risks for those who develop diabetes in pregnancy. Diabetes mellitus and its classifications are a source of confusion for everyone, but all classes and types have one thing in common: too much glucose (sugar) in the bloodstream. This is always due to either an inability to produce enough insulin in the pancreas, as with juvenile onset diabetes (Type I), or an inability of the cells to take up glucose and use it because the insulin is ineffective or being destroyed, as in adult onset diabetes (Type II).

With gestational diabetes, the problem seems to be related to the placenta, as with preeclampsia. In GDM, certain placental compounds either destroy insulin (placental insulinase), or cause the mother to make more sugar available in the bloodstream in other ways (placental lactogen). This leads to higher levels, which can pass down a gradient to the fetus and make it larger than normal. GDM usually goes away after pregnancy, but these women are at greater risk than the general population of developing AODM (Type II) diabetes later in life.

712

Q *Are some people more likely to get it than others?*

A Women who are overweight when they begin their pregnancies, have given birth to babies over nine pounds in the past, have had a prior still-birth, have one or more first-degree relatives with diabetes, and are thirty-five years of age and over all have an increased risk of developing GDM.

713

Q *How is gestational diabetes diagnosed?*

A (See Section 3: Prenatal Care, Glucose Screen)
Gestational diabetes is diagnosed with an oral glucose screen (OGS), in which an exact amount of sugar is given to you in a drink (usually 50 grams) and your blood sugar level is tested one hour later. If the reading is greater than 135 to 140, you may have diabetes. (Twenty percent of people flunk the screen, but only 4 percent actually have GDM.) To confirm findings, you then take a three-hour glucose tolerance test. Fasting blood sugar and then one-hour, two-hour, and three-hour values are drawn. If two out of three are abnormal, you meet the criteria for GDM. ACOG recommends all women diagnosed with GDM be screened 6-12 weeks after delivery as well with at least a fasting blood glucose.

714

Q *Are there other problems besides the risk of a large baby?*

A Yes. GDM is associated with an increased risk of developing pre-eclampsia, polyhydramnios (increased amniotic fluid), urinary tract infections, birth defects (for preexisting Type I DM), respiratory distress syndrome (RDS), hyaline membrane disease or premature lung disease, and stillbirths.

Amniocentesis with fluorescent polarization tests such as TDx and FLM II are appropriate to determine lung maturity in the diabetic before elective delivery.[13]

715

Q *Is there anything I can do to avoid diabetes?*

A Probably not. But there are certain things you can do to avoid a bad outcome:

1. If you have Type 1 diabetes before pregnancy, you should work with your doctor for tight control over it before conception. Many studies concur that birth defects are elevated only in those individuals with preexisting diabetes that is out of control at conception. Get a blood test called glycosylated hemoglobin (Hgb A-1C) before you conceive. It will help determine how stable you have been on your insulin regimen and help determine the risk for problems with your pregnancy.

2. Get early and regular prenatal care.

3. Monitor your blood glucoses as instructed by your doctor, especially the first one in the morning (fasting blood sugar, or FBS), and glucose levels measured one to two hours after each meal.

   Use a glucometer which will measure blood glucoses from a finger-stick drop of blood. Aim for the following levels: 60 to 90 at fasting levels, 130 to 140 one hour after eating, and less than 120 two hours after eating.

4. Test your urine for ketones. When your body uses fat for energy instead of sugar, ketones in your urine will rise and serve as a warning that your sugars are too high.

5. Adjust your insulin with your doctor's input after reviewing your home blood glucose record. With GDM, this may often only be a dose of NPH insulin in the morning. For preexisting diabetics, most can be managed with a combination of NPH and regular insulin twice a day.

6. Adhere to your diet. Many GDM patients will not need insulin if they eat a balanced diet. Some will only need the help of oral agents to lower blood glucose such as metformin (Glucophage) or glyburide (Glyburide), generally considered safe in pregnancy. This will usually be spread out into many small meals throughout the day, as well as a bedtime snack, to avoid hypoglycemia (low glucose) during the night.

7. Exercise. Regular exercise decreases the amount of insulin required to move glucose into cells. Discuss the timing, type, and amount with your doctor.

716

Q *Will I need to do anything different than what you've described above?*

A You will have closer surveillance than most pregnant women. Your doctor will want to see you more frequently, possibly draw an additional Hgb A-1C at some point, and order a second trimester ultrasound to rule out any serious defects. Toward the end of pregnancy, he or she will order tests to ensure that the baby is okay. These tests include electronic fetal heart rate monitoring with NSTs and/or specialized ultrasound exams with BPPs. (See Section 3: Prenatal Care, Tests of Fetal Well-Being)

Kick counts are an easy, helpful way to monitor fetal well-being at home. Healthy babies move about the same amount each day and sick babies sometimes start to move dramatically less. Let your doctor know if you feel movement has dropped off markedly. A specific way to count the number of kicks per hour may be suggested to help you with this. (See Section 3: Prenatal Care, Tests of Fetal Well-Being)

Amniocentesis may be recommended to insulin-dependent diabetics to help determine when the baby's lungs are mature, should delivery be indicated before term.

717

Q *My friends told me I would have to have a C-section if I've got GDM. Is that true?*

A Every case is different. Sometimes estimates of very large fetal weight, or poor performance on one of the tests of fetal well-being, might indicate the need for a C-section. Most GDM patients who are well in control may deliver vaginally and do not need to be delivered prior to their due date.

718

Q *Is my baby at risk for any special problems after birth because of the GDM?*

A Babies of GDM mothers tend to have increased risk for several newborn problems:

1. Low blood glucose. They've been producing their own insulin to handle your glucose. If your levels were high when the "sugar factory" gets shut down and the umbilical cord is cut, the baby's high insulin levels can overwhelm its own capacity to produce sugar and the baby's glucose levels will bottom out. This potentially can be associated with seizures and brain damage if untreated.
2. Low calcium and magnesium levels can also lead to newborn seizures.
3. Polycythemia (too many red blood cells) can make the blood too thick and also lead to jaundice. Neonatal jaundice (yellow discoloration to skin) can occur because the product of blood breakdown is poorly metabolized by the fetal liver.

Any or all of these conditions may require that your baby go directly to the nursery shortly after birth, no matter where you are in the bonding process. You should be emotionally prepared ahead of time for this possibility.

PRETERM LABOR AND DELIVERY

719

Q *What are my chances of delivering too early?*

A Overall, about 12.7 percent of babies born in the United States are born prematurely.[14] Premature delivery means having your baby anytime before the thirty-seventh completed week of gestation, or before thirty-five weeks from conception. Your chances could be even higher if you have any of the factors that increase your risk.

720

Q *What's all the fuss about? My brother was a preemie and he's fine.*

A Preterm birth accounts for 75 percent of all newborn deaths not related to birth defects. Premature babies tend to have slowed growth and development, and problems with hearing, vision, breathing, and nervous system development, which can lead to problems in school and in life. In 1992, more than 34,000 children in the United States died in their first year of life. Our infant mortality rate is 8.5 per woo live births, and problems of prematurity make up the majority of these deaths.[15]

As of 1994, 7.2 percent of all live-born babies in the United States weighed less than 2,500 grams (5 1/2 pounds). Very low birth weight, or less than 1,500 grams (3 1/3 pounds), accounted for 1.3 percent. There has been no improvement in these statistics in the last thirty years.[16]

Two huge difficulties—diagnosis and treatment—surround this condition (PTL), which accounts for the vast majority of morbidity and mortality of newborns and for health care expenditure in NICUs nationwide. Preterm labor can sneak up on you and, before you know it, you are so far dilated that none of our methods for treatment will work.

721

Q *What are the things that would put me at higher risk for PTL?*

A Preterm labor risk factors include:
1. History of preterm labor with this or an earlier pregnancy
2. History of preterm delivery in an earlier pregnancy
3. Multiple gestation (two or more fetuses)
4. Previous surgery on your cervix (cone biopsies more so than LEEP or LLETZ), which may "shorten" your cervix
5. Abnormalities of the uterus such as a septum, fibroids, or changes associated with DES exposure

341

6. Infections while pregnant, especially pyelonephritis (kidney infection)
7. Abdominal surgery with this pregnancy, for example appendectomy, gallbladder surgery, or surgery of the ovaries
8. Cigarette smoking or cocaine use
9. Second or third trimester vaginal bleeding (associated with possible previa or abruption)
10. Little or no prenatal care
11. IUD still in place with pregnancy
12. Death of the fetus
13. Induction or elective cesarean scheduled too early in error, based on inaccurate estimate of gestational age

722

Q *What might I feel that would indicate possible preterm labor?*

A Any of the following could be a sign of early preterm labor and should be brought to your doctor's attention:

1. Vaginal bleeding or increase or change in vaginal discharge
2. Pelvic or lower abdominal pressure
3. Constant low backache
4. Mild cramping that feels like menstrual cramps, but persists day after day
5. Tightness of your uterus so that it feels "hard" but not necessarily painful
6. More than five to six Braxton Hicks contractions per hour
7. Rupture of your membranes with a gush of fluid out of the vagina, which continues to leak

723

Q *I've heard that your cervix can change without the woman feeling any contractions. Is there a home monitoring device for uterine contractions?*

A Yes. Home uterine activity monitoring (HUAM) has been advocated by many as a way to detect contractions that may build to preterm labor and actually change your cervix, but without your feeling them. While doctors hoped that this technique would permit earlier intervention, thus preventing preterm birth, there is no convincing data of this effect, and the use of HUAM remains controversial.[17]

As of 1996, the American College of Obstetricians and Gynecologists (ACOG) could not advocate the use of HUAM on the basis of all the studies to date. "Data are insufficient to support a benefit from HUAM in preventing preterm birth. Therefore, the ACOG does not recommend the use of this system of care."[18]

Most significantly ACOG feels that any possible benefit from HUAM is severely limited by the ineffectiveness of current methods for stopping preterm labor.

724

Q *How is preterm labor diagnosed?*

A In reality, the same way labor is diagnosed—cervical change. If your cervix softens, moves forward, shortens (effaces), and/or dilates on pelvic exam or ultrasound prior to thirty-seven weeks with or without perceived contractions, you are in preterm labor (PTL). Just having uterine contractions that you can feel and that can be monitored does not, mean you are in preterm labor. The definition of PTL is the source of most of the confusion in determining which treatment approach works or doesn't work.

725

Q *What is Fetal Fibronectin?*

A Fetal fibronectin (Ffn) is a protein secreted in vaginal discharge between twenty-four and thirty-four weeks if preterm delivery is imminent in the next two weeks. A specialized cotton swab is placed in the vaginal fornix near the cervix and fluid collected. Within about six hours a lab can tell your doctor if Ffn is present, and if so he may wish you to be on bedrest, take tocolytic medicines such as terbutaline, or give you steroids to help mature the baby's lungs.

726

Q *What are the treatments for preterm labor?*

A The mainstay of treatment is hydration and decreased activity. Once in preterm labor, your doctor will hospitalize you. This stay may be short or very long, depending on the specific circumstances. But the common factor is that you will be lying down most of the time. Initially you will be hydrated with an IV. In that IV, you may be given medicines such as magnesium sulfate, or you may be given terbutaline subcutaneously. These medicines do seem to stop contractions, but not everyone agrees that they are better than bed rest and hydration alone for actually stopping preterm labor.[19]

Other medicines have been used, particularly those that block prostaglandins. (See Section 5: Drugs in Pregnancy, Antiprostaglandins) These include medicines such as aspirin and indomethacin. Unfortunately, these medicines may cause oligohydramnios (decreased fluid) and changes in the fetal heart such as premature closure of the ductus arteriosus. (See Section 4: Fetal Development)[20] Calcium channel blockers such as nifedipine and verapamil have also been tried.[21] Unfortunately, these medicines have been associated with decreased umbilical flow in some animals, as well as acidosis (falling pH) and decreased oxygen levels in monkey and ewe studies.[22]

Weekly injections of progesterone have been shown to help prevent preterm labor in women at high risk who have delivered a baby prior to 37 weeks gestation in the past.[23]

In 2011 the ACOG recommended consideration of IV magnesium sulfate in imminent premature deliveries for "neuroprotection," some data showing a decreased incidence of cerebral palsy in babies born between 24 and 31 weeks gestation. Your doctor may recommend this in the final 12 hours before a pre-term delivery whether unavoidable or induced for a medical reason.

727

Q *If a woman delivers prematurely, the treatment failed, right?*

A Right. But the rub is, how do you know when you've succeeded? Take oral terbutaline (Brethine), for example. Terbutaline has been used now for nearly twenty years for preterm labor, but it's not clear that it works, only that it stops contractions. In other words, if you are contracting, but not changing your cervix, you are not in preterm labor. You're having Braxton-Hicks contractions by definition. Terbutaline will stop these contractions at least briefly, as many thousands of women can assure you. Does that mean you have succeeded in stopping preterm labor? Probably not. Once you have changed your cervix, it is not at all clear that oral terbutaline helps. A recent meta-analysis of oral tocolytic therapy failed to support any role for oral terbutaline.[24]

728

Q *If I have a preemie, how long will my baby have to stay in the nursery?*

A This, as you might expect, depends a lot on how premature your delivery is. Many babies born over thirty-five weeks of gestation might get to go home in a few days with you, but not all. Under thirty-five weeks, you can expect the baby to be in the hospital about as long as it would have been to your original due date. So, a thirty-week preemie is likely to be in the hospital for up to two and a half months.

Many preterm babies cannot live without specialized support outside of the womb. These babies need the neonatal intensive care unit (NICU). Nurseries are categorized by the sophistication of their equipment and personnel as Level I, II, or III. Level I nurseries can usually only care for term healthy babies. Level II nurseries have some extra capabilities, and can usually stabilize very small or sick preemies while awaiting transport to a larger center. Level III nurseries are capable of handling any care needed by even the most extreme cases, but they are generally located only in cities of 100,000 people or more. A very few centers in big cities are called Level IV because they can perform ECMO, which means they can put very sick babies on heart-lung bypass equipment, or alternatively actually ventilate with liquid oxygen solution.

It is possible that either you, while in preterm labor, or your baby, after delivery, may require transport to one of these centers.

729

Q *What kind of problems might my preemie have right after birth?*

A Preemies have problems related both to small size and to underdeveloped organs. Premature lung disease or respiratory distress syndrome (RDS) is due to a lack of surfactant, a compound needed to keep the little air sacs open. (See Section 4: Fetal Development, Lungs) Some preemies may require that this compound be given down their endotracheal tubes. They may require a machine called a respirator or ventilator to help them breathe for a while until their strength improves and their lungs start functioning better on their own.

Preemies may also have trouble keeping their temperatures up (hypothermia), so they are kept under radiant warmers. They can have trouble regulating their sugar, magnesium and calcium levels as well, and these things are supplemented with IVs. This IV may often be through the umbilical vessels. (Umbilical artery or umbilical vein catheters are called UAC or UVC.)

Preemies can have trouble with sucking, swallowing, and digesting, so your baby may be fed by IV only and then eventually through a tube placed in the stomach via the nose or mouth (tube or gavage feeding). Preemies fed too early, or just spontaneously, may develop necrotizing enterocolitis (NEC). NEC is a condition in which the bowels are not able to digest food due to necrosis (death) of cells in their lining, which in turn is due to inadequate blood and oxygen to that area. In its worst forms, NEC may be lethal.

Preemies, even if only a few weeks early, frequently develop jaundice due to the immaturity of their liver. This yellow coloring to the skin goes away over time. It may be treated with exposure to ultraviolet light, which helps break down the bilirubin that accumulates as a result of red blood cell breakdown. (See Section 4: Fetal Development, Liver)

730

Q *Is there a medicine I can take to help mature the baby's lungs?*

A Yes. Betamethasone is given as an intramuscular injection that is repeated eighteen to twenty-four hours later. It has been shown to be remarkably effective in decreasing the incidence and severity of premature lung disease, or respiratory distress syndrome. This may also be administered orally as Dexamethasone—four milligrams three times a day, for two days.

In fact, the benefit from steroids administered to women at high risk for imminent preterm delivery has been so startling that the sole benefit of tocolytic (something that stops contractions) drugs may be to eke out two to three days more gestation so that the steroids have time to do their work.[25] As of 2010 ACOG recommends a single course of injected corticosteroids for all women at risk of pre-term delivery within 7 days between 24 and 34 weeks.[26]

731

Q *Are there long-term problems for preemies?*

A With the advent of synthetic surfactant and modern NICUs, many more very tiny babies are surviving. The smallest have the highest rate of long-term problems. These problems may include chronic breathing difficulty (bronchiectasis), hearing difficulty, visual problems, and neurological problems such as cerebral palsy (CP), as well as developmental problems and learning disabilities. These problems are often unavoidable. Still, the vast majority of preemies do not have these serious problems with the excellent care available today.

732

Q *Will I be able to hold my preemie?*

A Very small babies may need immediate support to survive, but stabilization usually takes only a brief time. Ask your nurses and the neonatologist (pediatrician who specializes in newborns) when you can hold the baby.

NICUs may look scary at first. Babies may have tubes down their windpipe while on ventilators to assist breathing. They may have several intravenous lines, including ones in their navel and hands. They will usually have many wires attached to monitor the heart, breathing, and oxygen levels.

Despite all the equipment attached to your baby, he or she needs to hear your voice and feel your touch. NICU personnel will help you get over your fear very quickly.

PREMATURE RUPTURE OF MEMBRANES (PROM)

Preterm PROM

733

Q *What is PROM?*

A The terminology is confusing. Premature rupture of the membranes (PROM) literally means that the amniotic sac ruptures spontaneously before the onset of labor. This occurs with about one-third of all normal labors. However, the term is usually employed to indicate preterm premature rupture of the membranes. While the problem only occurs in 2 to 5 percent of pregnancies, it has been estimated to account for about 20 percent of all perinatal deaths (just before and just after delivery).[27]

734

Q *What increases my risk for preterm rupture of membranes?*

A Ascending infection from the vagina and cervix often plays a major role.[28] Women with STDs such as gonorrhea, syphilis, chlamydia, and trichomonas, or with overgrowths of Gardnerella vaginalis and Group B Strep have increased risk of PROM.[29] It has also been associated with multiple gestation, i.e., twins, triplets, etc., previous preterm PROM, previous cesarean section, and a history of incompetent cervix with or without previous cervical surgery.

735

Q *Why is PROM such a significant cause of babies dying?*

347

The main reason is that PROM is associated with preterm labor and delivery, which very preterm infants often do not survive. Additionally, if the membranes are grossly ruptured before about twenty-four weeks so that there is little or no fluid around the baby (severe oligohydramnios), the lungs frequently fail to develop (pulmonary hypoplasia). Even if labor doesn't occur until months later, for example at thirty-four weeks, the lungs may have failed to develop, and life outside the womb will not be possible.

Finally, the intact membranes protect mother and baby from infection. PROM may be caused by, or lead to, infection in the uterus. This leads to labor, and often the baby is not only premature, but infected. No combination is more lethal for the fetus.

736

Q *What do we do if I have preterm PROM?*

A This is another area of extreme controversy in obstetrics. In general, if rupture occurs prior to thirty-four weeks of gestation, but there is no obvious sign of infection such as fever, elevated white blood cell count, or uterine contractions then management is "expectant," meaning you will be placed on bed rest, often in the hospital if you are beyond twenty-five weeks. There you will be monitored with intermittent NSTs and serial ultrasounds. ACOG recommends as of 2010 that a single course of corticosteroids be administered to patients with PROM between 24-34 weeks, the benefits being felt to outweigh the risks.[30] If you fail to go into labor by thirty-four weeks, many doctors would induce you at this point, fearing infection more than prematurity. C-section would be chosen for previas and breeches.

737

Q *What if I do have obvious signs of infection, or if I'm already in preterm labor?*

A This subject is controversial. For decades, the axiom has been to not try and stop contractions when present in preterm PROM. The risk of sepsis (overwhelming infection) in the mother was felt to be too great if efforts were made to stop the uterus from contracting.

In all likelihood, with grossly infected membranes (chorioamnionitis), no force on earth will stop labor. However, some doctors advocate delaying it for up to seventy-two hours with intravenous antibiotics and medicines such as terbutaline or magnesium sulfate while steroids are given. Most studies have shown that these efforts are doomed to failure and it would be better to allow delivery to occur.[31]

PROM at Term

738

 What if my membranes rupture when I'm due, but I don't go into labor?

About one in three term patients will rupture their membranes before going into labor. The vast majority will subsequently go into labor on their own in the next twenty-four hours. Several studies in the 1950s led clinicians to believe that allowing twenty-four hours to pass without delivery put you at a much increased risk of infection. Consequently, doctors have induced patients with oxytocin (Pitocin) shortly after ROM, believing they would shorten the time until delivery.

Recently, some studies have shown that far from helping, Pitocin induction has only caused an increase in cesarean rate by as much as three times and has made no difference in infection rates.[32] However, not all investigators agree.

739

Are there other options besides just waiting or inducing with Pitocin if my cervix is "unfavorable"?

An unfavorable cervix means one that is unlikely to respond well to Pitocin. We know that attempted induction with an unfavorable cervix has been associated with an increased C-section risk. Recently we have been using prostaglandin gels and suppositories (Prepidil; Cervidil; Cytotec) to ripen the cervix for subsequent Pitocin induction six to twelve hours later. Often the suppository alone will induce labor. Results have been encouraging.[33]

UMBILICAL CORD PROLAPSE

740

My friend lost her baby when the cord prolapsed. What happened?

Umbilical cord prolapse is one of the few absolute obstetric emergencies. Very rarely, when the membranes rupture either spontaneously (SROM) or are ruptured by the doctor artificially (AROM), a loop of umbilical cord may pass out of the partially open cervix and then out of the vagina. This can compress the cord and cut off oxygen to the fetus.

If the baby's head or butt (breech position) are presenting, and are at least entering the pelvic inlet (See Section 6: Prepared Childbirth, Terminology), then the presenting part acts like a cork and the cord cannot slip by If, however, the head or butt is very high, the baby is lying across the uterus (transverse lie), or the baby is a second twin, the cord may shoot out if the membranes rupture suddenly.

Not much can be done about prolapse of the cord, other than an immediate C-section. Very rarely, a breech extraction (pulling on the baby's legs) of a second twin, for instance, might be possible. If prolapse occurs outside of the hospital labor and delivery area, it is often fatal for the fetus.

POST-TERM PREGNANCY

741

Q *What happens if I go past my due date? This is my first baby and I've heard that its more likely for me to be late.*

A First, you are not more likely to be "late" with your first pregnancy. The term "due date," which has always been a source of confusion, refers to the day at the middle of a bell-shaped curve from thirty-eight to forty-two weeks. This means that you have a fifty percent chance of delivering before and a fifty percent chance of delivering after this date (assuming you have made it to thirty-eight weeks, that is, if you exclude the ten percent risk we know you had of delivering before thirty-seven weeks).

Second, nothing happens if you go past your "due date," except that you probably get a little harder to live with. Going past your due date is referred to as postdates. Going past forty-two weeks is called post-term and constitutes a very different situation. Less than 10 percent of all pregnancies will fit into this category.

742

Q *Why do some pregnancies go so long without labor beginning?*

A Most of the time the reason is unknown. Doctors think that, rarely, there may be an enzyme deficiency that is inherited as a sex-linked recessive trait (See Section 1: Before Pregnancy, Tests Before Pregnancy) called placental sulfatase deficiency (affectionately known in the business as another variant of "SUS," or stupid uterus syndrome). In women with this condition, the placenta is missing an enzyme that converts a hormone made by the fetal adrenal gland known as DHAS to estradiol and estriol. This conversion is a prerequisite for labor.

Antiprostaglandins such as aspirin, indomethacin, naprosyn, and ibuprofen may all contribute to failure of labor to begin as well.

743

Q *Will my doctor let me go two weeks past my due date?*

A How long your doctor may let you go past your due date depends on several things, including the reliability of the calculation of your dates, the "ripeness" or readiness of your cervix, your parity (the number of babies you've had before), the estimated fetal weight, and the presence of other factors such as hypertension or diabetes.

744

Q *I know I'd be going crazy, but other than that, why do anything at all?*

A With time beyond about forty-two weeks, placental function begins to deteriorate and amniotic fluid decreases rapidly. This leaves the cord open to an increased risk of compression. Fetal jeopardy and even stillbirth, as well as fetal distress in labor, seem directly related to decreased fluid and cord compression.[34] Meconium is also present in the fluid about 30 percent of the time compared to only 19 percent at term. Meconium aspiration syndrome is three times as likely at 1.6 percent versus 0.6 percent of deliveries. In post-term babies, almost 20 percent have shoulder dystocia (trouble delivering the shoulders because of size) as opposed to only 8 percent at term. Macrosomia (a weight of more than 4,500 grams) is more than three times as likely beyond forty-two weeks, at 2.8 percent versus 0.8 percent of delivery at term. Thus, after forty-two completed weeks, danger for the fetus increases rapidly.

745

Q *If it gets more dangerous for the fetus past forty-two weeks, and thirty-eight weeks is term, why not just induce everybody at term?*

A In general the answer is that God still does it better than we do! Despite the recent advent of Cytotec and prostaglandins for ripening the cervix as a precursor to Pitocin augmentation, intervening before the uterus is chemically ready leads to a significantly higher cesarean rate. This is more likely to be the case with first pregnancies, since subsequent pregnancies tend to dilate the cervix at least to some extent by term. (See this section: Induction)

746

Q *What can I do between forty and forty-two weeks to help safeguard my pregnancy?*

A All doctors seem to agree that being aware of fetal movement is particularly important after your due date. Kick counts may be recommended daily. Different criteria are used by different doctors and many women are not very aware of fetal movement during the daytime. However, in the evening when things quiet down, you should lie on your side and count the number of times the baby moves in two hours. Remember, movements won't be vigorous kicks since the baby-to-fluid ratio is markedly increased at this point. Movements are more likely to be twists and turns.

A good average is about ten movements in two hours. If after the first hour the baby is moving very little or not at all, try moving the baby yourself. You won't hurt him or her. A good shove ought to cause the baby to wake up and move about. Some advocate drinking something with sugar or caffeine to stimulate the baby, but not everyone agrees that this works. If there are still no, or very few, movements, call your doctor and come to Labor and Delivery to be monitored.

The other thing you can do is have sex. It seems that sexual intercourse provides the opportunity to expose your cervix to the natural prostaglandins that occur in the ejaculate. If you also happen to use a good lubricant such as Astroglide, increasing the chance that you actually *enjoy* the experience, orgasm causes uterine contractions. If nothing else, you might have a good laugh trying to find a reasonable position. (Of course, refrain from intercourse if that's what your doctor has recommended.)

Lastly, keep well hydrated. Really try and drink those eight to ten ten-ounce glasses of water each day, even if you think you'll explode.

747

Q *Are there any tests that my doctor might do when I'm postdates?*

A There is also much debate about what tests should be done, which are predictive, and when these tests should be started. Some doctors would advocate kick counts only until forty-two weeks, and then a combination of nonstress tests (NSTs) and biophysical profiles (BPPs). (See Section 3: Tests of Fetal Well-Being) Until recently, many doctors did no evaluation prior to forty-two weeks at all.

With a reliable date, most doctors nowadays get nervous after forty-one weeks. You are likely to have a BPP done right around forty-one weeks and then either NSTs or repeat BPPs done at least once more from forty-one to forty-two weeks. Assessment of amniotic fluid is viewed by the majority of experts to be more predictive of outcome than the NST, which has virtually no place by itself in the evaluation of postdates, and certainly post-term pregnancies. When the results of any of these tests become worrisome, or your cervix improves along with descent of the head, your doctor may recommend induction.

At Parkland Hospital in Dallas, all women are induced at forty-two weeks or sooner if amniotic fluid is markedly decreased on a sonogram or if the patient has markedly decreased fetal movement. With induction trials stretched over three days (willingness to abandon an induction attempt as failed one day and to reinitiate another trial within three days), 90 percent of women are induced successfully. The C-section rate has not increased and the fetal death rate has been reduced. Similar regimens work elsewhere as well.[35]

STILLBIRTH

748

Q *What causes stillbirth and what are my chances of having it happen in our pregnancy?*

A Stillbirth is the death of the fetus while it is still in the uterus at anytime after twenty weeks gestation. If it is discovered prior to labor, it is called a fetal demise until the actual birth occurs. Many of the severe medical and pregnancy complications described in Sections 8 and 9 can very rarely lead to stillbirth, but even so, it occurs in only about seven out of one thousand births in the United States. At or near term, the rate is significantly less.

"Stillbirth" is usually pictured as that unthinkable horror where the baby stops moving, you ignore it for a time, and then come in to be reassured, only to discover that the baby has died. While this does occur, it is exceedingly rare when prenatal care has been sought from early on and the usual testing leads one to believe there are no major problems with the fetus. When it occurs at term, it is most often unexplained. For example, the common perception that "the cord around the neck" leads to stillbirth is erroneous. One in three healthy live newborns have the cord around the neck. (Babies in utero breathe through the umbilical cord, not the neck.)

Morbid obesity, more than 14 days past due, multiple gestations, type A diabetes, lupus, renal disease, age over 40 and untreated hypertension are the greatest risk factors.[36] But when stillbirth occurs in low risk pregnancies it may in fact be analogous to Sudden Infant Death Syndrome (SIDS), which occurs in the newborn period—something occurs on a very basic level that causes the heart to stop functioning. As yet, no consistent explanation for stillbirth in the otherwise healthy pregnancy has been found. You should ask that the placenta be closely examined by a pathologist who is familiar with stillbirth, since this may occasionally lead to some answers. It is true that after forty-two completed weeks, the risk of stillbirth rises rapidly, and this too could be related to placental dysfunction or decreased amniotic fluid. Stillbirth may very rarely be associated with both bacterial and viral infections. These include bacteria such as Group B strep,

E. Coli, Ureaplasma urealyticum, found in the vagina, and viruses such as coxsackie, parvo, and cmv, which could reach the fetus through the blood. Syphilis, toxoplasmosis, leptospirosis, listeria and Lyme disease have all been associated with extremely rare cases of stillbirth. Perhaps twelve out of a thousand stillbirths are caused by such infections.[37] (See post-term pregnancy; kick counts; and references below on coping with pregnancy loss.)

749

Q *Is there anything that we need to know or do to help us survive a stillbirth?*

A Entire books are devoted to pregnancy loss, but there are a few very important considerations. As difficult as it may seem, strive to both see and hold your baby after birth. You will never get another chance to say goodbye. Have photos taken and keep them until you're ready to look at them. You will want them later. Cry with your husband whenever you need to; he will be as devastated as you are. Don't blame God. The people who try to comfort you by telling you this was "part of the plan" mean well, but they are misguided. God neither kills newborns nor gives leukemia to a three-year-old as a test. Bad things happen and you don't necessarily deserve them.

Expect to be "numb" at first, but to have intense feelings a few days to weeks later. You will recover, but the loss will always be there. Forgive your friends and acquaintances. They will feel awkward and at a loss. Simply recognize their loving intentions.

Finally, if after several months you continue to somehow "blame yourself," turn to your clergy or grief counselor to help you resolve these issues before another pregnancy. Also know that the chance of it happening again is only 8/1,000.

INDUCTION OF LABOR

750

What does "induction" of labor mean and how does it differ from "augmentation"?

A Induction of labor means that some action is taken to bring about regular uterine contractions that lead to the progressive effacement and dilation of the cervix. Augmentation means that labor has already begun, but is not progressing adequately for any number of reasons.

751

Q *Why would someone need to be induced?*

A There are many reasons, but here is a partial list of relative, not absolute, indications:

1. Premature rupture of membranes (PROM) either at term or preterm
2. Hypertensive disorders including chronic hypertension and preeclampsia
3. Chorioamnionitis (membrane infection)
4. Suspected fetal jeopardy, such as IUGR (slowed growth) and oligo-hydramnios (decreased fluid)
5. Maternal medical problems (diabetes, renal and pulmonary diseases)
6. Fetal demise
7. Logistic factors (history of precipitous labor less than three hours, distance from hospital, psychosocial indications)
8. Post-term pregnancy

To this list might also be added successful external cephalic version (ECV) of a breech after thirty-seven weeks with a favorable cervix, which is significantly thinned out and starting to dilate.

752

Q *Are there times when induction is the wrong thing to do?*

A Reasons to not do something are called contraindications in medicine. Absolute contraindications to induction are few, but include placenta previa, transverse lie of the fetus, prolapsed umbilical cord, prior classical (vertical) uterine incision at cesarean, or previous full-thickness myomectomy (surgical removal of fibroids), and active genital herpes.

Relative contraindications are those in which the doctor must think very carefully about induction, and the condition may require special attention. Relative contraindications include twins or more, polyhydramnios (too much fluid), maternal heart disease, worrisome fetal heart rate patterns when not in labor, more than three previous deliveries, very severe hypertension, breech presentation, and the presenting part floating above the pelvic inlet.[38]

Elective inductions may be performed after 39 weeks gestation. These are generally easier and more successful if not a first delivery, and induction before 39 weeks should be done only with evidence from amniocentesis of fetal lung maturity.[39]

753

Q *How is labor induced?*

A I've heard of everything from castor oil to Mexican food, to riding over the railroad tracks under a full moon at midnight. None of these has been shown to be clearly effective. Having sex is about the only thing you can do on your own (well, almost on your own) that seems to have some beneficial effect.

Methods your doctor is more likely to employ include stripping the membranes, prostaglandin gel or suppository insertion, amniotomy, and the administration of oxytocin as intravenous Pitocin.

754

Q *What is stripping the membranes? I've heard that it hurts.*

A Stripping the membranes (called "sweeping" in Europe) during an office examination has long been advocated by many obstetricians. This involves a usually uncomfortable pelvic examination where the examiner's first two fingers are advanced into the cervix as far as possible. The membranes are then swept away from the uterine wall in hopes that enough prostaglandin will be released as a result to initiate contractions.

Studies have clearly shown both that this works[40] and that it doesn't work.[41] The procedure takes only a few seconds and may hurt a little or a lot, depending on the individual and on the state of the cervix.

755

Q *What are these magic gels and tablets I've heard about for induction?*

A It's not quite magic, but prostaglandin gels, suppositories and tablets (Prepidil; Cervidil) are significant additions to our armamentarium. Cytotec (Misoprostol) is another agent currently used but unrelated to prostaglandins for ripening the cervix. Your doctor may recommend using these six to twelve hours before attempting induction by rupturing the membranes or with the intravenous administration of Pitocin, or both. The prostaglandin effaces (thins) the cervix, and sometimes even initiates labor over this time period. Usually you will feel either no pain or menstrual-type cramps over the six hours following insertion.

Clinical studies in over five thousand women in seventy trials strongly support the efficacy of these prostaglandin E_2 preparations.[42]

Cytotec is labeled by the manufacturer as contra-indicated in pregnancy because it causes abortions in the first trimester. Despite this, the American College of Ob/Gyn feels its use for medical induction is safe and effective.[43]

756

Q *What is an amniotomy and how does it work?*

A Amniotomy is the artificial rupture of the bag of waters by manually placing a disposable small plastic instrument similar to a crochet hook through the cervix and "snagging" the membranes. The resultant tear allows the amniotic fluid to leak out which will continue until delivery.

It apparently works by stimulating uterine muscle contraction. Amniotomy decompresses the uterus a little and thus shortens the muscle fibers, but also releases the prostaglandins that are in the membranes stimulating contractions.

Most studies looked at amniotomy to augment rather than induce labor but one large study did support its efficacy for induction.[44]

757

Q *I've heard from an attorney I know and in my prepared childbirth class that oxytocin is dangerous. What is the problem with it?*

A Oxytocin (Pitocin) is an extremely powerful and effective hormone that causes the uterus to contract. It was first synthesized in 1953. Its reputation as dangerous comes from the decades of its use in an uncontrolled fashion. For example, less than thirty years ago, this medicine was administered in chewing gum; it was given as an intramuscular injection; it was administered intravenously. Initially, it was monitored simply by "eyeballing" the drip rate with a known concentration in the bag. Dosing was approximate, and small overdoses for certain individuals led to tetanic contractions, meaning that the uterus tightened, shutting down oxygen to the placenta, and it stayed that way for long periods.

The advent of extremely accurate control pumps for IVs has markedly improved the safety of oxytocin administration as well as other medicines, such as the anticoagulant heparin and the cardiovascular drug dopamine.

758

Q *Is it true that induction with Pitocin hurts much more than natural labor?*

A Absolutely not. They both hurt quite a lot. Uterine contraction intensity can be measured exactly with intrauterine pressure catheters (IUPCs). We know that Pitocin-induced contractions are no stronger than natural contractions. It is true that the rate of onset of painful contractions may be faster than with natural labor, but often the opposite is true.

The simple truth is that anyone who has received Pitocin either wasn't in labor to begin with, or their contractions were ineffective. Going from no labor to labor hurts. Likewise, going from an ineffective labor that may hurt a lot, to a more effective labor that hurts even more, is a challenge as well. In both circumstances, Pitocin is blamed unfairly. A woman who compares a first delivery that was induced, with a second that came on naturally, will view Pitocin negatively, but she would have viewed any first labor compared to the ease of subsequent ones in the same light.

759

Q *How long will an induction with Pitocin take?*

A That depends on several factors, such as the number of previous deliveries, the "ripeness" of your cervix, and the size and position of your baby. There is no limit to the latent phase of labor (dilated less than four centimeters) with an induction. Progress of one centimeter per hour is considered sufficient in the active phase (dilated more than four centimeters). (See Section 7: Normal Labor and Delivery)

760

Q *What if my cervix never changes, despite Pitocin?*

A There is no time limit on the latent phase. Your doctor may decide that some random time of contracting, perhaps twelve hours, is enough if he or she is still unable to rupture your membranes. In this case, you may be asked to come back in the next day or two to try again, or you and the doctor may decide to perform a C-section, depending on your circumstances.

If you reach the active phase of labor, then indications for C-section will be the same as if you were undergoing a natural labor. (See this section: Cesarean Section; Section 7: Normal Labor and Delivery)

761

Q *Can I eat breakfast before I come in for an induction?*

A Eating solids in labor or immediately before is usually discouraged. Nobody wants to be cruel, but if you needed emergency general anesthesia, you have a small chance of aspirating (breathing in stomach contents while vomiting). Since aspiration pneumonias can be lethal, it's a better idea to stick with liquids. Ask your doctor about your circumstance; if labor might take more than sixteen hours, you may be allowed to eat solids, but it is not likely. Popsicles, ice chips, hard candies, and lollipops are all fine in labor.

762

Q *If I'm induced, when could I have an epidural?*

A (See Section 6: Pain Management; Section 7: Epidurals)
The older rule was that you may have an epidural when you have reached the active phase of labor (dilated about four to five centimeters and at -1 to 0 station). This will vary from institution to institution, doctor to doctor, and is also dependent on what medicine is placed in the epidural catheter. (See "walking epidural" in index.) Several recent studies suggest epidurals may be given at any time once labor is established.

CESAREAN SECTION

763

Q *What exactly is a Cesarean section?*

A Cesarean section is the surgical removal of the fetus through the abdomen. A "primary C-section" means the first one, as opposed to the self-explanatory "repeat C-section." Its development as a safe technique for both mother and fetus has changed the face of obstetrics more than any other development in human history. As recently as the end of the nineteenth century, the maternal death rate was greater than 85 percent (8,500/10,000) from cesareans; now it stands at about 0.01 percent (1/10,000).[45]

After about 1900, the introduction of sterile technique, reliable general anesthesia, and proper suturing of tissue planes were significant advances. Later, additions of blood transfusion and, after World War II, antibiotic therapy, improved the mortality rate to 1/1,000. With better techniques, antibiotics, disposable equipment, and regional anesthesia, the death rate is down to 1/10,000 cases.[46] Incidentally, the overall maternal mortality rate in the US has never been reported below 1/10,000, implying that Cesarean has a lower maternal death rate than vaginal in general.[47]

764

Q *Why have C-sections become more common in recent years?*

A The major changes responsible for this trend began about 40 years ago in the late 1950s. Prior to around 1960, the C-section rate was lower than 5 percent in the United States. It was performed only for maternal indications such as placenta previa, failure of induction in severe pre-eclampsia, and inability to deliver due to absolute cephalopelvic disproportion (CPD), documented with X-rays. In this context, CPD meant certain maternal death without C-section.

Several factors came together to shift the emphasis of C-section toward fetal indications after 1960. C-section became extremely safe about the same time that better methods were being developed to recognize the fetus at risk for asphyxia or physical injury at delivery. There are other contributing factors such as bigger babies being born and a greater percentage of deliveries being first-time pregnancies.

The development and continued refinement of ultrasound, continuous electronic fetal monitoring, and fetal scalp blood sampling all made detecting potential or at least perceived fetal distress a more frequent occurrence. Coupled with the astronomical rise in litigation related to anything other than a perfect outcome at delivery that began in the 1980s, these changes led to a common finding of cesarean rates of over 25 percent in many American hospitals.

The National Institute of Child and Human Development sponsored a Consensus Development Conference in September of 1980 to address rising rates of C-sections and found the following four circumstances to be responsible for 90 percent of the increase: dystocia (baby doesn't fit through birth canal), 30 percent; repeat cesarean delivery, 25 to 30 percent; breech presentation, 10 to 15 percent; and fetal distress, 15 percent. These are percentages of the increase, not the incidences.[48]

Other reasons include reduced parity (about half of pregnant women are having their first babies). There has been a decrease in midforceps use as litigation skyrocketed, and thus a decrease in the experience of obstetricians trained in the technique. Other studies show economic factors as well. Vaginal births after cesareans (VBACs) are lowest at private hospitals, with family income greater than $30,000, for those with private insurance, and in low-volume hospitals.[49] Silbar found a statistically significant trend toward larger babies that contributes to the absolute CPD rate as well.[50]

Finally, more women are simply choosing to have a first baby by C-section in hopes of avoiding the changes to the vagina and pelvic floor support that can result from repeated vaginal births.

765

Q *Is the C-section rate still climbing?*

A Technically, yes. While several forces, including insurance pressure and more liberal use of vaginal birth after cesarean (VBAC), served to slow the rise and briefly reverse it in the mid to late 1990s,[51] insurance pressures have now vaporized and rising recognition of the true risks to VBAC and the very low risk to scheduled C-section have fueled a renewed increase in C-section rates not only in the US, but in many places in the world.

More aggressive use of induction agents such as Cytotec and Pitocin and more relaxed standards in terms of time permitted in each stage of labor (active management of labor) may slow the rise somewhat by reducing the number of C/S performed for dystocia, failure to progress, or CPD, which all loosely mean the same thing, i.e., "baby no fit!"

766

Q *Our Lamaze teacher told us that epidurals increase the C-section rate. Is that true?*

A (See also Section 6: Epidurals; Section 7: Pain Management)
I firmly believe that the appropriate use of regional anesthesia, given at the right time, in the right dose, with the right drug, in the right way, will not increase an individual's risk of cesarean section, forceps, or lengthen the time to delivery.

While this is a hotly debated issue in obstetrics and anesthesia,[52] recent studies completed in 2005 have tended to support giving epidurals at any point in labor, given the proper techniques and medicines.[53]

767

Q *Is it true that continuous electronic fetal monitoring contributes to the increasing C-section rate?*

A (See also Section 6: Monitors)
It is probably true. EFM was instituted without any widespread trials to document its efficacy at lowering perinatal morbidity and mortality. While

it makes sense that it would, given that fetuses in distress do have fetal heart rate changes, recent data suggests that the only effect of EFM may be to raise the C-section rate.

A large recent study at UTSW in Dallas showed what had been long suspected all across the country. Continuous EFM did not improve fetal mortality and morbidity. In other words, use of EFM did not significantly statistically alter outcome. Even more distressingly EFM did do one thing—it raised the primary C-section rate for "fetal distress."[54]

Another study has shown that the pressure monitors may also contribute to the increasing C-section rate. Doctors who did not know the actual intrauterine pressures were less likely to perform a C-section than those who knew the correct data and followed established guidelines.[55]

768

Q *What are the indications for cesarean section today?*

A Indications for cesarean section include the following:

1. Active phase arrest (failure to dilate or descend in the active phase over two hours with documentation of adequate contractile force)
2. Stage II arrest (failure to deliver the baby after two hours of pushing without, or three hours of pushing with, an epidural)
3. Fetal distress in labor
4. Breech presentation
5. Transverse lie
6. Placenta previa
7. Placental abruption
8. Umbilical cord prolapse
9. Multiple gestation
10. Fetal jeopardy prior to labor as indicated by prenatal testing
11. Previous classical-incision cesarean or previous full-thickness uterine incision for myomectomy (removal of fibroids)
12. Extreme prematurity
13. Macrosomia, with floating head and fear of shoulder dystocia
14. Elective

769

Q *How will I know if I have to have a C-section?*

A If you fit any of the indications above, a C-section is likely. A decision to do a C-section in labor will be fully discussed with you at the time, unless an emergency C-section must be performed because of extreme, sudden fetal distress, as occurs with abruption or cord prolapse.

770

Q *Can't my doctor do an ultrasound ahead of time to see if the baby is too big?*

A Third trimester ultrasound is notoriously poor at estimating fetal weight with error margins of 10 to 15 percent in the hands of an experienced operator. Besides that, the fetal head is designed to mold and shape itself to the maternal pelvic inlet. Remarkably large babies can and do fit out of remarkably small women because of the pliability of the fetal head. (See also Section 6: Female Reproductive Anatomy and Terminology)

771

Q *How long does a C-section take?*

A In the hands of an experienced operator, about 20 minutes. Repeats after multiple previous C-sections may take a little longer because of scarring. Almost always, the incision on your abdomen will be a Pfannenstiel (bikini) cut. Even in a dire emergency, this incision may take only a few seconds longer than a vertical skin incision, which starts below your navel and ends just above your pubic bone. Occasionally, massively obese patients are better handled with a vertical skin incision due to concerns about wound infection below a large pannus (fat pad hanging down). Rarely, a situation will be extremely urgent, and with an assistant unavailable, the easily performed vertical incision is more appropriate.

772

Q *What determines the type of incision on my uterus?*

A Most cesareans can be performed with a low transverse incision. This incision goes across the bottom part of the uterus and leaves a stronger scar. This permits vaginal birth after cesarean (VBAC) for future deliveries.

Occasionally, especially with preemies, the lower uterine segment is too narrow to safely perform a transverse incision without getting into the huge blood vessels that course along either side of the uterus. In other cases, the fetus may be in a back down transverse lie, especially with twins or more, so that a decision to make a low transverse incision could be a disaster, with delivery impossible while the baby asphyxiates from decrease in blood pressure that accompanies the uterine incision. Some anterior placenta previas mitigate against transverse incision. Sometimes the bladder is so scarred from previous cesareans that it is not possible to move the bladder down normally to cut the incision in the uterus beneath it.

In cases such as these, a classical vertical incision should be chosen. Often an attempt is made to keep the incision in the lower part of the uterus (low vertical incision) but, for practical reasons, it usually extends up into the thicker active muscular section.

773

Q *Will I be awake and can my husband be with me?*

A You will be awake for any scheduled C-section and most sections done in labor. The vast majority of these will be done under epidural anesthesia. If a cesarean is needed while you are in labor, and you do not have an epidural in place, you may either be awake with an epidural placed at the time, be awake with a short-acting one-shot spinal anesthetic, or you may have to be put to sleep. There are emergency circumstances such as uterine rupture, abruption, and severe preeclampsia or eclampsia with HELLP syndrome, in which either there is no time to place an epidural or even the quicker spinal, or they are contraindicated.

In almost all American hospitals, your husband can be with you if you are awake. There is no reason for your spouse to be there if you are asleep, and most institutions will not permit him or any family members in the room if a general anesthetic is in use.

774

Q *What are the advantages and disadvantages of cesarean section?*

A *Advantages:* Since all cesareans should be clearly indicated, the major advantage is preserving the health of you and your baby. Scheduled cesareans have the additional advantage of being just that—scheduled. You can have all your plans in place with respect to your other children, grandparents, work, friends, and even who's going to feed the dog.

Disadvantages: Some women feel that "missing out" on the natural process is a disadvantage; others feel emphatically the opposite way. Certainly, the hospital stay may be a little longer and some women think that recovery is longer with a cesarean. Full recovery to all normal activities takes four to six weeks. (Most women who think recovery is longer or tougher with cesarean have either not delivered vaginally, or at least not had a large episiotomy.) The insurance industry views the increased costs associated with cesarean as a distinct disadvantage as well.

775

Q *What are the risks and complications of a cesarean?*

A Complications include a rate of infection in the wound or uterus that is lower than 4 percent, reversible injury to the bladder in about 1 in 400 cases, excessive blood loss requiring transfusion in about 4 to 6 percent of cesareans, and blood loss severe enough to require hysterectomy in fewer than 1 percent.

776

Q *How many C-sections can one person have?*

A There is no set number. Risks of problems with a weakened uterine scar and bleeding do increase with each repeat, and particularly after three repeats.

777

Q *What is a uterine "window"?*

A Jokingly referred to as a "womb with a view," a uterine window is an area of the lower uterus that is so thinned out from previous uterine scars that it is no more than one or two cell layers thick. In this circumstance, you can see right through the uterine wall to the baby. The concern is if you go into labor, you might be at increased risk for uterine rupture.

778

Q *What is uterine rupture?*

A For about a hundred years, the adage "once a section always a section" held sway in medical opinion. The reason for the expression was during labor, a scarred uterus was known to occasionally burst open and lead to expulsion of the fetus into the abdominal cavity, often with death of both mother and fetus. The actual incidence of "uterine rupture" is hard to determine because of the definitions involved, but it is felt to be between 1/2 and 1 percent. (See also this Section: VBAC)

779

Q *How do I prepare for a scheduled cesarean section?*

A If your cesarean is scheduled in the morning, do not eat or drink after midnight the night before. Some scheduled cesareans may be later in the day, in which case the restrictions on eating are the same, but you may have liquids until six hours beforehand.

Plan to bring with you all the things you would for a normal delivery. On arrival you will sign in, be taken to a labor room where you will change clothes, have an IV inserted and then sit up to have your epidural placed. After you start to feel numb, your lower abdomen will be shaved and a Foley catheter inserted in your bladder. Once the "level" of anesthesia is deemed adequate, you will be moved to the operating room. Your husband and another support person may come with you, cameras and all!

Generally your husband will be seated at the head of the OR table next to you so he can hold your hand, scratch your nose, etc. He will then be allowed to stand and see the actual delivery and give you the blow by blow since there will usually be a screen obstructing your view. If all goes well, you will be able to hold your baby after just a few moments of suctioning under the warmer! (See Section 6: Prepared Childbirth, What to Bring)

780

Q *If I have a scheduled repeat cesarean, how soon can I set the date?*

A Scheduled repeat cesareans are performed whenever we know statistically that the baby is unlikely to have any prematurity-related problems. The American College of Obstetrics' guidelines require that elective CS be scheduled no sooner than 39 completed weeks of gestation by best criteria.[56]

CPD

781

Q *What is CPD?*

A (See also Section 7: Failure to Progress)
Cephalopelvic disproportion (CPD) is the single largest reason given for cesarean, even more than previous cesarean. The word itself means "head/pelvis disproportion." In short, your baby is too big or is in the wrong position (such as persistent occiput posterior, or face up) to fit through the birth canal. (I call CPD "BNF" for baby no fit.)

When you fail to dilate or the baby fails to descend over the course of two hours after you have entered the active phase (dilated more than four to five centimeters), you either have CPD or inadequate contractile forces. After Pitocin augmentation is given, if you still fail to make progress, some doctors would recommend a C-section for CPD. Likewise, if you fail to move the baby down at all in the pushing stage (Stage II) over two hours without or three hours with an epidural, then you are in a Stage II arrest, and a C-section will be recommended for CPD.

Malpresentation: Breech and External Version

782

Q *What is meant by a malpresentation?*

A Basically, any presentation other than head down (vertex, or cephalic) is considered a malpresentation. Breech, whether complete (Indian-style), frank (feet up by ears), or footling (one or both feet hanging down), is an indication for C-section. Breeches occur at term about 4 percent of the time. At thirty weeks, however, about 40 to 50 percent of presentations are breech.

Transverse lie or shoulder presentation occurs when the baby lies across the uterus. It occurs in about 0.3 percent of all deliveries and is also a malpresentation indicating a need for C-section. This may be random, or related to a uterine anomaly such as a septum or fibroids, placenta previa, prematurity, or grand multiparity (more than four deliveries) with a relaxed, floppy uterus.

Face presentation occurs when the baby's neck is extended and the backward-tilted head enters the pelvis in such a way that the face (usually the mouth) appears at the vagina. While it occurs in only 0.2 percent of deliveries, the mentum (chin) posterior position cannot possibly be delivered vaginally and a cesarean is required. Most face presentations end in cesareans because they occur more often in women with contracted (smallinlet) pelvises and with big babies.

Brow presentation is a slight variant of the face presentation. Delivery is not possible with this position unless the baby is tiny and the pelvis is huge.

783

Q *If the baby is in breech position when I come for my visit at thirty-six weeks, can he or she be turned around?*

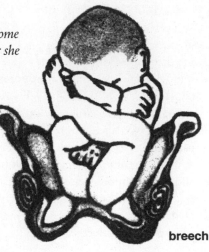

breech

A About 4 to 5 percent of babies are in breech position at thirty-seven weeks. Because of the potential for injury at birth with a vaginal breech, many doctors will recommend a scheduled cesarean section. The risk of fetal injury with breech vaginal delivery is extremely small, but it exists and legal concerns are a sad but real phenomenon in today's world. There has been controversy for at least forty years over how to handle the breech presentations at term.

Currently, the American College of Obstetricians and Gynecologists (ACOG) recommends that all women with breech babies be offered a trial of external cephalic version (ECV) to turn the baby around, in the absence of contraindications. An ultrasound will determine if there is adequate fluid, where the placenta is, what the orientation of the fetal spine is, and in what position the extremities are. Sometimes the position of the cord can be determined as well.

Your doctor will discuss the findings with you and together you will decide if a trial ECV is the right thing for you. The technique is described below.

784

Q *How often does external cephalic version actually work?*

A The overall success rate for ECV is about 70 percent at thirty-six weeks and beyond. Success rates are higher earlier in gestation, but a higher number then revert to breech before the onset of labor. Success rates are lower after thirty-eight weeks, and for this reason, ECV should be attempted as close to thirty-six to thirty-seven weeks as possible. Success rates are also lower in obese women. (See Section 9: Obesity) ECV tends to be more successful, the more babies you've had in the past.

About 15 percent of successful ECVs will revert to breech before labor and about 15 percent of failed ECVs will become vertex (head down) before labor.

785

Q *How is an external cephalic version performed?*

A Because there is a 1/400 risk of needing an emergency C-section, ECV should probably be performed in a Labor and Delivery unit with an operating room immediately available. You will be asked to disrobe and lie on your back. The bed will then be tilted with the head down and the foot raised in a position known as Trendelenburg. An ultrasound will determine the position of the baby, spine, and amount of amniotic fluid.

Next, the doctor will empty an entire bottle of Aquasonic gel (or other lubricant), which may have been warmed, onto your tummy. This will then be slathered around evenly while your doctor checks the position of the fetus. One hand will then be placed just above your pubic bone, and the baby's buttocks will be eased out of the pelvis. The doctor's other hand will be used to pull the fetal head into a forward or backward roll. This procedure takes several minutes and is moderately uncomfortable, but tolerable.

786

Q *What are the risks associated with external cephalic version?*

A External cephalic version risks are few, but noteworthy. In about 40 percent of cases, there will be relatively severe and prolonged fetal heart-rate decelerations during and shortly after the ECV attempt. Rotating the fetus will put pressure on the fetal head, especially if the fetus spends several minutes lying across the uterus. This pressure fires the vagus or tenth cranial nerve and slows the fetal heart as a defense mechanism. The same thing occurs to a certain degree with pushing in normal labor. These changes are transient and almost never require intervention.

In 1/400 cases, an emergency C-section will be performed because of abruption (tearing away) of the placenta or presumed umbilical cord compression.

787

Q *Why can't I just deliver the baby in breech position vaginally?*

A (See also Section 8: Malpresentation)
Whether you deliver a baby in breech position vaginally will have to be discussed on an individual basis with your doctor. In most cases, babies in breech position are delivered by elective C-section if ECV fails.

Several factors mitigate against vaginal breech deliveries. An estimated weight of more than 3,600 grams, a contracted pelvis (small inlet) as determined by pelvic measurements on exam and/or CT scan or an MRI, a hyperextended fetal head (looking up), failure to enter labor without induction, footling breeches (feet hanging down first), or prematurity all are relative contraindications to vaginal delivery. In premature breeches, the head is much larger than the butt. As a consequence, the bottom, abdomen, and chest might fit through the dilated cervix, but then entrap the head, leading to decreased oxygen supply and, rarely, death.

Placenta Previa

788

Q *Does placenta previa always require a cesarean delivery?*

A Total or complete previa, in which the placenta lies directly over the cervix, does mandate cesarean delivery. Marginal or partial previas may sometimes be watched in labor, recognizing that both heavy blood loss and abruption can occur. (See this section: Placenta Previa)

Prematurity

789

Q *Do little preemies have to be delivered by cesarean?*

A Usually not. However, this is another controversial area. Premature babies, especially those under thirty-four weeks, tend to develop bleeding in the brain. This is called intraventricular hemorrhage (IVH), and for many years, some experts felt it was due to compression of the fragile little head with vaginal delivery. Subsequent studies have shown the route of delivery to be irrelevant to the incidence of IVH.

Little preemies are often in malpresentations, however, especially breech. With preemie breeches under thirty-four weeks, cesareans are usually chosen to avoid the risk of fetal head entrapment. At this gestational age, the butt is smaller than the head. The fear is that the butt will dilate the cervix only so far, slip through, and the head could then be trapped, leading to asphyxia and death.

Fetal Distress

790

Q *Does fetal distress always mean a C-section to save the baby and avoid cerebral palsy?*

A Not necessarily. If the fetal heart rate changes are such that delivery is felt to be urgent and you are in the second stage at below +1 station, then a forceps or vacuum delivery may be attempted. Fetal distress of a lesser degree may also be addressed with intrauterine resuscitation (mother moves to lateral position, addition of oxygen by mask and increase in IV fluids with Pitocin either decreased or stopped for the moment).

Cerebral Palsy (CP) in which the baby may demonstrate permanent neurological damage including full or partial spastic paraplegia (jerky, irregular movements which persist into adulthood making use of arms, legs, and even speech difficult) has been consistently shown NOT to be associated with fetal distress in labor, the labor process or the route of delivery, as was once believed. Instead it is felt to be almost always the result of a fetal arterial ischemic stroke occurring earlier in pregnancy. [57]

Vaginal Birth After Cesarean (VBAC)

791

Q *Didn't they used to say, "Once a section, always a section"? What changed?*

A Yes, they used to say that. What changed was the realization that the policy of mandatory repeat cesarean, which stemmed from the fear of catastrophic rupture of the previous scar often accompanied by death of both the mother and the fetus, was based on a history of vertical or classical uterine incisions. This is a large, up-and-down incision that goes through the thick, muscular layer of both the upper and lower portions of the uterus.

Low transverse uterine incisions have been used since the mid-1920s, but it wasn't until the quadrupling of the cesarean rate that occurred between 1965 and 1980 that people began looking at letting women purposely deliver vaginally after a previous lower uterine incision. (See this section: Cesarean Section)

792

Q *Is VBAC becoming increasingly popular?*

Yes. There seems to be a steady trend toward increasing VBAC rates and falling cesarean rates. Cesarean rates have fallen slowly since 1989, but they vary widely from one state to another. The average total rate in 1995 was about 24 percent. The highest rates of C-sections are in the South, the lowest rates are in the West, and intermediate rates are in the Northeast and Midwest. Louisiana had the highest total C-section rate (27.7 percent), and the highest primary rate (19.6 percent); Alaska had the lowest total rate (15.2 percent), and Wisconsin the lowest primary rate (10.6 percent). VBAC rates parallel these inversely.[58]

793

Which women are, and which women aren't, candidates for VBAC?

At the moment, VBAC is technically still indicated for all those who wish to deliver vaginally, but had a previous low transverse incision cesarean section.[59] VBAC may be indicated for selected patients who have had two lower transverse cesareans as long as the second was a scheduled repeat.

VBAC is contraindicated (not a good idea) for those with a previous classical incision, multiple gestations, and breech presentation. There is little data on VBAC after previous myomectomy (surgery to remove fibroids), but VBAC is considered contraindicated by most. Macrosomia (big baby) on clinical exam or ultrasound is not considered a contraindication as it has been in the past. This is due to our complete inability to accurately predict estimated fetal weights near term.

794

What are the chances of success with a VBAC?

Overall, about 60 to 80 percent succeed at VBAC.[60] Women who had their first C-section for a nonrepeating cause such as breech, fetal distress, or placenta previa are likely to succeed. Those who had sections for macrosomia (big baby), active phase arrest (dilated four to ten centimeters), and failure to descend (pushing), are less likely to succeed. In fact, the degree to which you were dilated at the time of your first cesarean is directly related to VBAC success. A recent study at New York University concluded that those who got completely dilated but were unable to push the baby out with the first pregnancy had only a 13 percent chance of successful VBAC.[61]

795

Q *Is it true that you can't have an epidural if you have a VBAC?*

A No. We would prefer that you have an epidural. Originally it was felt that an epidural might obscure the pain of a rupturing uterus, one of the clinical warning signs. Subsequently it has been clear that true catastrophic ruptures, rare as they are, are almost always accompanied by falling blood pressure, rising pulse, evidence of fetal distress, and a uterus that suddenly stops contracting. There are plenty of clinical indicators in place and, with an epidural, an emergency can be handled quickly and potentially more safely than with a rushed general anesthetic given in an emergency.

796

Q *I am now over 41 weeks and planning to have a VBAC but my doctor doesn't want to induce me. Is Pitocin dangerous when attempting VBAC?*

A (See Section 8: Induction)
Both induction and augmentation with oxytocin have been reported with VBAC. One meta-analysis of several trials showed no association between use of oxytocin and uterine rupture in attempted VBAC, but another case-controlled study did correlate at least higher oxytocin infusion rates with rupture of the uterine scar.[62]

797

Q *Can I be given prostaglandin gel to ripen my cervix when attempting a VBAC?*

A As of 2006, most training programs forbid the use of any induction agent with VBACs, whether Cytotec, Prepidil, Cervidil, or any method to augment labor.[63]

798

Q *How many times can I have a VBAC?*

A As many times as you like. Risks of increased bleeding and malpresentation such as breech slightly increase after the third baby, but that is true for anyone.

799

Q *Can I still attempt a VBAC after more than one cesarean?*

A Current recommendations are that a VBAC may be attempted after no more than two cesareans, where the second cesarean was not a failed VBAC but an elective repeat. In reality, by 2006, few practitioners were allowing VBAC after two successive C-sections.

800

Q *Isn't it true that a lower uterine segment transverse incision could still rupture?*

A Absolutely. The risk is about 0.5 to 1 percent in most studies. However, the risk of uterine rupture with a repeat cesarean has been quoted at about 1.8 percent, or slightly higher.[64] This has been reconfirmed with a meta-analysis of multiple different trials in 1991.[65] However, none of these studies distinguished between simple scar separation and clinically significant rupture.

801

Q *How is it possible that the rupture rate is greater for repeat cesareans than for vaginal trial?*

A This is an excellent question. The greater rupture rate for repeat cesareans probably reflects terminology and definitions used for the diagnosis. A uterine scar separation, which means a "window" where it appears that only the amniotic membranes are keeping the fetus inside, is easily seen at a repeat cesarean. Such a window, or separation, must be actually palpated (felt) with a hand in the uterus (called uterine exploration) after a successful VBAC. With no excessive bleeding, uterine exploration may be overlooked. With no epidural, it may be purposely overlooked because of the pain involved. Separation with both a successful VBAC or a repeat C-section would normally be asymptomatic, without significant uterine bleeding or fetal distress.

Additionally, recent data from the University of North Carolina comparing VBACs with repeat cesareans suggests a major complication rate almost twice as high for mothers attempting a trial of labor rather than a scheduled C-section.[66] Criticism of this study is that the failed VBACs who had cesareans subsequently had their morbidity and mortality grouped in the VBAC category rather than the cesarean. This, however, is probably appropriate when comparing VBAC trials to elective, scheduled repeat cesareans.

802

Q *If the uterine scar separation rate is about 1.5 to 2 percent, do we know the true, catastrophic, clinically significant rupture rate?*

A The true catastrophic rupture rate is probably around 0.33 percent MU (3.3/1,000), or about 1/330. A review of 6,138 women in Dublin, Ireland, revealed fifteen true uterine ruptures (excluding scar separations) from 1986 to 1992. Thirteen of these were in the 3,940 VBAC attempts, or 1/304. This is a catastrophic rupture rate of 0.33 percent.[67]

We have experienced several catastrophic uterine ruptures with VBAC attempts in our own practice with no maternal deaths, but with significant maternal and perinatal morbidity. Several recent studies have shown that when this complication occurs with a VBAC attempt, it can be disastrous for the fetus and end in a hysterectomy for the mother.[68]

803

Q *Can I do a VBAC if my first uterine incision was a low vertical?*

A Just recently obstetricians around the United States have been permitting VBAC attempts in some women with low vertical uterine incisions (which has nothing to do with the skin incision). This may be only in a circumstance where the doctor performed the first procedure and knows with certainty that the incision did not extend up into the thicker, muscular, active segment, which would make it truly a classical incision and not suitable for VBAC trial.[69]

OBSTETRIC HEMORRHAGE

804

Q *What does it mean when someone hemorrhages?*

A Hemorrhage is a dramatic term often misused by the public to mean any bleeding. In obstetrics, hemorrhage implies life-threatening blood loss of catastrophic volume, usually over a very short period of time. The most common time for dangerous amounts of blood loss is immediately after and within twenty-four hours after delivery.

Traditionally, a blood loss of more than 500 cc (0.5 liters) has been defined as postpartum hemorrhage. Observational studies have shown both that the doctor's estimate of loss is often only half of the actual loss, and that average blood loss, in fact, usually exceeds 500 cc at delivery.

805

Q *How common a problem is obstetric hemorrhage?*

A Obstetric hemorrhage remains one of the greatest challenges facing doctors and their patients. Even in recent years, it is responsible for about 15 percent of all nonabortion pregnancy-related deaths. However, tremendous strides have been made in its treatment, with the maternal death rate falling about tenfold from 1950 to 1985, and fifty-fold since 1900.[70]

Currently about 1.5 to 2 percent of pregnancies require transfusion, but about 6.8 percent of women having cesareans require transfusion, recognizing that the reason for the C-section may be associated with an underlying cause of increased blood loss such as abruption or previa.[71]

806

Q *What causes too much blood loss after delivery?*

A Postpartum hemorrhage is the most common source of serious blood loss in pregnancy, and accounts for about 25 percent of all deaths due to bleeding. Predisposing factors include any cause of an overdistended uterus that fails to contract well after delivery. This failure to contract is called uterine atony (atony means "no muscle tone").

When other areas of the body are injured, they depend on clotting factors, platelets, and vasospasm to stop bleeding. The immediate postpartum uterus has huge open venous sinuses in the walls and will only stop bleeding if strong uterine contraction collapses these vessels and stops their flow. Causes of atony would include twins or triplets, polyhydramnios, large clots accumulated shortly after delivery, or retained portions of the placenta. Some general anesthetics can contribute to uterine atony. Lastly, a uterus that is just plain worn out (muscle fatigue from a long labor, a very rapid and tumultuous labor, or from oxytocin or prostaglandin stimulation) may fail to contract after delivery.

807

Q *What are the treatments for a uterus that won't stop bleeding after delivery?*

A Three primary medicines are used to get the uterus to contract after the baby and placenta are delivered. Intravenous oxytocin is either continued, or initiated, at a much higher rate than would be used to induce labor. Methergine, a potent smooth muscle constrictor, and thus blood vessel and uterine stimulant, may be given intramuscularly, and followed up with oral administration. Hemabate, a form of prostaglandin F2 alpha may be given intramuscularly to contract the uterus as well. Hemabate has the side effects of diarrhea and fever, for which the patient can be pretreated with Tylenol and Lomotil.

808

Q *What do you do if these medicines don't work?*

A The problem is then approached surgically in one of four ways: tying off some pelvic vessels called the hypogastrics (hypogastric artery ligation); whip-stitching the back wall, or placental bed of the uterus, with multiple large sutures to pull the blood-filled sinuses closed; removing the uterus (hysterectomy); or performing a therapeutic uterine artery embolization, in which an interventional radiologist threads a catheter into the vessels supplying the bleeding area of the pelvis and releases little silicone spheres that block off the vessel. Embolization may only be available in the largest medical centers.

809

Q *What are the most frequent causes of bleeding that lead to emergency hysterectomy?*

A Emergency hysterectomy is infrequent, but it is occasionally lifesaving. The causes for hysterectomy are in descending order: uterine atony (43 percent), placenta accreta (30 percent), uterine rupture (13 percent), and extension of uterine incision into large vessels or vagina (10 percent).

810

Q *Why isn't uterine artery embolization used more frequently than it is?*

A Uterine artery embolization is a fantastic technique and has proved to be lifesaving for some patients. Several small studies attest to its effectiveness in the 1990s.[72]

The fact is that the number of radiologists skilled in this technique with adequate facilities readily at hand is still growing slowly. In rural areas, hysterectomy is undoubtedly faster and often the patient's only chance for survival. Large university centers may be able to mobilize quickly for this procedure. Recently at Presbyterian Hospital in Dallas, an embolization took less than twenty minutes. Including transport time, the bleeding was stopped less than thirty minutes from the decision to try it. While the patient received four units of blood, she maintains her fertility.

811

Q *What other types of obstetric hemorrhage are there?*

A Placenta previa, placental abruption, placenta accreta, uterine rupture, ectopic pregnancy, molar pregnancy, and bleeding from spontaneous miscarriage are also causes of life-threatening hemorrhage. Third trimester bleeding is associated with nearly four times the risk of preterm delivery as well. In addition, placental abruption, HELLP syndrome, and amniotic fluid embolus may all be associated with DIC, or diffuse intravascular coagulation, which can lead to internal bleeding as well. (See Section 9: Coagulation Disorders)

812

Q *How frequently do each of these causes of hemorrhage occur?*

A Causes of obstetric hemorrhage are as follows in descending order with incidence per number of deliveries in parenthesis. In late pregnancy: previa (1 in 200), abruption (1 in 120), preeclampsia-related (1 in 20). During delivery and postpartum: cesarean (1 in 6), obstetric lacerations in the vaginal area (1 in 8), uterine atony (1 in 20), retained placenta (1 in 160), uterine inversion (1 in 2,300), and placenta accreta (1 in 2,500).

813

Q *Can I donate my own blood before delivery just in case I need a transfusion?*

A Autologous donation gained popularity during the early 1980s when people became more concerned about HIV infection. Giving your own blood to be stored and used should you need it makes sense for some scheduled surgeries in nonpregnant women when you are known to be at high risk for hemorrhage. However, studies have shown that in pregnancy, less than 40 percent of women who needed transfusions could have been identified at high risk; this constitutes only about 0.6 percent of the pregnant population.

Consequently, organized obstetrics has frowned on autologous donation. Most have found it is not cost-effective, and in any event, minimum guidelines severely limit its usefulness. A minimum of eleven grams per deciliter Hgb or 34 percent Hct is required, and donation must be between forty days and seventy-two hours prior to delivery. Several arguments mitigate against autologous donation in pregnancy: catastrophic bleeding almost always requires more than two units of blood; most doctors would not recommend allowing more than one unit to be autologously donated; cost is prohibitive, in any event, with several hundred dollars per unit often being required, and this is not covered by insurance.[73]

814

Q *What about asking for a donation from a relative who has compatible blood?*

A Designated donor blood is still an available program for most blood banks nationwide. However, designated donor blood is no more or less screened than the general population's donations. Blood is tested for HIV, hepatitis B-E, as well as various other blood-born infectious agents.

You may have a warm spot in your heart for a relative, but you may not know everything there is to know about that person's private life. In general, bank blood should be considered no greater a risk for infectious disease than designated donor blood.

815

Q *How much blood would I have to lose to need a blood transfusion?*

A In normal pregnancy, you increase your blood volume by 30 to 40 percent. This means you have an extra one to two liters of blood circulating at delivery. (See Section 2: Blood) You've got to lose a lot of blood to need a transfusion. However, during delivery, you can lose a lot of blood very rapidly. Assuming normal blood volume at the onset of labor, a loss of about 2,000 cubic centimeters will leave you with a blood count of about 15 percent Hct and 5 percent Hgb. This is barely enough blood to keep oxygen delivered to tissues at adequate levels.

Even with a very low count, if the bleeding is essentially stopped and the underlying problem is resolved, you can be discharged to bed rest, fluids, and iron supplementation. Only if you are unable to perform simple tasks such as walking to the rest room or if you are continuously dizzy and/or have a severe headache with rapid pulse and rapid respiratory rate will your doctor plan to transfuse you. A transcutaneous oximeter, or pulse oximeter, may be clipped to your finger and a reading of your oxygen levels taken painlessly. A Hct of less than 15 percent and a pulse oximeter of less than 89 percent usually will warrant transfusion, but every case must be individualized.

MULTIPLE GESTATIONS

Twins are placed at the end of Section 8 because all of the potential complications associated with carrying and delivering twins are described earlier in the book. Descriptions of unfamiliar terms may appear earlier in this section.

816

Q We just had our first obstetric visit and our vaginal ultrasound had a little surprise finding—twins. We're excited and petrified. What do we do first?

A Calm down twice as much as normal, and just get used to the idea of doing things twice. Luckily you have some time to adjust, because prior to twenty weeks of gestation just about everything you've found in this book applies to you in the same way. Approaches to all the physiological changes, from morning sickness to exercise to dietary requirements are just the same. While you will be at increased risk for several potential problems later in gestation, you certainly don't need to be petrified.

817

Q How often are twins born in the United States?

A Overall, twins occur naturally in about one in eighty pregnancies, but this is changing rapidly as the number of pregnancies resulting from the use of fertility drugs increases. Triplets occur naturally in about 1 in 6,400 pregnancies, and quadruplets 1 in every 512,000 pregnancies.[74]

818

Q What is the difference between identical twins and fraternal twins?

A Identical twins are monozygotic twins, meaning that they come from one egg, penetrated by one sperm. The egg divides shortly thereafter. Fraternal twins, or dizygotic twins, come from two eggs fertilized by two different sperm. Identical twins are the same sex, and fraternal twins may or may not be.

Advanced reproductive technologies such as in vitro fertilization (IVF), and the use of medicines such as Pergonal and Fertinex markedly increase the risk of twins and, to a lesser extent, triplets and quadruplets. Women from thirty to forty also have a higher risk of twins naturally than any other age group. African Americans have a higher risk of twinning than whites, who in turn have a higher risk than Asians.

Fraternal twinning does run in families, but only on the maternal side.

819

Q What is a vanishing twin?

A Vanishing twin is the term applied to early missed abortion of one of multiple fetuses. Roughly 15 percent of pregnancies will abort in the first or early second trimester, and twins are no exception. About 15 percent of the time, when a vaginal sonogram at less than nine weeks reveals two sacs and two fetuses, a repeat sonogram at later than twelve weeks reveals only one of each. It is unusual for a twin miscarriage of one fetus to complete itself with heavy bleeding and passage of tissue. Instead, the fetus that succumbs is simply reabsorbed, with no apparent ill effect on the remaining fetus.

820

Q *I'm 35, pregnant with twins, and need advice about whether to have amniocentesis, an alpha fetoprotein 3 test, or no test. What do I need to know?*

A (See also Section 3: Amniocentesis/CVS; Alpha Fetoprotein 3)
If your twins are from different eggs (fraternal or dizygotic twins), then your risk of genetic problems such as trisomy 21 or Down's syndrome is roughly twice what it would be normally for your age. That means that instead of about 1 in 270 to 350, your risk is closer to 1 in 135 to 175. It also means that both sacs would need to be sampled when an amniocentesis is done, so that your true risk of miscarriage may be considerably increased from about 1 in 800 to as high as 1 in 400.

While most multiple gestations that result from taking fertility drugs such as Clomid or Serophene, Pergonal, and Fertinex will be dizygotic (nonidentical) twins, those that occur spontaneously have about a one-third chance of being identical (monozygotic or single egg).[75] Monozygotic twins occur in about 1 in 250 births worldwide. Amniocentesis with identical twins would only require tapping one sac, but of course knowing that they are identical with certainty isn't possible at the second trimester ultrasound, although it may be suspected by the thinness of the dividing membrane.

Alpha fetoprotein 3 (AFP3) testing is available for mothers with twin gestations. Originally, the norms were not as reliable for multiples as for singletons, but the data has improved in recent years, and you could certainly choose this route initially.

As discussed earlier in Section 3: Amniocentesis, a full discussion with your doctor about relative risks and benefits of prenatal genetic testing is particularly warranted with twins.

821

Q *How do we know if our twins are identical?*

A You don't. If the babies are of the same sex, they have a chance of being identical, but only special genetic testing after birth can determine that with certainty. Probably the best way is to wait and see if they look alike. You can get a hint by examining the placental membranes, but not always a definitive answer. (See Section 4: Placental Development)

822

Q *What are the increased risks of having twins, other than those above, such as miscarriage and genetic risk?*

A Now, be calm, but this is a partial list of increased complications associated with multiple gestations:

1. Preterm labor and delivery
2. IUGR and low birth weight (discordance if only one affected, i.e., unequal growth)
3. Twin-twin transfusion (one steals blood from the other)
4. Pregnancy-induced hypertension (preeclampsia)
5. Anemia, blood loss at delivery due to atony and/or cesarean
6. Placenta previa or placental abruption, and attendant blood loss
7. Cord accidents with prolapse, entanglement, or vasa previa (entanglement of cords occurs only with very rare single sac identical twins)
8. Polyhydramnios
9. Malposition of fetuses (breech, transverse lie)
10. Overall increased perinatal morbidity and mortality (54 in 1,000, compared with 10.4 in 1,000 in singletons)

823

Q *When does my pregnancy start to be different from carrying one baby?*

A Twin gestations get bigger quicker. In fact, at about thirty-two to thirty-four weeks, you will measure the same as mothers of singletons at term.

At twenty weeks, your doctor will start helping you plan for some possible lifestyle changes. First of all, you will be at increased risk for preterm labor, and your doctor may want you to decrease exercise significantly from twenty-four weeks on. Some have recommended complete bed rest with hospitalization from this point on, although most evidence would not support such a drastic move.[76] Certainly sex, strenuous exercise (except swimming), prolonged periods without rest, distant travel especially for more than an hour in the car, should all be discouraged. Drinking large amounts of fluids and lying down for several hours during the day are beneficial.

Some doctors advocate preventive treatment with oral Beta-mimetics such as terbutaline. (See Section 5: Tocolytics; Section 8: Preterm Labor) Evidence is conflicting, but recent reports indicate that it is unlikely for these medicines to work preventively in twins.[77]

Other doctors advocate home uterine activity monitoring (HUAM) so that a patient may obtain a daily record of the number of uterine contractions she is having in an hour, but may not be sensing. The theory is that as a pattern of increasing little contractions (uterine irritability) develops, intervention with intravenous hydration and medicines (tocolytics) may begin sooner and thus be more effective.

Data about the effectiveness of this approach is controversial. As of 1996, the American College of Obstetricians and Gynecologists (ACOG) could not advocate its use, concluding that "data was insufficient to support a benefit from HUAM in preventing preterm birth."[78]

824

Q *When will I have to stop work?*

A Every case really must be individualized with twins. Much may depend on your type of work and what your doctor thinks of your cervical examinations. After twenty-four weeks, your doctor may wish to do a two-finger pelvic examination every week to two weeks. Early changes that seem to be warning signs might precipitate a recommendation that you quit work and begin modified bed rest. Remember, just because bed rest was not necessarily shown to work preventively does not mean it won't help once preterm labor has begun to change your cervix.

825

Q *Is there anything we can do about the increased risk of preeclampsia with twins?*

A That is not clear. Certainly lots of oral fluids and bed rest, once the process becomes evident, are helpful in slowing it down. (See this section: Preeclampsia) There is no evidence that avoiding salt intake actually helps avoid the preeclampsia process, although it may help symptomatically by reducing swelling.

Whether or not minidose aspirin is helpful for preventing pre-eclampsia is unclear at this time. For many, the potential benefits outweigh the risks, and 82 milligrams of aspirin daily are prescribed from the time that the diagnosis of twins is made.

826

Q *What about the risk of placenta previa and abruption with twins?*

A The risk of previa is increased simply because the placenta or placentas take up more room and thus are more likely to cross partially or wholly over the cervix. With an overdistended uterus and an increased risk of preterm labor, premature separation (abruption) of the placenta is increased as well.

There is nothing other than avoiding sex that you can do to avoid the problems associated with previa. However, "forewarned is forearmed," and your knowledge of placenta previa may lead you to not only practice abstinence, but get bed rest in the late third trimester, ensure your proximity to a hospital, or even schedule an early cesarean. (See this section: Placenta Previa; Placental Abruption)

827

Q *Will I definitely have to have a cesarean?*

A Absolutely not. However, your chances of needing a cesarean are markedly increased by your other increased risks of previa, abruption, discordant growth (one baby much bigger than the other), IUGR, premature labor, and malposition (breech or transverse lie).

You can expect about a 45 to 50 percent chance of a cesarean, with another 5 to 10 percent chance for emergent cesarean of the second twin following vaginal delivery of the first.

828

Q *How often will the first (presenting) twin be head down or cephalic?*

A About 70 to 75 percent of the time, the first twin will be head down, but only about half the time will that be the one that weighs the most. If the second twin is breech and larger, there is some concern about the possibility of the head becoming stuck because the first twin inadequately dilated the cervix. If the first twin is breech, there is concern about cord prolapse, entrapment of the later-appearing head if it is larger than the butt (more likely the smaller the baby is), and, very rarely, locked twins in which the chin of the first breech baby locks against the chin of the second cephalic baby, and delivery is impossible.

Finally, the second twin is always considered an unstable lie, meaning that after the birth of the first twin, anything can happen, and the second twin may use its new spacious uterus for some serious acrobatics.

829

Q *What is a breech extraction?*

A After a first head-down fetus delivers vaginally, the second twin becomes an unstable lie as described above. If this baby stays in breech position or gets into serious fetal distress with sudden rupture of membranes and cord prolapse, for example, the obstetrician may reach his or her entire hand and arm into the uterus, feel for the baby's legs and grasp them, and then literally drag the fetus from the womb. In the hands of an experienced operator this may usually be done safely, but it is generally reserved for emergencies.

830

Q *Should I have an epidural for a vaginal twin delivery?*

A Yes. Should an emergency arise in labor and your vaginal attempt become the wrong thing to do, an epidural will allow a safer, quicker transition to cesarean. It will also allow for breech extraction as well as manual exploration to remove the placenta, if needed. An overdistended uterus is also more prone to uterine atony and severe postpartum hemorrhage. Therefore, having an epidural in place may allow for vigorous bimanual massage of the uterus to help it contract without extreme pain, as well as for postpartum surgical intervention, should that become necessary.

831

Q *Should I just schedule a cesarean for my twins and let go of trying to deliver vaginally?*

A Again, this issue is up to you and your doctor. Certainly in some circumstances, such as breech/breech, breech/vertex, breech/transverse, and transverse/transverse, this is the prudent course. Vaginal delivery with the first twin cephalic has been shown over and over to be safe, even for the second noncephalic twin who weighs over 1,500 grams. [79]

There are about a million things to prepare for with twins, so check out the resources and Websites at the end of this section.

LATER CHILDBEARING

832

Q *I'm thirty-nine years old. Is it true that I'm "high risk" because of my age?*

A No. Although being a little closer to the end of your reproductive years may have given you additional time to develop chronic health problems such as diabetes, kidney disease, high blood pressure, obesity, and thyroid disease, in the absence of these, you may expect to do as well as any twenty-nine-year-old.

833

Q *Even if I'm healthy, don't I have some increased risks?*

A Yes. You do have an increased risk of genetic abnormalities such as Down's syndrome (trisomy 21). (See Section 1: Chromosomal Errors) For instance, your risk of any chromosomal error is about 5.2/1,000 at age thirty-five, but 15.2/1,000 at age forty and 47.6/1,000 at forty-five.[80] You may evaluate your fetus for these problems by having a chorionic villi sampling before eleven weeks or an amniocentesis between about fourteen and eighteen weeks. (See Section 3: Amniocentesis)

In general, women over thirty-five are likely to have early miscarriages and low-birth-weight babies, and slightly more are likely to have stillbirths. Statistically, women over thirty-five, just as women under 18, are a little more likely to have a cesarean with their first pregnancy, and to develop preeclampsia. Women over 40 will usually be induced before their due date and have increased sonograms in the last trimester.

834

Q *I'm thirty-eight and newly married. We want to have a family, but we want some time to ourselves first. Is there any reason why we shouldn't wait another couple of years to get our family started?*

A Yes. Your family may never get started. Despite press stories about a woman having a baby at age fifty-five in Los Angeles, your fertility significantly decreases as you approach and pass through your early forties. Not only do you have more time to develop problems such as endometriosis, but you may begin to have irregular periods, indicating inconsistent ovulation. Furthermore, even with regular ovulation, your eggs may become less penetrable, and thus more difficult to fertilize, as you grow older.

Women over forty may have perfectly normal pregnancies, but you should not purposely choose to delay childbearing too long. If you can complete your family before the ages of thirty-eight to forty, it is still advisable to do so.

835

Q *I'm forty-one and the regional vice president of a large computer software company, but I'm also a newlywed and planning a pregnancy soon. I'll be able to handle a baby and my job, won't I?*

A With the loving support of a mate who is equally determined to bring a new life into the world and raise the child responsibly, you may be able to succeed in being both a mother and an executive simultaneously. You are more likely to have adequate financial resources and more likely than a younger woman to face problem-solving maturely.

However, the mature woman may also have unique issues to face. You may feel comfortable only when you're "in control," and an awful lot of things related to pregnancy and child rearing will be out of your control. Your life will change dramatically when you have a baby. People with children know that it changes for the better, but you need to fully expect these changes. Your time and mobility are about to be re-prioritized and you, your employer, your family, and your spouse need to understand that ahead of time.

PRECIPITOUS LABOR
(RAPID—LIKE ON THE INTERSTATE)

836

Q *My last labor was only four hours from start to finish. What if I don't make it to the hospital?*

A Precipitous labor is defined as a total labor of less than three hours. It is not common with first babies, but it is increasingly common with subsequent deliveries. While your doctor's cervical examination after thirty-seven or thirty-eight weeks cannot predict when you will go into labor, occasionally it helps with predicting a rapid labor. With a history of very rapid labors, your doctor may be willing to induce you. (See this section: Induction)

837

Q *What if I literally don't make it to the hospital? What should I do?*

A If you're at home and either your water breaks and you suddenly feel extreme pressure, or your contractions that started irregularly only thirty minutes ago suddenly are right on top of each other, call your doctor at once. If you are waiting for him or her to call back, or if you feel that you can't make it to the hospital, call 911 and try to stay calm.

The vast majority of times that this circumstance arises, you will have already delivered one or more babies in the past. Remember, women had babies at home routinely until halfway through this century. Home delivery is not recommended (See Section 1: Home Delivery), but 95 percent of the time, you will have no problem.

838

Q *What do I need to do to deliver at home, or in the car, if necessary?*

A If you are at home, either lie on the floor on a sheet with several pillows under your hips, or lie down in bed. If you are at home alone, try to pant between contractions, and only bear down as you would with a bowel movement when you have the urge to do so.

As you feel the baby's head spread your labia, ease the head out with your hands, while you are curled up, knees bent and apart.

After the baby delivers, place it against your chest and dry it with a towel. You may leave the cord attached with placenta in place while you wait for help to arrive. If the placenta comes out spontaneously, wrap it in a towel and try to keep it on or near your chest at about the same elevation as the baby until there is no pulsation, or simply tie it off with a shoelace or piece of twine.

If your husband is with you, do the same as above, but position yourself near the end of the bed. As the baby emerges, have your husband put gentle pressure against the head so it doesn't "pop" out suddenly and cause a perineal tear between your vagina and rectum. After the head delivers, loop a finger under the cord if it is around the neck and pull it back over the head. Then, put a hand on either side of the head and gently move the head down toward the floor to help the shoulder ease under the pubic bone. Once the shoulder comes out, the rest of the baby quickly follows. Place the baby on the mother's chest and await the placenta. You may tie off the cord as above after a few minutes. After the placenta delivers, massage the top of the uterus, which is about the level of the navel, until you feel it "ball up" firmly. This, along with breast-feeding, will help to slow your bleeding.

All of this may be approximated in the backseat, or a reclining front seat, of a stopped car. Once the placenta is delivered, wait for the ambulance if you are at home, or continue to the hospital if the driver is in a condition to do so safely.

Suggested Reading

SUGGESTED READING

Friedman, Robhellle, et al. 1996. *Surviving Pregnancy Loss.*

Friedrich, Elizabeth. 1990. *The Parents' Guide to Raising Twins.*

Kauffman, Elizabeth. 1996. *Vaginal Birth After Cesarean, The Woman's Guide to VBAC.*

Mathes, Patricia. 1994. *Teen Pregnancy & Parenting Handbook.*

For any obstetric condition, ask for the patient information available from:

American College of Obstetrics and Gynecology. 1995.
    ACOG Website: http://www.acog.com
    Main Switchboard: 800-673-8444, (206) 638-5577
    Order Desk: 800-762-2264 (Patient Education Pamphlets)

American Diabetes Association
    1660 Duke Street
    Alexandria, VA 22314
    1-800-DIABETES
    Website: http://www.diabetes.org/takeaction/theADA

TWINS

International Twins Association: Promotes the spiritual, intellectual, and emotional growth of your twins. (612) 571-3022

Mothers of Super Twins (MOST): Provides information, resources, and understanding to families of multiples. (516) 434-6678 MOST, P.O. Box 951, Brentwood, NY 11717

Mothers of Twins Club (MOTC): Local nonprofit organizations in every major city in the country. Usually your hospital can help you get in touch or check the local phone book.

The National Organization of Mothers of Twins Clubs, Inc. (505) 275-0955 NOMOTC, P.O. Box 23188, Albuquerque, NM 87192-1188

Center for Loss in Multiple Birth (CLIMB): Provides support for those who have lost one or more of their babies. (907) 746-6123 CLIMB, P.O. Box 1064, Palmer, AK, 99645

Books

Alexander, T.P. 1987. *Make Room for Twins*, New York: Bantam Books.

Gromada, K. 1985. *Mothering Multiples: Breastfeeding and Caring for Twins,* LaLeche League International.

Kushner, Rabbi Harold. 1989. *When Bad Things Happen to Good People.* New York: Schocken Books.

Novotny, P.P. 1988. *The Joy of Twins,* New York: Crown Publishers.

Magazine

Also look into *TWINS,* which is a bimonthly magazine full of resources and ideas. Order at (888) 55-TWINS, (888) 558-9467, or write to 5350 S. Roslyn, Suite 400, Englewood, CO 80111-2125
Web site: http://www.TWINSmagazine.com
E-mail: TWINS@businessword.com

WEBSITES

Cesarean Section

http://www.childbirth.org/section/section.html
http://www.babycenter.com/refcap/pregnancy/childbirth/160.html
http://www.nlm.nih.gov/medlineplus/cesareansection.html

Gestational Diabetes/Diabetes in Pregnancy

http://www.nlm.nih.gov/medlineplus/diabetesandpregnancy.html

Preeclampsia/Hypertension in Pregnancy

http://www.nlm.nih.gov/medlineplus/highbloodpressureinpregnancy.html
http://www.nlm.nih.gov/medlineplus/highbloodpressure.html

Pregnancy and Infections

http://www.nlm.nih.gov/medlineplus/infectionsandpregnancy.html

Preterm Labor

http://www.marchofdimes.com/pnhec/188_1080.asp
http://www.nlm.nih.gov/medlineplus/prematurebabies.html
http://www.babycenter.com/refcap/pregnancy/ pregcomplications/1055.html

VBAC

http://www.vbac.com/
http://www.childbirth.org/section/VBAC.html
http://www.pregnancyweekly.com/pregnancy_information/vbac.htm

Section Nine

Medical Complications

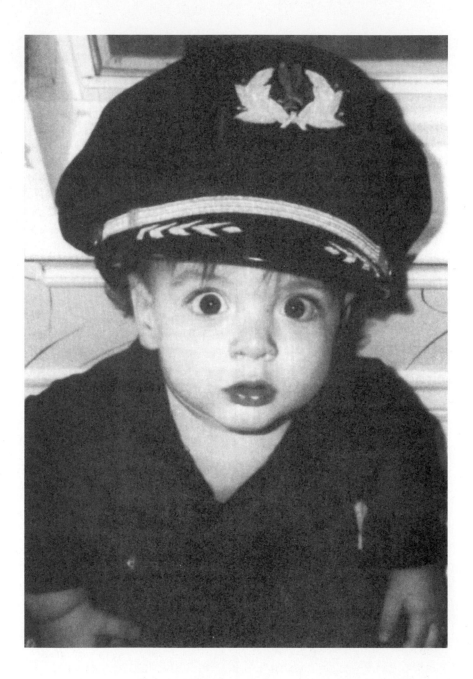

INTRODUCTION

Obstetrics deals mostly with young and generally healthy women. It is a fact of nature that reproduction occurs in our species during those years when the mother is most likely to attract a mate, survive long enough to protect her essentially helpless young, and be free of serious disease that would otherwise have already been fatal or at least compromised her ability to get pregnant and deliver successfully.

Recent changes in Western society have encouraged or at least led to childbearing in older groups of women. There is little intrinsically different about pregnancy in a forty-year-old than in a twenty-year-old, except for the increased risk of chromosomal errors such as Down's syndrome and other trisomies. However, delaying childbearing until early middle age does allow for time to develop any of a number of chronic diseases.

It is far beyond the scope and intent of this book to fully discuss the ramifications of each and every chronic disease on pregnancy. Fundamental questions that any woman would be likely to ask about some of these diseases are answered here. Women who have these conditions will have a better knowledge of them and will require more detailed information than they will find here. Your doctor, working in concert with an internist or the appropriate specialist, will need to address your specific condition, and in the detail you require.

HIGH RISK

839

Q *How do I know if I'm "high risk"?*

A The term "high risk" has neither an adequate definition nor, because of this ambiguity, any usefulness. Every pregnancy has its own set of problems. Every pregnancy can start without any difficulties and then end up with multiple complications. The designation "high risk" serves no purpose but to adversely affect the patient's outlook.

All Board Certified obstetricians are competent to handle any obstetric circumstance. There are certain procedures, such as targeted high-resolution ultrasound, amniocentesis, and intrauterine transfusion with cordocentesis, which are better handled by Board Certified perinatologists. Perinatologists are obstetricians with usually two additional years of training, often largely in basic science research, who have chosen to limit their practices first to obstetrics, and second to consultation with other obstetricians about less common medical and obstetric complications of pregnancy.

In large university centers, the perinatologist handles "high risk" patients transported from outlying areas. Therefore, they may develop more expertise in situations in which the obstetrician is knowledgeable but less experienced due to the infrequency of the problem.

Referral for consultation to a perinatologist is usually appropriate when your obstetrician would like to get another opinion, or you develop a problem with which he or she has little experience. Your obstetrician may either stay in control of your case or suggest that you transfer your care completely to the perinatologist.

Many hospitals with perinatologists on staff have guidelines that mandate consultation in the event of certain diagnoses.

INFECTIONS

Viral and Parasitic Infections

840

Q *Can viral infections harm my baby?*

A Viral infections and parasitic infections that humans may contract during pregnancy number in the thousands. While any systemic infection could potentially increase the chance of early miscarriage, there are certain specific viruses known to adversely affect the fetus before, during, and/or after birth. If the fetus is infected at birth, it constitutes a congenital infection. The most important viral infections include varicella (chicken pox), rubella (German measles), cytomegalovirus (CMV), herpes, and parvovirus 19 (Fifth's disease). Toxoplasmosis is usually considered with this group, although it is a parasite and not a virus.

841

Q *What are the TORCH titers I've heard mentioned?*

A TORCH is an acronym for five of the major congenital infections whose antibody titers are often drawn together in a panel. They include toxoplasmosis, syphilis (in the "o" spot for "other"), rubella, cytomegalovirus, and herpes.

The word "titers" refers to blood tests for antibodies. If you have recently been exposed to a viral or parasitic disease, your body will produce these immunoglobulins which are special proteins that attach to the foreign invader and help destroy it. Recent infection leads to IgM antibodies; previous infection leads to IgG antibodies. The presence of IgG antibodies usually means you have defeated this infection in the past and are now immune.

Varicella (Chicken Pox)

842

Q *If I contract chicken pox during my pregnancy, what problems can it cause for my baby?*

A Chicken pox (varicella) is a DNA viral infection of the herpes group, which is spread by the respiratory route. (Herpes zoster is the recurrent form of the same infection and may cause skin lesions and nerve pain, but may not be spread by the respiratory route, nor is it a cause of congenital infection.) A fetus infected with varicella due to a susceptible mother contracting the virus is at slight risk for multiple anomalies, including scarring of the skin, malformed limbs, malformed fingers and toes, eye and brain abnormalities, and mental retardation. The actual risk is small, but it is largest in the first trimester, when it approaches 10 percent.[1]

Infection beyond sixteen weeks seems to pose little or no risk for the fetus until just prior to delivery. About 15 percent of newborns whose mothers acquired chicken pox in the five days before delivery became infected, and 30 percent of those died as a result of their severe viral pneumonias.[2]

843

Q *Is chicken pox dangerous for me in pregnancy?*

A Yes. If you are not immune to varicella, infection in pregnancy, although rare, can be extremely dangerous. Although earlier reports were even worse, recent studies suggest a maternal death rate of about 10 to 20 percent from varicella pneumonia in pregnancy.

Acyclovir (Zovirax), and more recently valcyclovir (Valtrex), are being used to treat mothers with chicken pox. The Michigan Medicaid Recipient Study reviewed 478 newborns exposed to acyclovir in the first trimester. There was no evidence of an association between acyclovir and birth defects.[3]

Varicella vaccine recently became clinically available. It contains live virus, however, and should be avoided both during pregnancy and for three months prior to pregnancy.

844

Q *My son came home from school with chicken pox, but I know I had it as a child. Is my fetus at risk?*

A Varicella infection (called wild virus) imparts lifelong immunity. If you are certain you were infected as a child, you do not have to worry. If you are not certain and your mother can't remember, then your doctor can draw blood and check your antibody titer. If your IgG Ab titer is high enough, you are immune.

If you have never been infected and you are exposed to chicken pox, you can be given Varicella Zoster Immune Globulin (VZIG). It has been available for a number of years, but it is expensive and not readily available outside of large cities; however, it can be flown in. It should be given within ninety-six hours of exposure. If administered in time, it seems to somewhat reduce the severity of both maternal and newborn infection. It should be used only for those who know they are susceptible.

Rubella (German Measles)

845

Q *I thought everyone born since the 1960s got vaccinated for rubella as a baby. Are there many people who aren't immune?*

A Although the Federal Government did make a big push to get everyone under the "rubella umbrella" with vaccination, there are several holes in the system. First, rubella vaccine given prior to January 1979 did not always provide lifetime protection. Second, lots of children were not vaccinated, despite the rules. Third, there are many people born outside the United States who have arrived here unvaccinated.

The vaccine is a live virus and it is recommended that pregnancy not be allowed within three months of vaccination. Nevertheless, hundreds of exposures to the vaccine in the first trimester have been reported, but never a case of congenital rubella.

Rubella causes a mild illness in children five to nine years old, with low-grade fever, rash, and joint soreness. If, however, you acquire rubella during the first trimester of your pregnancy, there is a 20 percent chance that the fetus will contract the congenital rubella syndrome. (Fifty percent are affected if exposure occurs during the first eight weeks.) The syndrome includes cataracts, deafness, and congenital heart defects among other less common problems. Risk with exposure after the twelfth week of gestation is negligible. The infection in adults is difficult to detect: a mild rash starts on the face about two to three weeks after exposure. Because of this difficulty, recent vaccination is strongly suggested and antibody testing should be offered to anyone vaccinated with the old preparation prior to 1979 who is contemplating pregnancy.

Cytomegalovirus (CMV)

846

Q *What is cytomegalovirus and what can it do to the fetus?*

A CMV is another DNA virus in the herpes virus family that was once thought rare. It is now known to be the most common cause of congenital intrauterine (crosses the placenta) infection, with about 0.5–2.5 percent of all babies infected by the time they deliver. About 5 percent of these may have some long-term neurological problem. About 0.25 to 1.75 per 1,000 live births have neurological deficits. The full-blown CMV inclusion disease only affects about 1 in 10,000 to 20,000 newborns.[4] Another 5 percent of all infants are infected by virus in the cervix, in breast milk, or from transfusions, rather than across the placenta, but these infants do not develop problems related to the virus.

Of those infants that acquired the virus in utero (the 0.5 to 2.5 percent mentioned above), 90 percent are asymptomatic. Still, 10 percent of these will develop later problems. Of the 10 percent who have CMV symptoms

(0.05 to 0.25 percent of all births, or about 1 in 400), hearing loss is the most common problem. Mental retardation, developmental delay, seizures, learning difficulties, blindness (chorioretinitis and optic atrophy) and calcifications in the brain constitute the other more common severe problems. Less commonly, CMV causes liver and splenic disease, jaundice, and clotting problems.[5] Much more severe disease is seen in those whose mother acquired the virus in the first and early second trimester.

847

Q *Can I get CMV?*

A About 50 percent of all females of reproductive age are susceptible, or nonimmune. In fact, up to one-third of all pregnant women have live CMV virus in the cervix or urine. About 6 percent of all congenital fetal infections occurred in women considered previously immune, so recurrent disease, as well as primary infection, is a problem. Maternal infections are asymptomatic and essentially impossible to detect unless everyone is tested. If screening is desired, IgM antibodies imply recent infection and IgG immunity, as with other viruses such as rubella and varicella.

If you work in a neonatal intensive care unit (NICU), where CMV infections are frequently seen, you may wonder if it is safe for you to work there while you are pregnant. Both Swedish and American studies have demonstrated that nurses in nurseries have no greater rate of turning positive (IgM seroconversion) than the rest of the population. This may be related to care with hand-washing between baby contacts.[6]

Women exposed to infant or toddler urine and saliva should have their CMV titers tested when they are not pregnant. If found to be nonimmune, they should consider minimizing this exposure during pregnancy. Universal screening, such as with rubella, is not recommended, since no effective vaccine or treatment currently exists.

Parvovirus B19 (Fifth's Disease)

848

Q *What is all the fuss about? I teach fifth grade and can't go a single day without running into somebody terrified about Fifth's disease.*

A Parvovirus B19 seems to be on everyone's mind. Since 1975, it has been known as the causative agent of erythema infectiosum (Fifth's disease). It's also called slapped cheek disease because of the bright red, warm rash that occurs on the cheeks, and is accompanied by a low-grade fever; several days later a rash appears on the extremities. It usually occurs during the winter and early spring, but is still the fifth most common childhood rash behind chicken pox, measles, mumps, and German measles. In pregnancy, the virus likes fetal red blood cells and is very rarely associated with fetal anemia and fetal hydrops, or heart failure.

In the United States, 50 to 75 percent of women are immune. If you have been exposed, you may have titers drawn to prove or disprove your immunity. If you prove to be nonimmune, you may simply follow up on the fetus with an ultrasound about eight weeks after exposure which can detect fetal hydrops. If your fetus is affected, it may be treated successfully with intrauterine transfusion, or if exposure occurs after thirty-two weeks, delivery and transfusion after birth. Recent studies have even shown possible spontaneous recovery if infection occurred after twenty weeks.[7]

It is unlikely that you will have known anyone whose baby had a problem with Fifth's Disease. The initial studies done on the effects of parvovirus exposure during pregnancy were retrospective (looking backward). Not all variables were accounted for, numbers were small, and percentages of actual transmissions grossly misleading. The Center for Disease Control in Atlanta did a large prospective study of 3,526 exposures and found a slight, but not statistically significant, increased risk of fetal death before twenty weeks, and nothing thereafter. They found no increase in preterm labor, similar birth weights to noninfected infants, and no increase in birth defects whatsoever.[8]

Toxoplasmosis

849

Q *Everyone talks about toxoplasmosis and cats as a risk for my baby. How much of a real problem is it?*

A Toxoplasma gondii is an intracellular parasite whose only natural, definitive host (the one it reproduces in) is the cat. The life span of parasites is complicated, but the oocyst form exists in cat feces. Another form of the parasite, the cysts, can exist, rarely, in undercooked meat, especially lamb.

Classically, the three effects seen in the clinically infected newborn are hydrocephaly (water on the brain), intracerebral calcifications, and blindness due to chorioretinitis.

If you've had an indoor-outdoor cat for any number of years, your chances of being immune from previous infection is high; as high as 90 percent immunity was found in Paris, for example. Of the 10 percent or so susceptible, only about 2 in 1000 (0.2 percent) pregnant cat owners acquire the infection during pregnancy, as evidenced by antibody titer changes. If infected, only 30 percent of these 0.2 percent (or 0.06 percent of fetuses) are infected. Now, only 30 percent of those 0.06 percent (or 0.018 percent) are clinically affected. This is out of the susceptible pregnant cat owners, which may constitute only 10 percent of the population.[9] You can understand why doctors don't actually see the problem very frequently. *Only about 0.0018 percent (1.8 in 100,000) of the fetuses of pregnant cat owners will get sick from toxoplasmosis.*

You may request testing to see if you are immune. To avoid getting toxoplasmosis, just wash your hands after changing the litter box or have someone else do it, and cook your lamb chops thoroughly. (See Section 5: Antiparasitics for treatment)

Herpes Simplex

850

Q *What is genital herpes?*

A Genital herpes is a herpes simplex (HSV) infection in the vulvar area. It usually involves either the inner lips of the vagina (labia minora) or the outer lips (labia majora). The virus is acquired through intercourse or oral sex with an infected partner. First episode primary herpes begins as multiple small blisters in the genital area; these blisters become open, burning ulcerations that are extremely tender to the touch. Initial infections resolve after about ten to twenty days.

Forty percent of people, however, will have recurrences. These may occur only once every few years, or every other month. In between outbreaks, the virus lives up in a nerve ganglion near the spinal column. Particularly in times of stress, the virus travels down the nerve to the skin in the same area every time. Typically these outbreaks are much less severe, and are called secondary episodes. It has only recently been learned that many women acquire the virus silently, with no symptoms the first time, but then later have "recurrences," which to them, are their first outbreaks. These are called first episode non-primary outbreaks and are less severe, just like known secondary outbreaks.

Even if you have had just two sexual partners, you may be at risk for this disease. Genital herpes is one of the commonest reasons to visit the gynecologist. A 1992 study showed that about one-third of middle-class women had antibodies specific to herpes type II, the kind that infects the genitals 90 percent of the time. However, of these women, it is now estimated that two-thirds acquired the infection without symptoms.[10] Remember the math of sexually transmitted diseases: you may have had only two partners, but if each of them had two, and each of those had two (and so on), you could easily have been exposed to the equivalent of more than sixty-four partners in a very short time.

851

Q *What can happen to a newborn infected with HSV at birth?*

A Neonatal herpes is potentially a disaster. Because of the baby's incomplete, immature immune system at birth, HSV can become a systemic infection devastating almost every organ system. The neonatal mortality rate is higher than 50 percent.

852

Q *I have genital herpes and my last outbreak was about five months ago. Do I need to have a C-section?*

A Current recommendations are that in the absence of a currently visible lesion in the genital area, a C-section is not warranted. Weekly cultures from thirty-six weeks on in women with no symptoms should be abandoned, even though there is reason to believe that 0.5 percent of pregnant women are shedding the virus without lesions present, because it appears that well over 95 percent of neonatal herpes infections are from women with first episode primary outbreaks.

If you've had herpes in the past, you still have some risk, but it is markedly reduced. It seems that your IgG antibodies cross the placenta and provide a large measure of protection to the fetus. Less than 5 percent of women who deliver vaginally with a recurrent lesion will infect their newborn, but that's still enough to warrant a C-section.

There is a way to decrease your chances of recurrence as you get near delivery. Recent data from UTSW in Dallas demonstrates that acyclovir given in the last six weeks of pregnancy was safe and effective at preventing recurrences and lowering the C-section rate.[11] It is reasonable to assume that valcyclovir may be used in a similar fashion. The CDC as of 2011, recommends that ALL pregnant women receive the inactivated influenza vaccine.

853

Q *I get "fever blisters" from time to time. Is it okay to use topical Zovirax on them?*

A Fever blisters, or cold sores, are felt to be caused by the herpes simplex type I virus (HSV). It is safe in all trimesters to use topical acyclovir or Zovirax on the vermilion border of the lip.

Canker sores or aphthous ulcers, found on the inside mucosal surfaces of the mouth, are not the same as fever blisters. The cause is unknown, but there seems to be little benefit to topical antiviral drugs. Two percent viscous xylocaine gel may be used sparingly when sores are so painful as to interfere with eating and sleeping. Recent studies show up to 80% of genital lesions may actually be HSV I due to the prevalence of oral sex.[12]

Hepatitis

854

Q *I'm confused by all the different kinds of hepatitis. What types are there?*

A Hepatitis is a viral infection whose primary target is the liver. Types A through E have now been identified. Only A (HAV) and E are transmitted by the fecal-oral route, that is, by contaminated food handled by unwashed hands. These two types never cause long-term damage. Types B (HBV), C (HCV), and D (HDV) are all transmitted by sex, contaminated needles, and blood transfusion. Type B (HBV), the former "transfusion" hepatitis, may also be transmitted at delivery. Types B, C, and D all may cause chronic liver disease, with Types C and D having rates as high as 50 to 70 percent. (Chronic liver disease, incidentally, can kill you.) HCV is now known to cause the majority of transfusion hepatitis cases.

855

Q *Didn't my doctor screen me for one of these?*

A The HBsAg blood test is now routine in the United States at initial pregnancy visits. HBsAg is a protein from the outer coat of the virus and is shed by the liver into the blood. Its presence on a screen means you have had HBV in the past (or have been vaccinated). If you are HBsAg-negative, you are not considered at risk for infecting your fetus, unless you acquired the virus within thirty days before the test, in which case it would not yet be positive.

The HBeAg is a protein from the core of the virus and can also be found in the blood. If HBeAg is present, the patient is infectious. If HBeAg is absent, but the antibody to it is present (HBeAb), the patient is noninfectious. In pregnancy, HBsAg-positive women with "e" antigen present will always infect the fetus; with "e" antigen absent, infection is much less likely.

856

Q *What needs to be done if I am HBsAg-positive?*

A HBV is not associated with birth defects or increased fetal loss. However, the newborn is at risk of having received the virus from an HBsAg-positive mother. Transmission rates are low in asymptomatic carriers. If a woman is HBeAg-positive, even asymptomatic carriers have high transmission rates to the fetus.

You will receive further testing to determine how your liver is working and if you are infectious. Your baby will receive hepatitis B immune globulin (H BIG) as well as hepatitis B vaccine (Recombivax HB) within twelve hours of delivery. The vaccine should be repeated at one and six months of life to prevent chronic liver disease in your baby.

Other Viruses (Influenza, Measles, Mumps)

857

Q *I had the flu in the first trimester. Could I have hurt my baby?*

A Influenza infection may lead to more severe disease in you during pregnancy, up to and including a lethal pneumonia, although the incidence of this is extremely small. There is no reliable evidence that influenza viruses are associated with increased rates of congenital defect, premature labor, growth restriction, or stillbirth.[13] The effect on miscarriage is less clear. Any febrile (with fever) illness may be associated with a slightly higher risk of spontaneous abortion.

858

Q *I know about rubella and chicken pox, but what about mumps and measles?*

A Mumps and measles (rubeola) are both common childhood illnesses, and are also required vaccinations in the form of the MMR shots given to children as toddlers. Nevertheless, mumps occurs more commonly in pregnancy than either measles or chicken pox. However, mumps has not been associated with increased rates of IUGR, prematurity, stillbirth, or any congenital defects in humans. There is about a twofold increased risk of miscarriage if mumps is acquired in the first trimester.

Measles, on the other hand, is extremely rare in pregnancy. It is not associated with an increased miscarriage rate, but is clearly associated with an increased risk of prematurity. No teratogenic effects of measles have ever been proven.

Sexually Transmitted Diseases (STDs)

Herpes
    (See Viral Infections) Syphilis

859

Q *I've heard about syphilis, but I didn't think we had to worry about it anymore since we have penicillin. Is it still a problem?*

A It's still a problem. Syphilis is a sexually transmitted disease (STD) caused by the *Treponema pallidum,* a special kind of a bug called a spirochete. It can be a chronic infection, which, if it is left untreated or is inadequately treated, can lead to slow but lethal destruction of the central nervous system. Although syphilis dramatically decreased from the mid-1940s until about 1960, it has been on the rise since then. Very recently, there has been a dramatic rise in congenital syphilis in newborns. In over 90 percent of the cases, those who are afflicted live in poverty and are African Americans or Latinos. The increase is thought to be due to treatment of another STD, gonorrhea, with a drug that does not eradicate syphilis at the same time; an increase in exchange of sex for drugs; and an increase in reporting.

860

Q *How would I know if I had syphilis or if my partner did?*

A Blood tests for syphilis include the screening RPR and VDRL tests, and also the confirmatory FTA-ABS and MHA-TP tests. The RPR test is required for pregnant women in all states.

Syphilis causes a painless ulcer on the genitals, with a raised border, on average about three weeks after exposure. This is primary syphilis. The lesion is obvious on the penis, but more often than not, the woman's lesion is up inside on the cervix or vaginal wall. Usually, the lymph nodes in the groin will be enlarged and easy to feel. The lesions go away in about a month and the secondary phase begins. Symptoms now include raised red rashes on the palms and soles, whitish patches on the mucous membranes of mouth and vagina, and enlarged lymph nodes throughout the body. These symptoms resolve in about a month, as well, and the asymptomatic latent phase begins.

If untreated, one-third of patients will develop tertiary syphilis, whose symptoms include aortic dissection and valve disease (heart disease), as well as neuromuscular coordination problems and eventually brain involvement, with insanity ensuing.

861

Q *If I had syphilis during pregnancy, what can it do to my baby?*

A Syphilis, either primary, secondary, or latent, can lead to Treponema pallidum crossing the placenta to the baby as early as six weeks of gestation. The risk is much higher with primary or secondary phases, leading to a 50 percent transmission rate and at least a 50 percent perinatal death rate, 35 percent of which is stillbirth.[14]

Survivors may be blind and deaf, and they may also have problems with their liver, spleen, and bones. If these problems are untreated, victims go on to have central nervous system disease and heart disease.

Treatment in pregnancy consists of Benzethine Penicillin G, 2.4 million units, given by intramuscular injection. If disease is suspected for more than one year, repeat every six weeks for three total doses. Penicillin-allergic patients should be desensitized with an oral regimen. Doxycycline, taken at 100 milligrams twice a day for two weeks is effective, but its use in pregnancy has always been contraindicated until recently. (See Section 5: Drugs in Pregnancy)

Gonorrhea

862

Q *What is gonorrhea?*

Gonorrhea (GC), colloquially referred to as "the clap," is a gram-negative diplococci bacteria that causes a purulent (pus filled) discharge with very painful urination in men, and a painless, sometimes noticeable discharge in women. In nonpregnant women, GC can be one of several bacteria that ascends to the fallopian tubes and causes pelvic inflammatory disease (PID), which can lead to chronic pain with sex and to infertility.

863

Q *Can I get PID when I'm pregnant?*

A Technically, no. The gestational sac prevents GC from moving up and entering the fallopian tubes. However, GC can lead to amniotic fluid infection with premature rupture of the membranes (PROM), prematurity, growth retardation, postpartum endometritis (uterine infection), and newborn sepsis.

While GC is usually asymptomatic with respect to the genitals in pregnancy, disseminated GC (DGI) is the most common presentation. This means skin lesions that start as little blisters and progress to pustules scattered on the undersurfaces of the arms, palms, and fingers. DGI may also include arthritis, since the bacteria embolizes to the joints, or endocarditis as an infection sets into the heart valves.

Opthalmia neonatorum (newborn eye infection) has been the traditionally recognized threat. GC infects the cornea as the baby passes through the birth canal, and this leads to scarring and blindness.

The erythromycin antibiotic ointment placed in your child's eyes shortly after birth is for prevention of this problem. (Silver nitrate was used in the past.)

If you have a cervical culture that is positive for gonorrhea, you can be treated in pregnancy. A one-time intramuscular injection of 250 milligrams of Ceftriaxone and 500 milligrams of erythromycin orally four times per day for seven days is adequate treatment for lower genitourinary tract involvement.

Chlamydia

864

Q *What is chlamydia?*

A Chlamydia trachomatis is an intracellular bacteria which, often in concert with gonorrhea, is the causative agent of the sexually transmitted tubal infection known as pelvic inflammatory disease (PID). It may live without symptoms in the female cervix. While it may cause no symptoms in women, it may also cause a cervical-vaginal discharge, postcoital (after sex) bleeding, a condition similar to bladder infection with burning on urination (urethritis), or severe abdominal pain as with PID. Chlamydia causes burning on urination and a penile discharge in the male (nongonoccocal urethritis, or NGU).

In developing countries, chlamydia is the cause of "trachoma," which is considered the leading cause of preventable blindness in the world.

Chlamydia is thought to be present in the cervix about 5 percent of the time in American women. Because it is an STD, certain groups of pregnant women have a higher incidence of this disease. These include prostitutes, unmarried women, those who have contracted other STDs, women less than twenty years old, those whose partners who have NGU, women who receive late or no prenatal care, those who experience cervical discharge, women having bladder symptoms with culture-negative urine (sterile pyuria), and residents of socially disadvantaged communities. In these groups, as many as 30 percent of sexually active females may be culture-positive for chlamydia.[15]

865

Q *Is chlamydia more dangerous in pregnancy?*

A Yes. It is certainly more dangerous in that it can devastate your newborn. As many as 70 percent of newborns born through an infected cervix will develop infections. Fifty percent will have severe eye infections in the first two weeks, and 20 percent will contract pneumonia within the first three to four months of life.[16]

Many studies on the effects of chlamydia in pregnancy have reached conflicting results on whether or not *Chlamydia trachomatis* is associated with prematurity, premature rupture of membranes (PROM), low birth weight, and increased perinatal mortality. Routine screening in early pregnancy has also remained controversial. Certainly, women in the high-risk groups listed above should be screened.

As with gonorrhea, state laws require the administration of an erythromycin antibiotic ointment in your baby's eyes shortly after birth. If conjunctivitis resulted anyway, systemic treatment with erythromycin seems to work well and it prevents the development of pneumonia.

Chlamydia can be treated in the pregnant woman when discovered with erythromycin base 500 mg each day for seven days. Alternatively, women may be treated with amoxicillin 500 mg three times per day for seven days with 98 percent eradication of the chlamydia from the cervix.[17]

After the first trimester, chlamydia may be treated with four pills of Zithromax taken all at once.

Condyloma Accuminata, or Venereal Warts (HPV)

866

Q *What are venereal warts?*

A Venereal warts (Condyloma accuminata) are growths that may occur on any portion of the vulva, perineum, and anus, as well as on the cervix. As implied by the name, they are sexually transmitted manifestations of infection with any one of over twenty serotypes of human papilloma virus (HPV), thought capable of infecting the skin and mucous membranes of the female genital tract. (There are over sixty total serotypes of the virus.)

Condyloma tend to grow very rapidly during pregnancy. The highest prevalence is in women sixteen to twenty-five years old, but the warts may be seen at any age during the reproductive years.

867

Q *How is condyloma transmitted?*

A Like all the other STDs, vaginal or anal sex with an infected partner leads to transmission of the virus 65 percent of the time on first contact. The latent (dormant) period varies from three weeks to eight months, with an average of 2.8 months before the warts appear.[18] Warts are dangerous in two ways:

1. They signify the presence of HPV in your genital tract, certain serotypes of which are known to be the cause of most cervical cancers.

2. The warts can, *rarely,* transmit the HPV virus to your newborn, possibly resulting in benign growths on your child's larynx (voice box) years later.

However, transmission to the fetus is so rare that the Center for Disease Control does not recommend a cesarean to prevent transmission.

868

Q *Are the warts treatable in pregnancy?*

A Yes. Trichloroacetic acid (TCA) may be applied safely and effectively in pregnancy. Large lesions may need to be excised or vaporized by laser under anesthesia. Podophyllin, a common treatment in nonpregnant women, cannot be used in pregnancy. It has been associated with fetal deaths and maternal nerve problems, and it is also considered a first trimester teratogen. Likewise, 5-fluorouracil should be avoided in pregnancy. Systemic interferon A has recently been used to treat condyloma, but little experience exists on its use in pregnancy. A new drug, Aldara, became available in 1997. (See Section 5: Drugs in Pregnancy, Antivirals)

Human Immune Deficiency Virus (HIV)

869

Q *I only found out I was HIV-positive six months ago, and now I'm six weeks pregnant by accident. Will HIV harm my pregnancy?*

A Probably not. HIV is the cause of acquired immune deficiency syndrome (AIDS), which may be acquired through intercourse, anal intercourse, blood and blood product transfusion, and contaminated needles from illicit drug use. At any one time there are about seven-thousand to eight-thousand ongoing pregnancies in the U.S. in which the mother is HIV-positive. Many states now have laws mandating HIV testing at least twice during pregnancy.

There is little evidence that HIV affects pregnancy other than transmission to the fetus. Several reports have suggested it causes higher-than-normal rates of abortion, preterm labor, and low-birth-weight babies, but not higher than in HIV-negative drug addicts.[19] Other studies have shown no effect of HIV whatsoever on any outcome.[20]

If you are HIV-positive, no one knows for sure what the chances are for your baby to be infected; numbers vary between 15 and 50 percent. Recently, several experts have suggested that about 30 percent of babies of untreated mothers is average.[21] But the large European Collaborative Group reported only a 14 percent untreated rate of transmission. Transmission, when it occurs, is thought to be about 80 percent across the placenta and about 5 to 20 percent via a contaminated cervix and vagina.

AZT has been shown to be effective in blocking transmission to the fetus and should be instituted if you are HIV-positive. (See Section 5: Antivirals)

Vaginal Infections

Yeast

870

Q *I heard that yeast infections were more common in pregnancy. Is that true, and are they dangerous?*

A Candida albicans and Torulopsis glabrata account for, respectively, about 80 percent and 15 percent of vaginal yeast infections in pregnancy. About one-fourth of all pregnant women have candida present in the vagina, and about 15 percent develop symptomatic infections in pregnancy. Even women who have never had a yeast infection may acquire one in pregnancy due to the high estrogen levels and an increase in vaginal glycogen.

Yeast infections in pregnancy do not appear to be dangerous. You can use over-the-counter medicines for yeast, but make sure a yeast infection is what you have. Monistat, Femstat, Gyne-Lotrimin, Vagistat, and other medicines are safe in all trimesters. (See Section 5: Drugs in Pregnancy) Yeast infections may often be confused with bacterial vaginosis (BV) caused by Gardnerella vaginalis. Yeast primarily causes itching, with variable amounts of a whitish discharge, and little odor. BV primarily causes a fishy, amine odor, a yellowish gray discharge, and little itching. Burning with sex is common to both, but the odor associated with BV is worsened by sex.

Bacterial Vaginosis (Gardnerella)

871

Q *Is bacterial vaginosis common in pregnancy, and is it dangerous?*

A Bacterial vaginosis, or Gardnerella, is even more common than yeast infection in pregnancy. The symptoms are described above, with odor and discharge being much more prominent than itching. Recent data has linked BV to pregnancy complications including preterm labor, PROM, and postpartum uterine infections.[22]

Treatment has recently switched from oral metronidazole as primary therapy to Metrogel Vaginal Gel used twice per day for five days. It may be effective if it is used only once per day for five days as well. Alternatively Cleocin Vaginal Cream may be used, once per night for seven nights. Both appear to be safe in all trimesters. (See Section 5: Drugs in Pregnancy, Antibiotics)

Trichomoniasis

872

Q *What is trichomonas, and how did I get it?*

A Trichomonas vaginalis is actually a trichomonad, or small flagellated parasite. Infection with this parasite causes a very itchy, foul-smelling vaginal infection that is often accompanied by pain with urination. Trichomonas is felt to be sexually transmitted virtually all of the time. Males often have no symptoms.

Most studies have found this disease to be associated with a higher incidence of pregnancy complications. The National Institutes of Health (NIH) Infection and Prematurity Study showed a significant association between maternal Trichomonas infection and low-birth-weight (LBW) babies, as well as with PROM.

Trichomonas may be treated in both you and your partner with a one-time dose of two grams or four 500-milligram tablets of oral metronidazol (Flagyl) for both you and your sexual partner. (Ask your doctor to prescribe enough pills for your partner as well, if he has no known allergies.) High-dose oral therapy such as this should be withheld, if possible, until after ten completed weeks of gestation.

Mycoplasmas

873

Q *Are there any other vaginal infections to worry about?*

A There are a few others, but they are not particularly worrisome. Mycoplasmas are divided into the respiratory infections like the kind that causes "walking pneumonia" and the genital mycoplasmas, which include Ureaplasma urealyticum and mycoplasma hominis. They are a little different from bacteria because they have no cell walls. The colonization rate of the mycoplasmas increases markedly from prepuberty to the age when sex has begun. Number of partners even affects the colonization rate, with up to 95 percent of women having Ureaplasma urealyticum in their vagina normally.

You may not know that you have a mycoplasma infection because the mycoplasmas seem to rarely cause symptoms unless they are present with another infection, such as Gardnerella. However, some doctors feel that the mycoplasmas can be responsible for some bacterial vaginosis without the presence of *Gardnerella*. The mycoplasmas could be dangerous in several ways:

1. Association with increased miscarriage rate (cause and effect not clearly shown)
2. Either form may be associated with cases of chorioamnionitis, which can lead to PROM and preterm labor
3. Possible association with low birth weight

However, a recent, large, multicenter study showed no association with any of these things in 4,934 women colonized with Ureaplasma urealyticum.[23]

Group B Strep Infections

874

Q *I've heard that strep infections are dangerous. Is this "strep" as in "strep throat"?*

A Beta-hemolytic streptococci are common bacteria that cause a multitude of human infections. They are grouped A through E, but A, B, and D are the only ones which infect humans.

Group A strep is the type of bacteria that causes "strep throat' It is also the cause of the old "childbed fever," and before the introduction of penicillin after World War II, this postpartum uterine infection was the second most common cause of maternal death after hemorrhage. With modern antibiotics, it is almost nonexistent as a cause of serious morbidity and mortality.

875

Q *Is this the type of strep that everyone's worried about causing pneumonia in the newborn?*

A No. Group B strep is the one you've been hearing so much about. Group B strep (GBS) lives in the vagina or rectum without causing symptoms (called colonization) in about 20 to 40 percent of all pregnant women. However, this bug may cause cystitis (bladder infection), endometritis (infection of uterine lining), amnionitis (infection of the amniotic fluid), and wound infections.

GBS can cause infection in the newborn, including severe pneumonia, meningitis (infection of the brain and spinal cord), and sepsis (infection in the blood). It may be acquired as the baby passes through a vagina colonized with GBS. Even though up to 40 percent of women are colonized with GBS, only about 2 in 1,000 newborns become infected in the United States; nevertheless, this still represents about 7,600 cases per year, with a mortality rate of 5 to 20 percent in the first 90 days of life. Those with early infection, in which symptoms occur within the first seven days of life, are more likely to die than those with late infection, who become symptomatic after the first seven days.[24]

876

Q *Why can't we just treat the one-third of women who have Group B strep with oral penicillins and get rid of the strep infection in the vagina?*

A That would be great, except these aren't infections, they're colonizations. That means that the bug likes living in your vagina, and your immune system tolerates its presence. You could be treated for ten days, get rid of the bacteria for a brief time, and it would come right back. Then you could pass the bacteria on to your baby at birth.

Preventing Group B strep (GBS) in newborns is a very complex issue. Some doctors advocated screening all pregnant women with cultures, but a few questions remained. What week of gestation should it be done? How does the doctor interpret false negatives, since a woman can be positive one week and not the next? Others advocated treating every woman with intravenous antibiotics in labor, but some women will have serious drug reactions and the cost will be immense. The American Academy of Pediatrics (AAP), the American College of Obstetricians and Gynecologists (ACOG), and the Center for Disease Control (CDC) all had different perspectives on the best approach.

A recent meta-analysis of seven trials (computer compilation of data) revealed a thirty-fold reduction in the incidence of newborn GBS if women with positive screening cultures received intravenous antibiotics in labor.[25]

The current ACOG recommendation is to screen all pregnant women with a vaginal culture at thirty-five to thirty-seven weeks of gestation. If the culture is positive, penicillin G or Ampicillin is given intravenously in labor to prevent newborn infection. ACOG has also recommended alternatively that the same treatment in preterm PROM less than thirty-seven weeks, rupture longer than eighteen hours, previous birth of child with Group B strep, and fever in labor of higher than 100.4 degrees Fahrenheit is an acceptable approach to decreasing the incidence of this disease in newborns.[26]

Other Infections

877

Q *My sister was diagnosed with Lyme disease last year. Can this affect her pregnancy?*

A Lyme disease is caused by the tick-born infection with the spirochete (same group as syphilis) *Borrelia bergdorferi.* This causes a multisystem infection that starts with the classic red target rash, may proceed to a meningitis stage with severe headache and stiff neck, and then progresses to pulmonary and arthritic complications over time. Diagnostic serum antibody tests are available, as is the case with the common viral diseases discussed above.

No one has proved it causes birth defects, but congenital and trans-placental infections have been documented.

Treatment consists of 500 milligrams of oral amoxicillin four times per day for ten to thirty days or, if the woman is allergic to penicillin, 250 milligrams of oral erythromycin four times per day for ten to thirty days. Two milligrams of intravenous Ceftriaxone for fourteen days is given for neurological disease or arthritis.

CHRONIC HYPERTENSION

(See also Section 8: Obstetric Complications, Preeclampsia)

878

Q *I'm thirty-seven years old and I've had hypertension for several years, but I've never been pregnant. Will my hypertension be a problem?*

A Chronic hypertension complicating pregnancy means high blood pressure (consistently over 140/90 untreated) that was present before pregnancy, or diagnosed in pregnancy before twenty weeks of gestation.

The vast majority of chronic hypertensives have uneventful, normal pregnancies. In fact, most chronic hypertensives have improving blood pressures throughout most of the pregnancy. Somewhere between 10 and 30 percent, however, will develop superimposed preeclampsia with proteinuria (protein in the urine), worsening blood pressure, and significant edema (swelling). They are then subject to all the dangers of the preeclamptic pregnancy as described in Section 8: Preeclampsia.

879

Q *Should I stay on my blood pressure medicine now that I know I'm pregnant?*

A Your doctor may continue, stop, or start with a different drug, depending on your circumstance. Do not stop your medicine without calling your doctor beforehand.

All of these medicines are discussed in Section 5: Antihypertensives.

880

Q *I've always been told never to stop my blood pressure medicine. How could stopping it be an option?*

A Pregnancy is a very special circumstance. Remember that the placenta is a low-pressure "sink." Those who do not become preeclamptic will actually drop their blood pressure from the middle of the first trimester through several weeks after the end of the second trimester.

An excellent study by Sibai and colleagues looked prospectively at a randomized study in which pregnant women with hypertension were either not treated at all, treated with Aldomet, or treated with the beta-blocker labetalol. Surprisingly, there were virtually no differences in the three groups in terms of maternal complications or perinatal outcome. Eleven percent of the untreated group did require treatment initiation for blood pressure higher than 160/110 at some point during pregnancy. Only the development of superimposed preeclampsia was associated with increased morbidity for mother or fetus.[27]

881

Q *So should I be taking any medicine for chronic hypertension in pregnancy or not?*

A Most experts agree that, for patient safety, treatment of blood pressures that are higher than 160/110 is indicated, and that this may decrease the incidence of superimposed preeclampsia, which is clearly dangerous. Blood pressures below that level at the start of pregnancy may either be treated with methyldopa, or observed. Your treatment will need to be individualized by your physician.

HEART DISEASE

Arrhythmias

882

Q *I'm twenty-eight weeks pregnant and sometimes I can feel my heart racing like a trip-hammer! I usually feel a little short of breath, too. It's scary, but is it dangerous?*

A Episodes of fast heartbeat are called tachyarrhythmias and are quite common in pregnancy. No one knows exactly why they occur more frequently in pregnancy. It may be due to lower potassium levels, or it may be related to hormonal changes. In any event, they are almost never dangerous as long as you had no underlying heart disease before becoming pregnant.

Usually these arrhythmias are supraventricular tachycardias (SVT), in which the upper chambers of the heart beat very rapidly for brief periods, and some or all of the impulses are transmitted to the lower chambers as well. You may feel as though your heart is pounding, in addition to its fast rate. The subjective sensation of shortness of breath is never accompanied by a true oxygen deficit when you remain conscious. You can usually stop these episodes with the following simple vagal maneuvers (things that fire the tenth cranial nerve and slow the heart).

Valsalva maneuver: Hold your breath and bear down for fifteen to twenty seconds as though you were having a bowel movement.

Try splashing ice-cold water on your face.

Finally, feel your pulse in the front part of your neck just below the jaw, then rub on one side only. (Cartoid massage.)

Usually these tricks are all that is needed. If the episodes are happening many times per day and you feel either dizzy or actually faint, you may need a medicine such as digoxin, nifedipine, or atenelol. Recently, intravenously administered adenosine has been used successfully for SVT that fails to correct in any other way, but this failure will be rare. Discuss your symptoms with your doctor, who will determine whether such medicines are justified.

883

Q *What other rhythm problems could I get?*

A All the others are very rare without underlying heart disease. Rarely, atrial flutter, or fibrillation, is seen with symptoms similar to SVT. In atrial flutter, the upper chambers (atria) of the heart beat so fast and shallowly that they don't move blood as quickly as normal. As a consequence, a blood clot can form in one of the atria. The blood thinner heparin may be used for people who have this condition all the time. It is most often associated with uncontrolled hyperthyroidism.

Other problems, such as slow rates (bradyarrhythmias), are rare; they are associated with underlying heart disease and are best managed by a cardiologist. Although pregnant women with pacemakers are rare, these devices have been used successfully in pregnancy.

Mitral Valve Prolapse

884

Q *I have mitral valve prolapse and the dentist always gives me antibiotics. Do I have to do anything different in pregnancy?*

A Mitral valve prolapse (MVP) is seen in 5 to 20 percent of normal women of childbearing age. The valve between the left atria and left ventricle tends to "pop" back into the atria, which causes the classic mid-systolic click when the ventricle contracts; it may be heard with a stethoscope. Rarely are there associated symptoms, but anxiety, palpitations, shortness of breath, fainting, and unusual chest pain can be encountered.

Use of beta-blockers such as atenelol is appropriate for severe symptoms. As of 2010, ACOG no longer recommends you receive antibiotics in labor for prevention of endocarditis, the risk of infection being lower than the risk if the antibiotic side effects.[28] Other heart valve lesions are rare in pregnancy. Atrial Septal Defects (ASD), mild Ventricular Septal Defects (VSD), Mitral Insufficiency, Aortic Insufficiency, and surgically corrected Tetralogy of Fallot usually pose little danger in pregnancy. Mitral and Aortic Strenosis however, may be extremely dangerous and are relative contraindications to pregnancy.

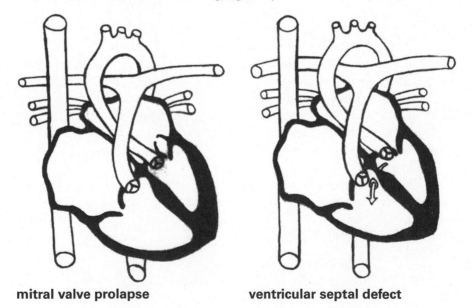

mitral valve prolapse   **ventricular septal defect**

Coronary Artery Disease (CAD)

885

Q *I had a heart attack at age thirty-one. Can I still have babies?*

A Yes. If your heart attack (myocardial infarction) did not produce heart failure, significantly weaken the function of the left ventricle as determined by echocardiogram, or leave you with unpredictable chest pain (unstable angina pectoris), your prognosis for a successful pregnancy is excellent. Rarely, a previous heart attack patient will need nitrates, calcium channel blockers, or beta-adrenergic blockers to control chest pain, but otherwise mild angina or a previous heart attack does not significantly affect pregnancy.

If you've had a heart attack in the past, depending on the severity of your heart condition, you may have virtually no restrictions or be so limited as to require bed rest throughout the entire pregnancy. (American Heart Association Classes 1-4). No limitation (Class 1) means exactly that. Mild limitation (Class 2) means that you can perform normal activities such as walking, climbing stairs, exercising, and having sex, with no resultant chest pain or serious shortness of breath. With moderate limitation (Class 3), you feel fine at rest and with minimal activity, but shortness of breath and chest pain are brought on by any exercise more strenuous than walking short distances. Severe limitation (Class 4) means you have symptoms even at rest.

You will have to follow the advice of your cardiologist and obstetrician in order to have a safe pregnancy. Pregnancy in the presence of a previous heart attack may require decreased exercise, absolute cessation of smoking, medications for hypertension or arrhythmia taken without fail, and strict adherence to a low-fat, moderate-sodium diet.

Cariomyopathy (heart failure due to muscle weakness) is a very rare, very severe problem which occurs around delivery or within thirty days afterward. Preeclampsia, obesity, and severe anemia are risk factors. Fifty percent die within the first year and heart transplant is the only definitive treatment.

BLOOD DISEASES

Anemias

Iron Deficiency

886

Q *My doctor told me I was anemic at twenty-eight weeks of pregnancy and put me on iron. Am I at more risk of needing a transfusion than others?*

A (See Section 2: Iron and Cardiovascular Changes)

Probably not. If you weren't anemic at the beginning of your pregnancy, your low Hct (hematocrit) at twenty-eight weeks is due to relatively more water in your blood, or hemodilution. Your body naturally retains water in order to expand your blood volume, and has one to two liters of extra blood by the time you deliver. Because your normal iron loss through menstrual periods doesn't occur during pregnancy, you hang on to most of the iron in your diet and vitamin supplements. This iron is put into bone marrow stores and then used from about thirty to forty weeks to turn water into blood.

Whether you need to start taking extra iron in addition to that in your prenatal vitamin as you approach thirty weeks depends on several factors: your hematocrit at the start of pregnancy, your current hematocrit, the amount of iron in your current diet and vitamins, and your ability to tolerate iron supplements with respect to constipation, diarrhea, or stomach cramps.

Your doctor will evaluate all of these factors and decide what is best for you. (See Section 2: Iron) Those patients who do NOT demonstrate iron deficiency anemia in the first trimester do not need iron supplementation other than what is found in most prenatal vitamins.[29]

Megaloblastic anemia

887

Q *I was anemic at the start of my pregnancy, but my doctor said he could tell from my blood tests that it wasn't due to lack of iron. He told me I needed more folate. Isn't that just to prevent spina bifida?*

A Folate (folic acid) can help reduce the risk of neural tube defects if it is taken between conception and about one month after conception, but it serves many other purposes as well. If your red blood cells appear bloated and larger than normal on a microscope slide, but your blood count is down, you may have megaloblastic anemia and not iron deficiency. This results from a dietary deficiency of folate and will be rapidly corrected with supplementation.

Hemoglobinopathies

888

Q *My doctor said I'm anemic because I inherited the problem, and it had something to do with being Italian. Could she be right?*

A Hemoglobinopathies are inherited abnormalities in the structure of the oxygen-carrying proteins inside your red blood cells. Examples include the alpha and beta thalassemias, as well as the sickle-cell syndromes, both the disease and the trait. Women with beta thalassemia minor, alpha thalassemia minor, and sickle-cell trait tolerate pregnancy well. Those of Mediterranean descent, such as yourself, have an increased risk of beta thalassemia.

Beta thalassemia is an inherited anemia, seen more commonly in descendants of those along the Mediterranean Sea. This includes Italian, French, Spanish, Greek, and Turkish people. Beta thalassemia minor, in which only one of two genes is affected, produces only a mild, hypo-chromic (pale-cell) microcytic (small-cell) anemia, which mimics iron deficiency but fails to respond to iron. Women with beta thalassemia minor tolerate pregnancy well.

Beta thalassemia major (Cooley's anemia), which involves both genes, leads to a severe anemia; children rarely survive to adulthood and are usually sterile even if they do, so its rarely seen in pregnant women.

Alpha thalassemia minor, found in those of Asian descent, also creates a mild anemia that is tolerated well in pregnancy. Alpha thalassemia major (Hemoglobin Bart) affects the fetal blood supply and always leads to stillbirth or newborn death. It is a common cause of stillbirth in Southeast Asia. There are no adult survivors with alpha thal major.

Other less common hemoglobinopathies include Hemoglobin C and C beta thalassemia, both of which result in mild to moderate anemias and do not appear to significantly affect pregnancy outcomes.[30]

889

Q *1 have sickle-cell anemia. Can I carry a pregnancy safely?*

A Even with the best of care, sickle-cell disease in pregnancy includes a risk of stillbirth or newborn death of about 20 percent, a 2.5 percent risk of death for you, and the prospect of multiple sickle-cell crises, in which oxygen to your bones is severely diminished, leading to episodes of excruciating pain. Sickle-cell is considered a relative contraindication to pregnancy.

Sickle-cell anemia is a disease affecting those of African descent. It is caused by a single amino acid error in one of the hemoglobin proteins. This leads to red cells that are more easily deformed, which are then destroyed more frequently in small blood vessels, in the spleen and in the liver. This leads not only to severe anemia, but also to destruction of the spleen and injury to the liver, bone, kidneys, lungs, and brain when associated with stroke. One in twelve African Americans carries the sickle trait (one gene), and thus the risk of sickle-cell disease in a black baby is 1/12 x 1/12 x 1/4, or 1 in 576. All of the sickle diseases, including sickle-cell anemia, sickle-cell hemoglobin C disease (SC disease), and sickle cell-beta thalassemia disease

(S-B-thalassemia), have increased rates of maternal morbidity and mortality, abortion, and perinatal mortality.

SC disease may lead to a similar clinical picture as sickle cell in the pregnant woman, although it is usually benign in the nonpregnant woman.[31]

If you are already pregnant and have sickle-cell anemia, you must stay well hydrated at all times, so drink lots of fluids. Second, your bone marrow works overtime to create red cells because your liver and small vessels are so busy destroying them. Your bone marrow needs folate in order to produce red cells, so at least one milligram of folic acid per day is a must. Get vaccinated against pneumonia.

Prophylactic (preventive) blood transfusions may be recommended, and they clearly decrease the number and severity of any sickle crises. If they truly help, the fetal outcome is controversial. You may need intravenous hydration, narcotic pain relievers, and oxygen during a crisis, which may mean you'll be in and out of the hospital.

Generally, starting at about thirty-two weeks, weekly nonstress tests will be performed, often alternating with a biophysical profile.

890

Q *I just have the sickle-cell trait. Am I at the same risks as someone with sickle cell disease?*

A No, you're not. Sickle-cell trait does not appear to adversely affect pregnancy except for an increased frequency of bacteria in the urine and thus of urinary tract infections. But you should be sure that your mate is tested before pregnancy is considered. If he carries either the sickle-cell trait or betathalassemia minor, your child's risk of disease will be one in four If your mate has the trait or carries a gene for an abnormal hemoglobin, prenatal testing via amniocentesis is available.

Other rare anemias such as Hereditary Sphorocytosis and G_6PD enzyme deficiency are usually well tolerated in pregnancy, but full discussion is beyond the scope of this text.

Clotting Disorders

891

Q *My sister says the doctors told her she had ITP. What does that mean?*

A Idiopathic thrombocytopenic purpura (ITP) is now recognized as a chronic condition of decreased platelets caused by autoantibodies. The body mistakenly attacks its own platelets, coating them with antibodies that the spleen then filters out and destroys. This leads to clotting failure and inappropriate bleeding.

Treatment is with oral steroids such as prednisone when platelets fall below 50,000 (more than 150,000 platelets is normal). In the 10 percent in whom this fails, removal of the spleen (splenectomy) is usually indicated. Treatment with high doses of immunoglobulins, as well as treatment with immunosuppressive drugs such as azathioprine and cyclosporine, have been used when steroids fail. Unfortunately, the degree of fetal thrombocytopenia does not correlate with the degree of severity in the mother. About 3 percent of the newborns of mothers with ITP will have severe disease and experience intracranial bleeding.

ITP does not normally require cesarean delivery and epidural anesthesia may be used safely with platelet levels over 100,000.

892

Q *What else can cause decreased platelets?*

A Thrombocytopenia (decreased platelets) is most common in pregnancy as a result of preeclampsia. (See HELLP syndrome) However, it may also accompany rapid blood loss with transfusion, as well as bleeding placenta pre-via, abruption, Diffuse Intravascular Coagulation (DIC) from sepsis (overwhelming infection), or amniotic fluid embolus; it may also result from a viral infection. Systemic lupus erythematosis (SLE) is also a cause of decreased platelets. Severe folate-deficient anemia has been associated with thrombocytopenia as well.

893

Q *What about hemophilia?*

A Hemophilia A, a deficiency of clotting factor VIII:C, is the most common type and is X-linked. This means that its occurrence in women (46XX) is extremely rare, since they have a second normal X chromosome which covers for the faulty one. Men (46XY) are affected, with only the one X, leading to the classic bleeding disorder. Hemophilia A is germane to pregnancy because an affected male must have factor VIII:C levels checked before circumcision is considered.

Hemophilia B (Christmas disease) has clinical symptoms similar to hemophilia A, but it is a deficiency of factor IX instead of VIII. It is extremely rare for women to be affected.

Von Willebrand's disease is the most common inherited bleeding disorder (1 in 1,000 women) and involves malfunction of factor VIII and dysfunctional platelets. The vast majority are heterozygous (have only one affected gene) and have less severe disease, but have the disease nevertheless, so that this is an autosomal dominant (AD) form of disorder. (See Section 1: Genetic Disorders) Activity of factor VIII:C should be tested before labor. Treatment is with factor VIII-rich cryoprecipitate if necessary.

Deficiencies of factors VII, XI, and XII also exist but are rarely seen in pregnant women.

894

Q *Aren't there diseases that actually increase the risk of clotting abnormally?*

A (See also Section 2: Miscarriage)
Yes. Antibodies such as lupus anticoagulant (LAC) can lead to excessive clotting despite its paradoxical name. Anticardiolipin (ACL) has also been associated with increased clotting problems such as deep vein thrombosis (DVT, or phlebitis) and resultant pulmonary embolism (blood clot to lungs). These antibodies have been associated with recurrent miscarriage as well.

Deficiencies of certain regulatory proteins such as Protein S, Protein C, and Antithrombin III have all been associated with recurrent miscarriage and blood clotting problems. "Sticky platelet syndrome" has the same effect.

All of the above may be treated with heparin and minidose aspirin.

Deep Vein Thrombosis and Pulmonary Embolus

895

Q *What is deep vein thrombosis?*

A Deep vein thrombosis (DVT) affects about 1 in 2,000, or 50 in 100,000, pregnancies. It is the formation of a clot in at least one of the large veins that return blood to the heart. The risk is roughly fivefold that in the non-pregnant woman; this is probably due to stasis (slowed flow) in the veins of the pelvis and lower extremities during pregnancy.[32]

The danger in DVT is that one of these large blood clots could break free (embolize) and return to the heart. From there, it may pass to the lungs and block blood flow so that you can't get oxygen, with death sometimes the result of a large clot. This is called a pulmonary embolus (PE). If DVT goes untreated, about 24 percent will develop PE, and 15 percent of those will die. It is the primary cause of maternal death today.[33]

Unfortunately, DVT frequently has no symptoms, especially if it occurs in the pelvic veins and not the legs. The thigh, calf, and the area right behind the knee are the most common sites in the legs. The area over the clot maybe extremely tender, reddened, warm to the touch, or swollen so that the circumference of the affected calf is substantially larger. However, all of these symptoms have been found to occur with equal frequency in limbs with and without thrombosis.[34] Amazingly, one study reported that 98 percent of DVT occurs in the left leg, once confirmed with Doppler ultrasound.[35]

896

Q *Does pulmonary embolus have symptoms?*

A Although DVT may have no symptoms, after an embolus occurs, you may experience shortness of breath, chest pain, fast heart rate, and a feeling of dread or severe anxiety. Patients with PE had the following incidence of symptoms in retrospect: fast respiratory rate or tachypnea (89 percent), shortness of breath or dyspnea (81 percent), pain on taking a big breath or pleuritic pain (72 percent), a feeling of dread or apprehension (59 percent), a cough (54 percent), and a fast heart rate or tachycardia (43 percent). The classic symptom of coughing up blood occurs only one third of the time.[36]

Respiratory rates less than sixteen almost rule out PE.[37] Transcutaneous oximeter readings taken from your finger that are greater than 90 percent also virtually rule out a significant PE, with 75 percent of PEs having a pO_2 (oxygen level) of less than 80 percent.[38]

897

Q *How is DVT diagnosed if the symptoms are inconsistent?*

A DVT may be diagnosed in the lower extremity by using a Doppler ultrasound flow study. The same technology as that used to take pictures of your baby in the second trimester may be applied to your leg. Sensitivities approach 99 percent with current technology.[39]

DVT in pregnant women is often in the pelvic veins. Magnetic resonance imaging (MRI) holds promise as the preferred method for detecting deep pelvic clots, but if no symptoms are present, it is unclear who needs this test. Venography with injected radiopaque dye in the foot veins was the standard test in the past, but it is painful, difficult to interpret, cannot be repeated, and may not fill all the relevant veins.

898

Q *How is a pulmonary embolus diagnosed?*

A A pulmonary embolus (PE) is diagnosed with the combination of symptoms and blood oxygen levels mentioned above, a normal chest X-ray, and a highly suspicious ventilation-perfusion scan (V/Q scan).

If one suspects a pulmonary embolus, the pregnant woman inhales a small amount of a radioactive substance, usually technitium (99mTc) or xenon 133, and a tiny dose of technitium is injected intravenously. The theory is that an embolus will block the vessels (perfusion) but not the ventilation (air spaces). The ventilation part of the scan was intended to help rule out pneumonias or collapsed areas as explanations for abnormal perfusion. As it turns out, recent data suggests the ventilation portion adds little, and furthermore, that V/Q scanning picks up 96 percent of emboli but has a huge false positive rate, with only 10 percent of women with positive results having a clot.[40]

In summary, of V/Q scans that are highly suspicious, about 88 percent will have an embolus, but only a minority of those who actually turned out to have an embolus had a high probability scan. So, pulmonary angiography, in which radiopaque dye is injected into a vein in the thigh, is used for all patients except those with a very suspicious scan or a very normal scan.

899

Q *How are DVT and PE treated?*

A DVT is treated initially with bed rest, elevation of the affected extremity, and intravenous heparin to full anticoagulation in the hospital. After the acute event is controlled, usually in seven to ten days, you would be placed on subcutaneous heparin or low molecular weight heparin. (Lovenox). Aspirin should be discontinued if it was in use before the clot, since after the diagnosis it just increases the risk of bleeding.

PE is treated in the same way, including intravenous heparin to full anticoagulation. Most patients would require ten days to two weeks of therapy. Subcutaneous heparin will then be necessary for the rest of the gestation, with oral coumadin to be started after delivery.

The new "clot-busting drugs," streptokinase, urokinase, and tissue plasminogen activator, which have been shown to accelerate destruction of large pulmonary emboli, unfortunately, have not been associated with a reduction in the fatality. They are, however, associated with markedly increased risks of severe bleeding problems and therefore are not used to treat PE in pregnancy.

900

Q *What is an amniotic fluid embolus? Is that different from a pulmonary embolus?*

A Pulmonary embolus does imply that the material traveling to the lung vessels is a blood clot. Amniotic fluid embolus is an extremely rare event in which amniotic fluid, vernix, and hair can all be forced into the large open veins in the wall of the uterus during delivery, travel to the lungs, and cause a condition very much like shock. Chemicals released in response to this foreign material in the lungs cause the lung to become leaky, and fluid fills the air spaces, causing adult respiratory distress syndrome (ARDS). As the patient drowns in her own fluids, this often triggers diffuse intravascular coagulation (DIC), in which all the clotting factors are consumed and bleeding from every possible site begins.

The process is hard to document unless proved at autopsy. But it occurs in probably less than 1 in 10,000 deliveries, and has a very high fatality rate. Treatment involves ventilation and fluid, blood, and blood component replacement. Care is largely supportive, but recovery is complete if it occurs.

LUNG DISEASES

Asthma
(See Section 5: Antiasthma drugs)

901

Q *I've had asthma since I was a child. Will pregnancy make it worse, and will I have to change what I'm doing now?*

A Asthma, or reactive airways disease, is a common accompaniment of pregnancy. There is an old adage that during pregnancy one-third get better, one-third get worse, and one-third stay the same. In general, almost any medicine you were on for asthma, including steroids, is safe to continue in pregnancy.

Asthma may also appear for the first time in pregnancy, and about 4 to 10 percent of all pregnant women have reactive airways to some degree.[41]

Although you may want to minimize the drugs you take, don't be afraid to take drugs for asthma that are considered safe. The true risks of asthma in pregnancy are almost exclusively restricted to those women who are undermedicated. Uncontrolled asthma has been associated with increased maternal risk of hyperemesis, preeclampsia, and third trimester bleeding. Increased fetal risks include growth restriction (IUGR), preterm labor and birth, low birth weight, and newborn hypoxia (decreased oxygen).[42] Moderate to severe asthma may require inhaled corticosteroids alone (like fluticasone), or combined with salmeterol (Advair) along with a rescue inhaler(Albuterol). Generally a low to medium dose inhaled steroid like fluticasone combined with salmeterol (Advair) is safe and effective in pregnancy.

902

Q *What should I do differently in pregnancy with asthma?*

A Strive to avoid your known asthma triggers, whether they are allergens or exercise. Avoid house dust, animal danders, mold spores, pollens, and tobacco smoke. Keep pets out of your bedroom. Encase mattresses and pillows in airtight covers, avoid vacuuming, keep humidity below 50 percent, close windows, and use air-conditioning whenever possible. Symptoms such as increased coughing, wheezing, and chest "tightness" may come and go, or get worse at night or during the day; always report them to your doctor. If you have hypertension, be careful to avoid using beta-blockers, such as propranolol that are noncardiovascular-selective. These drugs may worsen your asthma.

Get a flu shot even while pregnant. Keep up your allergy shots. Inhaled beta-agonists and inhaled cromolyn should be used for at least five minutes to an hour before desired exercise, including sex. (See Section 5: Antiasthma Drugs)

903

Q *How will my response to treatment be followed while pregnant?*

A Peak expiratory flow rates (PEFR) may be measured in the doctor's office or at home. PEFR is the greatest flow velocity that can be obtained with a maximum forced expiration after filling the lungs. This measurement correlates well with the FEVi measured on office spirometry. (FEVi is the volume of air expelled in one second with a forced expiration.) Predicted values for PEFR are 380 to 550 liters per minute. You should establish your personal best when well; if you fall off by 10 to 20 percent, your treatment scheme should be reevaluated.

904

Q *Should I be monitoring the fetus somehow?*

A With severe, steroid-dependent asthma, your doctor may recommend weekly NST or intermittent biophysical profiles (BPP) from thirty-two to thirty-four weeks onward. Others may simply recommend "kick counts" as a reasonable way to follow the health of your baby at home. (See Section 3: Tests of Fetal Well-being)

Cystic Fibrosis

905

Q *What is cystic fibrosis and how often does it happen?*

A Cystic fibrosis (CF) is the most frequent semilethal genetic disease in Caucasians, with a carrier frequency of 1 in 29, and an incidence of about 1 in 3,300 in the white population. The American Zuni Indian population has an even higher incidence: 1 in 1,500. It is extremely rare in African Americans, with a carrier frequency of 1 in 65 and an incidence of 1 in 15,300, and even more rare in Asians, with an incidence of 1 in 32,100.[43]

The disease leads to thickened mucus in the lungs, pancreas, and bowels. There is progressive obstruction of airways, susceptibility to pneumonias and bronchitis, and digestive problems due to thickened secretions from the pancreas.

As an autosomal recessive disorder, you must have both genes to be affected; therefore, if a woman with the trait mates with a man having the trait, the chances of having an affected offspring are one in four. Because there are over six-hundred different gene mutations associated with CE, and they are distributed differently in different ethnic groups, about 90 percent of white carriers may be identified through blood testing. About 97 percent of Ashkenazic Jews may be identified, and 94 percent of Native Americans, but only 57 percent of Latinos and 30 percent of Asians.[44]

Where once few children with CF lived to adulthood, now 80 percent live beyond their teen years. The disease has variable severities, and more than 40 percent now live beyond age thirty. This is largely due to improved antibiotics, better pulmonary therapy, and pancreatic enzymes that are easily available. Pregnancy may now be tolerated in selected CF patients with good baseline pulmonary function.

906

Q *I've never had any lung problems, but my first cousin has cystic fibrosis. Is there a way to find out if I carry the gene?*

A Recently, the gene locus for CF has been found on chromosome 7. There are many different mutations, although one of them (known as DF508) accounts for over 75 percent of cases. Carrier testing on a blood sample is possible using several complicated techniques. This will usually involve testing of other immediate family members as well. A woman known to carry CF who is pregnant by another carrier may have prenatal testing done with chorionic villi sampling or amniocentesis, and results have a high degree of accuracy, although not 100 percent.

Some have argued that all pregnant women or those planning pregnancy should be tested for carrier status because of the gene's frequency, but this does not have the force of ACOG (American College of Obstetricians and Gynecologists) policy at this time; however, it is the recommendation of a National Institutes of Health Consensus Panel, May 1997.

Tuberculosis

907

Q *I thought tuberculosis was a disease of the early twentieth century. It isn't still a problem, is it?*

A Unfortunately, tuberculosis (TB) is on the rise again in the United States wherever large populations of Mexican and Southeast Asian immigrants have settled. Breathing in Mycobacterium tuberculosis from an infected individual is the only known route of infection. The immune system then wraps up the bug in the lung tissue as a granuloma, which appears to stop the infection often for years, but it will show up on a chest X-ray.

908

Q *If the disease can be asymptomatic, who should get skin-tested for TB?*

A The five tuberculin units of PPD is the preferred skin test and should be given to:

1. Any HIV-positive person
2. Close contacts of those known to be infected
3. Foreign-born persons from countries known to have a high prevalence of endemic tuberculosis
4. Intravenous drug abusers and alcoholics
5. Medically underserved, low-income minority populations
6. Immunosuppressed individuals
7. Residents of long-term care facilities such as nursing homes and prisons

909

Q *What do I do if my skin test is positive and I'm pregnant?*

A (See Section 5: Antituberculosis drugs)
Get a chest X-ray. There is no risk to the fetus from even multiple chest

films. If the X-ray is negative, some doctors recommend withholding treatment with 300 milligrams per day of Isoniazid (INH) until after delivery; others recommend use in pregnancy but not until after twelve weeks of gestation.[45]

If the chest X-ray is positive, treatment with at least two drugs should begin, usually Isoniazid at 5 milligrams per kilogram and Rifampin at 10 milligrams per kilogram with pyridoxine (vitamin B_6) at 50 milligrams per day, for all nine months. Ethambutol, at 20 milligrams per kilogram per day, may be substituted for the Rifampin. All have been shown to be safe and effective in pregnancy.

Streptomycin should not be used in pregnancy because of the increased risk of severe deafness in 15 percent of those fetuses exposed.

Congenital tuberculosis (contracting the disease in utero) is extremely rare. It may be acquired across the placenta or through contact with maternal secretions. If the mother has been treated for at least two weeks, infection in the newborn is almost unheard of Infectious, untreated women should be isolated from their babies while treatment is initiated.

ENDOCRINE (HORMONAL) DISEASES

Insulin-Dependent Diabetes Mellitus (IDDM)
(See also Section 8: Gestational Diabetes)

910

Q *I have insulin-dependent diabetes and want to get pregnant soon. Is there anything I need to do?*

A Yes. Get your diabetes under very tight control. What the gestational diabetic does not have to contend with, but you do, is that birth defects are most strongly correlated with control at conception, and are fourfold higher in those that are poorly controlled.[46]

Glycosylated hemoglobin (HgbAl-C test) levels that are lower have been shown by some to be associated with lower birth defect rates, as have controlled studies comparing those who established rigid control before conception to those who sought care after six weeks.[47]

911

Q *Do I have other risks that the gestational diabetic does not have?*

A Yes. Type I, or insulin-dependent, diabetes that predates pregnancy is somewhat different from gestational diabetes (GDM), even when insulin is required. Type II, or adult-onset, diabetes is not a disorder of decreased insulin production, but of decreased effectiveness at the cell level throughout the body and is treated with diet and oral medications.

ACOG classifies GDM as Classes A through H, with A not requiring insulin. A-1 has a normal fasting plasma glucose, but an elevated reading one hour after a meal. A-2 has both an increased fasting and one-hour result. Classes B through H are all Type I. Class B is GDM that started over age twenty and has lasted for more than ten years; Class C started in the teens and has lasted ten to nineteen years; Class D started at older than ten years or has lasted less than twenty years and has changes in the retina of the eye; Class F has vascular disease involving the kidney; Class R has serious disease of the vessels in the retina; Class H has heart disease.

Risks of pregnancy depend somewhat on classification, but all Type I individuals are subject to a fourfold increased risk of preeclampsia as well as an increased risk of the following: miscarriage, birth defects, diabetic ketoacidosis episodes, very large baby, urinary tract infection, stillbirth, and fetal distress in labor, with the attendant risks of a cesarean and increased amniotic fluid (polyhydramnios). Ultimately, there is an increased risk of maternal death due to all of the above.

Perinatal mortality (stillbirth or newborn death) is highest (17 percent) when preeclampsia, pyelonephritis (kidney infection), or ketoacidosis is present, and lowest (7 percent) without these complications.[48]

You can minimize all these risks with tight control of glucose levels before conception, daily blood testing with a home glucometer to keep fasting levels below 105, and two-hour after-meal levels below 120. Frequent visits to the obstetrician and/or endocrinologist to keep insulin dosages adjusted is a must. Rigid adherence to diet and exercise guidelines will make glucose control easier. Weekly NST is recommended from about twenty-eight to thirty-two weeks.

Hospitalization after thirty-four weeks is usual, with frequent tests of fetal well-being performed at least twice a week. Amniocentesis for determination of lung maturity may be done at an estimated thirty-seven completed weeks. If exact dates are known, then delivery is encouraged as soon after thirty-eight weeks as possible.

Thyroid Disease
(See Section 2: Hormones; Section 5: Thyroid Drugs)

Hyperthyroidism

912

I've been on Synthroid for several years since being diagnosed with Grave's disease. Is there any danger to my pregnancy?

There is no danger as long as you continue your thyroid replacement as adjusted by your doctor. Grave's Disease is a common autoimmune disorder of women of childbearing age. If previously diagnosed and treated, thyroid replacement need only be monitored with thyroid-stimulating hormone (TSH) and T7 in pregnancy, and you may require a slight increase as pregnancy progresses.

913

My heart was beating like crazy all the time even when I was lying in bed, and I was twenty weeks pregnant. Now they tell me I have Grave's disease and I'm in thyrotoxicosis. Is my baby in danger?

Thyrotoxicosis means the constellation of effects caused by increased thyroid hormone. It is most often caused by Grave's, and certainly may occur in pregnancy. In Grave's disease, autoantibodies actually stimulate the thyroid to overproduce. Symptoms include increased resting heart rate, enlarged thyroid, exophthalmos (protruding eyes), and failure to gain appropriate weight.

Thyrotoxicosis is treated with propylthiouracil (PTU) or, less often, with methimazole, both of which cross the placenta. (See Section 5: Thyroid Drugs) These theoretically could cause hypothyroidism and goiter (enlarged gland) in the fetus (less than a 2 percent risk), but in light of the fact that untreated thyrotoxicosis can lead to preeclampsia and heart failure, the benefits clearly outweigh the risks. Surgical thyroidectomy may be used in the second trimester. The usual treatment for Grave's, which is thyroid ablation (destruction) with radioactive iodine is contraindicated in pregnancy, since it would destroy the fetal thyroid as well. About 80 percent of nonpregnant women treated with I (131) will eventually become hypothyroid and require thyroid replacement.

Rarely, hyperthyroidism has been caused by molar pregnancies. (See Section 8: Molar Pregnancy)

Hypothyroidism (Low Thyroid)

914

Is hypothyroidism in pregnancy a problem?

It's a problem if it happens to you, but it is only rarely seen in pregnancy, probably because hypothyroidism is commonly associated with the inability to ovulate and therefore with infertility. There are over twenty-five known causes of decreased thyroid function, but most cases in adults are caused by autoimmune thyroiditis known as Hashimoto's disease. Symptoms include fatigue, intolerance to cold, weight gain, constipation, muscle and joint aches, hair loss, dry coarse cold skin, hoarse voice, brittle nails, slowed reaction times, and slowed heart rate.[49]

Clinical hypothyroidism in pregnancy is associated with an increased risk of preeclampsia, placental abruption, low birth weight, and stillbirth. It is treated with oral thyroid hormone replacement.

More commonly, there are no symptoms, and only an increased thyroid-stimulating hormone level (TSH) will be noted on blood work. This means that the brain is working overtime to whip your thyroid into functioning, and it is also an indication of your need for thyroid replacement, even if your actual thyroid levels are normal.

915

Q *What is "cretinism"?*

A Cretinism is the term given to children born with congenital hypothyroid states that go uncorrected, leading to mental retardation. Cretinism was more common over a hundred years ago in the United States before the introduction of iodized salt. Iodine is the essential ingredient in the thyroid hormone. In fact, thyroid hormone comes in two forms known as T4 and T3. The real name for T3 is tri-iodothyronine. It is the absence of iodine in the diet that leads to maternal goiter (thyroid enlargement) because the thyroid enlarges as it attempts to compensate for its inefficiency at producing thyroid without iodine.

Today, there is mass screening of newborns for thyroid dysfunction, and immediate treatment in the 1 in 4,000 cases found seems to completely avert the mental retardation.

916

Q *I heard that many women are hypothyroid after they give birth. Why?*

A As many as 10 percent of women develop transient thyroid dysfunction in the months following delivery. It is probably a grossly underrecognized cause of postpartum depression, loss of memory, and an inability to concentrate in young mothers.[50]

Pituitary Adenoma (Prolactinoma)

917

Q *I was diagnosed with a prolactinoma when I was being worked up for infertility. My prolactin hormone levels were too high and we could see a little tumor in the pituitary. I got pregnant by taking Parlodel. Do I continue Parlodel in pregnancy?*

No. Bromocryptine (Parlodel) is a dopamine agonist, which means it functions like prolactin-inhibiting factor in the brain. If you got pregnant successfully, then your adenoma has been adequately "shrunk" to not need therapy in pregnancy. Only 1 to 2 percent of women demonstrate any enlargement of their adenomas while pregnant.[51]

Parlodel tends to make one nauseous and light-headed from time to time. A newer drug, carbegoline (Dostinex) is now available for the same indications and seems to cause less side effects. Furthermore, rather than taking it twice a day, you need to take it only one to two times per week.

(Note: A minority of prolactinomas are larger than ten millimeters in diameter and are much more likely to cause symptoms—headaches and visual field defects—than the more common micropituitary adenomas associated with infertility. These macroadenomas may need longer treatment with agents such as Dostinex, or with surgical or radiation therapy before pregnancy.)

While your prolactin levels increase, there is no significant evidence of dangerous growth to your adenoma while breast-feeding.

GASTROINTESTINAL DISEASE

Esophagus and Stomach
   (See also Section 2: Constipation and Other Complaints)

Hyperemesis Gravidarum
   (See Section 2: Morning Sickness; Section 5: Antinausea Drugs)

Heartburn (Gastroesophageal reflux disease, or GERD)
   (See Section 2: Constipation and Other Complaints)

918

Q My heartburn just gets worse. Is there anything more I can take besides antacids?

Yes, there are several things. Reflux of stomach contents into the lower esophagus is a very frequent occurrence in pregnancy and worsens as gestation progresses. It occurs because of the relaxation of the sphincter that normally closes off the top of the stomach. Relaxation is caused by increased progesterone levels in pregnancy.

Antacids such as Calcium TUMS, Maalox, and Mylanta may all be safely used in pregnancy. Use them not just with symptoms, but three to five times a day, especially shortly after meals. Sleep with the head of your bed slightly elevated, and avoid eating within two to three hours of bedtime. Avoid spicy foods and alcohol, and stay away from cigarettes. If your heartburn is severe and antacids don't relieve it, you can take 400 milligrams of cimetidine (Tagamet) twice a day, or 150 milligrams of ranitidine (Zantac) twice a day; both drugs are considered safe in pregnancy.

Peptic Ulcer

919

Q *Could I have an ulcer? I have midepigastric pain that just doesn't get better with antacids.*

A A peptic ulcer in pregnancy is possible but rare. Normally, gastric acid secretions decrease (heartburn is only from the reflux), bowel motility is reduced, and mucous secretion increased. If you already had peptic ulcer disease, there is a 90 percent chance that it will actually go away with pregnancy!

Vomiting Blood

920

Q *I'm only ten weeks pregnant, but I've seen some flecks of blood when I vomit. What is this?*

A Tiny amounts of bright red blood flecked in vomitus is not dangerous, and usually comes from minor irritation at the back of the throat. Large amounts of blood during or immediately following retching may be due to Mallory-Weiss tears. These small lacerations near the gastroesophageal junction usually respond to ice-water lavage, intravenous cimetidine or ranitidine, and oral antacids. Rarely, blood transfusion and endoscopy (in which a fiber-optic cable is inserted in your esophagus) is necessary.[52]

Constipation
(See Section 2: Constipation and Other Complaints; Section 5: Over-the-Counter Drugs, Constipation)

Inflammatory Bowel Disease (Crohn's Disease and Ulcerative Colitis)
(See also Section 5: Anti-inflammatories and Immunosuppressives)

921

Q *I was diagnosed with Crohn's disease about three years ago. What is the difference between Crohn's and ulcerative colitis?*

A Crohn's disease, or regional enteritis, is a segmental disease (multiple areas) of the small and large bowel characterized by intermittent bouts of abdominal cramping and diarrhea, often leading to fistulus tract formation between bowel and bowel or bowel and skin (particularly the perineum between vagina and anus), intermittent symptoms of bowel obstruction with vomiting and bloating, and repeated surgeries for relief of obstruction and resection (excision) of portions of the small bowel. There is also an association with arthritis. Its cause is unknown, but there is a genetic predisposition to it and an increased propensity to develop colon cancer that is six times the general population's risk.[53]

Ulcerative colitis (UC) is a similar disease, but is not segmental and seems to involve only the colon or large bowel. It usually starts in the rectum; it progresses upward and is associated with bloody diarrhea. Rarely, toxic megacolon may develop in which the colon dilates massively and emergency colectomy (removal of the colon) is required. Like Crohn's, it has been associated with a reactive arthritis, an inflammation of the eye (uveitis), and the skin disease erythema nodosum on the shins. Similarly, UC also has a genetic predisposition and an increased risk of colon cancer.

922

Q *How do pregnancy and inflammatory bowel disease affect one another?*

A In general, they have little effect on each other. Contrary to popular belief, flare-ups of ulcerative colitis are not more common in pregnancy. If the disease was in remission at conception, it is likely to stay that way in two-thirds of cases; if it was angry at conception then pregnancy outcome may be affected and flare-ups will be more severe.[54] A similar circumstance exists for Crohn's disease.[55]

The central caveat is that almost all the usual treatments—such as prednisone, infliximab (Remicade), or mesalamine (Asacol)—may be used in pregnancy. Sulfasalazine (Azulfidine) may be used throughout pregnancy, but if possible might be avoided after 36 weeks to avoid the kernicterus, which can be associated with sulfa drugs in the third trimester. (See Question 319) Only azathioprine (Imuran) is classified as Category D and should probably be avoided if possible due to its association with intrauterine growth restriction (IUGR) in human fetuses and limb defects in animal studies.

Appendicitis

923

Q *Can I get appendicitis in pregnancy?*

A Sure, but it isn't any more likely than when you are not pregnant. In other words, about one in one-thousand-four-hundred women are diagnosed with appendicitis in pregnancy.

It may, however, be more difficult to diagnose. The appendix moves up and out onto the flank as pregnancy progresses. Common symptoms such as anorexia (not hungry), nausea, and vomiting happen to pregnant people anyway. Other conditions, but particularly pyelonephritis (kidney infection), kidney stones, gallbladder disease, separation of the placenta (abruption), and myomas dying inside (degenerating fibroid) can mimic appendicitis. The white blood count, which normally rises with appendicitis, is slightly elevated in pregnancy to begin with.

You can be operated on in pregnancy, but the later in your pregnancy that the problem occurs, the more likely you are to have preterm labor and/or a fetal loss. In a large Swedish study, the fetus was lost more than 20 percent of the time when surgery occurred after twenty-three weeks.[56] Some studies show that maternal mortality may be increased because of surgical delay.

Gallbladder and Pancreas

924

Q *I had horrible pain in my stomach last week for twenty-four hours and six months pregnant. The doctor says I have gallstones, Is that dangerous for me or the baby?*

A Gallstones, or cholelithiasis, happen with much greater frequency in pregnancy than at any other time in life. Just like the rest of the bowel, the gallbladder, which lies just under the liver in the right upper quadrant of the abdomen, is sluggish in pregnancy. After a meal, it empties incompletely, probably because of high progesterone levels that relax the smooth muscle in the gallbladder wall. This is the same as what happens in the colon with constipation. Cholesterol stones make up almost all the gallstones seen in pregnancy.

Gallstones themselves are not dangerous to you or the baby. In fact, your need for surgery to remove the gallbladder only increases 1 to 2 percent per year, so that after twenty years of having gallstones, only about one in five people will have to have their gallbladder removed.[57]

Cholecystitis is inflammation of the gallbladder, with stones present and probably blocking the cystic duct (tube out of the gallbladder) about 90 percent of the time. In up to 85 percent of the cases, there is truly bacterial infection present. It occurs in about one in one-thousand pregnancies. About two-thirds of cases can he managed successfully with intravenous hydration and antibiotics.[58] If surgery is chosen, it is best to have it performed in the second trimester to diminish the risk of both abortion and preterm labor.

Other treatments for cholelithiasis, such as laparoscopic cholecystect-omy, are considered contraindicated in pregnancy by some; other doctors consider these treatments worth considering before twenty weeks gestation.

Pancreatitis, inflammation of the pancreas with severe mid-abdominal pain through to the back, may rarely complicate pregnancy. Blood tests for amylase and lipase can make the diagnosis. It is treated with IV hydration and pain medicine.

Liver

Hepatitis
(See Section 8: Viral Infection)

HELLP Syndrome (Hypertension, Elevated Liver Enzymes, Low Platelets)
(See Section 8: Preeclampsia)

Cholestasis of Pregnancy

925

Q *I've been itching terribly since about thirty-two weeks. Why?*

A You may be suffering from a relatively common (one in 500) pregnancy condition called intrahepatic cholestasis of pregnancy. Just like the bowels and gallbladder, the liver is another part of the gastrointestinal tract that gets backed up in some women. Bile salts collect in the center of the liver rather than all being excreted into the bowel via the hepatic duct. Subsequently, they leak back into the bloodstream and cause extreme, generalized itching.

Less often, bilirubin is increased as well, leading to jaundice (yellow dis-coloration of skin). Although there may be a tendency to inherit jaundice, the condition seems most closely linked to high estrogen levels.

Note: If blood pressure is normal and the urine has no protein, preeclamp-sia is ruled out. If liver enzymes aren't very high, then viral hepatitis is unlikely; and ultrasound can rule out a stone obstructing the common bile duct.[59]

Cholestasis and itching can be treated. Cholestyramine has long been the mainstay. Taken orally, it is intended to bind bile salts and block reuptake by the bowel. Unfortunately, it also blocks fat-soluble vitamin absorption, including absorption of vitamin K, which, over a long period could lead to bleeding tendencies. Additionally, several studies show the drug to be inef-fective at halting itching unless taken for very long periods of time.[60]

Dexamethasone, administered orally at a dose of twelve milligrams per day for a week, led to marked improvement in one study.[61]

Acute Fatty Liver of Pregnancy

926

Q *I know drugs and viral hepatitis can damage the liver, but what is acute fatty liver?*

A A very rare disorder of the liver, it occurs in about one in fifteen-thousand pregnancies and is often fatal to both mother and fetus. The cells in the liver are basically packed full of fat and thus cease to function. About half the cases are associated with preeclampsia. Symptoms include fatigue, nausea, vomiting, anorexia, stomach pain, and progressive jaundice. Diffuse intravascular coagulation (DIC) often complicates the picture, leading to uncontrolled bleeding.

Acute fatty liver is self-limited if delivery is achieved, and the mother survives about 75 percent of the time; the fetus survives about half the time.[62]

A similar clinical picture to acute liver failure is seen with massive Tylenol overdose during suicide attempts. N-acetylcysteine is the antidote.

URINARY TRACT DISEASE

(See also Section 2: Bladder and Kidneys)

Bladder

927

Q *Is it true that urinary tract infections are more common in pregnancy?*

A Yes. Bladder infection (cystitis) and kidney infection (pyelonephritis) are both more common in pregnancy. Bacteria in the bladder without any symptoms (asymptomatic bacteriuria) occurs about 5 percent of the time. Infections may be increased because of the slower flow of urine down the ureters (tubes from the kidneys) called urinary stasis. In some women, there is a reflux of urine in the bladder back up the ureters, which also promotes infection.

Urine is cultured as a routine procedure at your first prenatal visit, and asymptomatic bacteriuria is treated with a single dose of nitrofurantoin (Macrodantin), or sulfamethoxazole-trimethoprim (Bactrim DS).

Symptoms of pain on urination (dysuria), frequent urination, and the sense that you have to urinate immediately often herald the presence of cystitis. Treatment lasting three days with one of the above antibiotics is appropriate. Doctors are more likely to culture in pregnancy, since 40 percent of kidney infections are preceded by bladder infections.

Don't be unduly concerned if there is blood in your urine (hematuria). It is usually a sign of nothing more than a bad bladder infection. Occasionally in pregnancy, it may be the sign of a kidney stone or ureteral stone. (See below) Hematuria right after delivery, or after cesarean performed in the second stage of labor, is very common. It is usually from blunt trauma of the baby's head beating on the bladder, and it resolves by itself after less than twenty-four hours. Often a Foley catheter may be left in place in the bladder until the urine clears.

928

Q *Why can't some women urinate after delivery?*

A Inability to urinate (urinary retention) shortly after vaginal delivery may be due to epidural anesthesia or trauma to the lower urinary tract with accompanying swelling. The area around the urethra may be lacerated or swollen, as may any part of the vulvar area. Outward signs of swelling often accompany swelling in the base of the bladder, and compression of some critical nerves may make urination temporarily difficult or impossible. Overfilling or distention of the bladder may also be hard to sense in the presence of swelling, episiotomy pain, or tears around the urethra.

Ice packs to the area, intermittent catheterization, or Foley catheters left in place for twenty-four hours may be recommended after delivery if you have trouble voiding.

Kidneys

929

Q *My back has been killing me, and a friend said I could have a kidney infection. Is that right?*

A It could be right, but it's more likely that your back is killing you because you're pregnant. (See Section 2: Back Pain) One to 2 percent of pregnant women develop pyelonephritis (kidney infection), and it presents with upper back pain just below the shoulder blades, not lower back pain. Its most common symptoms are nausea, vomiting, and spiking fevers and chills. About 75 percent of the time, the disease occurs only on one side, right more than left; in about one-fourth of the cases, it is on both sides. On examination, when the doctor taps his fist lightly over the middle of your back, you typically hit the ceiling!

The bacteria Escherichia coli and Klebsiella cause more than 90 percent of the infections. Patients with pyelonephritis should be hospitalized, hydrated intravenously, and treated aggressively with the appropriate intravenous antibiotic. Fifteen percent of women will have bacteremia, or bacteria in their blood.[63]

Treatment is usually continued until you've had no fever for twenty-four hours and then continued after hospital discharge with oral medications for seven days.

Pyelonephritis is dangerous for the baby only because it may precipitate preterm labor; also, rarely, you can become very sick. About 2 percent of pregnant women with pyelonephritis develop adult respiratory distress syndrome (ARDS) due to an endotoxin (chemical released by the bacteria) that damages the lining of the lung and causes it to fill with water.[64] These same women may destroy a large portion of their red blood cells (hemolysis) and become anemic.[65]

930

Q *I had a kidney stone in my last pregnancy that passed on its own, but it was still extremely painful. Am I likely to get another one in my next pregnancy?*

A Kidney stones (nephrolithiasis) only occur in pregnancy about one in two-thousand times. However, a previous stone does increase your chances for another, but not necessarily in your pregnancy. Pregnant women seem to have fewer symptoms and pass stones more easily than either men or nonpregnant women. Usually the only danger is associated kidney infection or the extremely rare problem of complete obstruction.

This may be due to the physiological normal dilation of the ureter (tube from kidney to bladder) during pregnancy. Infection is the most common presenting symptom, as in pyelonephritis. Flank pain and hematuria occur less than 30 percent and 15 percent of the time, respectively, in one study.[66]

Diagnosis is made with ultrasound about two-thirds of the time, and by X-ray about one-third of the time. X-rays may include intravenous pyelograms (IVP) with contrast media (dye to show up the ureter on the film), or with plain films. Usually, treatment consists of intravenous hydration, pain medicines, and waiting. Urine is strained to look for the offending calcium salt rock (75 percent). About 50 percent of women pass the stone on their own, but at least one-third need a urologist to look in the bladder with a fiber-optic cable (cystoscopy), place plastic tubes in the ureters, or advance a small basket up the ureter to remove the stone. Rarely, surgery is required. Lithotripsy, in which the stone is destroyed by sound wave vibration is not used in pregnancy at this time.

931

Q *I had severe preeclampsia and my kidneys shut down. Why does acute renal failure happen?*

A Acute renal failure means the sudden cessation of function by the two kidneys. Twenty percent of all cases are related to pregnancy and almost all of these are related to preeclampsia, placental abruption, prolonged fetal death, or bleeding.[67] This is usually related to decreased blood supply to the kidneys, which leads to acute tubular necrosis, or damage to a specialized portion of the kidneys responsible for reabsorbing substances that are not supposed to be lost in the urine.

Treatment with appropriate blood replacement, avoidance of diuretic drugs, delivery of severe preeclampsia patients, and avoidance of drugs that constrict vessels, while treating low blood pressure, may all combine to reverse the effects of acute renal failure most of the time.

Chronic renal failure which has led to kidney transplant occasionally occurs prior to pregnancy. Despite a higher first trimester miscarriage rate, 90 percent of patients have successful pregnancies once they are past twelve weeks.

NEUROLOGICAL DISEASE

(See also Section 2: Muscles, Joints, and Nervous System)

Seizure Disorders

932

Q *My sister has grand mal seizures unless she takes her medicines. Can she get pregnant safely?*

A Yes. About 2.25 million Americans (about 1 percent) have "epilepsy," with the majority having complex partial seizures (60 percent), grand mal ton-icclonic seizures (30 percent), and petit mal or absence seizures (5 percent).[68]

Most women with seizure disorders have safe, successful pregnancies, with no increased risks of perinatal mortality, preeclampsia, preterm labor, or cesarean delivery.[69] It is true that there are legitimate concerns about the fetal effects of many medicines. (See Section 5: Anticonvulsant Drugs), but the benefits outweigh the risks in those people, such as your sister, with tonic-clonic seizures, and many others as well, depending on frequency and type of seizure prior to pregnancy.

933

Q *But aren't women with seizures more likely to have a baby with birth defects?*

A Yes. About 6 to 8 percent of babies born to women on antiseizure medicines have birth defects; the risk is about two to three times that of the normal population. All of the common medicines used, including phenytoin, phenobarbital, carbamazepine, valproate, and primidone, have been implicated in the cause of one or more defects. But the paramount management goal in pregnancy should be control of seizures, since they have the potential to be much more damaging to the fetus than the medications.

Most of the defects described are not incompatible with normal life and include cleft lip or palate and heart defects.[70, 71, 72, 73]

934

Q *What can I do to avoid neurological problems before I get pregnant?*

A Discuss your current medications with your obstetrician and your neurologist. If it is possible to narrow your drug use to only one medication, that would be a good idea, since there is some evidence to suggest multiple agents increase risk of birth defects. If you have not had seizures in more than three years, it may be possible to try and wean yourself off your medicine over one to two months while you are trying to conceive, but about half the people in this circumstance will have a seizure and need levels reinstituted.[74]

935

Q *I was told I have to take vitamin K during pregnancy if I have a seizure disorder. Why is that?*

A Vitamin K is essential for your liver and the baby's to make coagulation factors so that blood clots normally. Phenytoin (Dilantin), phenobarbital, and primidone (Mysoline) all interfere with vitamin K-dependent coagulation factors (Factors II, VII, IX, and X). Newborns of women taking these drugs should all receive one milligram of vitamin K (aquamephyton) intramuscularly at birth. Some doctors recommend treating pregnant women with oral vitamin K in the last trimester as well, or giving a single ten-milligram dose of aquamephyton intramuscularly to those in whom delivery is thought imminent. The theory is that this will help avoid bleeding into the newborn's brain, a condition called intraventricular hemorrhage (IVH).[75] This may also be done for any pregnant woman being treated for preterm labor who is likely to deliver under thirty-four weeks.

Taking folate is also a good idea, since all anticonvulsants interfere with folic acid metabolism. Because folate deficiency has been associated with neural tube defects and anticonvulsants, one milligram of folate supplementation may be taken in addition to your normal dietary intake.

936

Q *If I have a long labor and can't take my medicines, how can I avoid a seizure?*

A Therapeutic levels of both Dilantin and phenobarbital may be checked with a simple blood test. If the levels are normal in the last week or so before delivery, then the normal daily dose of Dilantin may be given intravenously in labor if necessary. A single dose of 60 to 90 milligrams of phenobarbital will cover labor and delivery.

Tegretol is not available intravenously. If a patient normally on Tegretol feels she is about to have a seizure, then. Dilantin may be loaded intravenously at 10 milligrams per kilogram, with a maximum of 50 milligrams per minute.

937

Q *Will I need more of my medicine while pregnant?*

A Probably. Blood levels should be evaluated every trimester and appropriate changes made. Especially important is the fact that blood levels may rise rapidly within the first few weeks after delivery as fluid shifts occur. Levels should be checked one week after delivery and dosage may need to be reduced rapidly if it was increased during the pregnancy.

938

Q *Can I breast-feed on my anticonvulsant?*

A Yes. All of these medicines pass into the milk in small amounts, but all have been approved by the American Academy of Pediatrics for breast-feeding. Breast-feeding should be stopped if signs of excessive sedation are seen, but it should be stopped gradually to avoid potential withdrawal in the newborn.[76]

939

Q *Will my baby have an increased risk of epilepsy?*

A Most evidence would suggest it will. The normal risk for any child developing epilepsy is about 1 percent. Children of women with seizures of unknown cause, however, have about a 4 percent risk of developing epilepsy.[77]

Multiple Sclerosis (MS)

940

Q *My secretary was just diagnosed with multiple sclerosis. What is it exactly?*

A Multiple sclerosis (MS) is the most common of the demyelinating diseases. This means that the sheaths that surround the nerves of the central nervous system (those in the brain and spinal cord) are gradually destroyed by an unknown inflammatory force leading to the death of the nerve cell or neuron. This process occurs randomly and intermittently, with starts and stops (exacerbations and remissions).

Usually it affects young adults initially, and thus women of childbearing age. Attacks are only a few days of weakness in a specific muscle group, or feelings of numbness distributed over wide areas that change from episode to episode.

Classic symptoms of MS include vision changes due to inflammation of the major nerve trunk to the eye and the optic nerve (optic neuritis). Other problems include joint pains (dysarthria), shakiness when making a specific, controlled movement (intention tremor), limb weakness, spasticity of muscle groups, and bladder dysfunction.

Diagnosis is made nowadays by magnetic resonance imaging (MRI). Changes in the brain on the MRI include the appearance of plaques, which are areas in which the myelin sheath has been stripped away.

Consensus would be that MS really doesn't affect pregnancy. While women may have exacerbations in pregnancy, they do not seem to occur with any greater frequency than they do in the nonpregnant state. About one-third of women with MS will have an exacerbation over nine and a half months. Some say these recurrences are slightly increased in pregnancy, and others claim they are reduced; everyone agrees that exacerbations do flare up more frequently in the first six months after delivery.[78]

Exacerbations may be treated with anti-inflammatory agents such as the steroid prednisone.

941

Q *I have MS. Is it likely my baby will develop this disease?*

A Unfortunately, the answer is "yes." Children of MS mothers have a fifteen-fold increased risk of MS developing as they reach young adulthood.

Spinal Cord Injury

942

Q *I was paralyzed in an automobile accident. Now I'm engaged, and we are planning to have children. Will there be any special problems with my pregnancy?*

A Spinal cord injury, usually from trauma in the reproductive age group, does not have any adverse effects on pregnancy. There are, however, a few exceptions. Constipation due to lack of activity may be worsened, and urinary tract infections may be more common as well, particularly if self-catheterization is required.

Labor is usually easy, painless, and often quicker than average. Lesions below thoracic vertebrae 12 (112) allow labor contractions to be felt normally; above that number, they are painless. In order to avoid emergency deliveries, serial cervical examinations should begin at 28 weeks. Elective admission after thirty-seven weeks is reasonable.[79]

Stroke (Cerebrovascular Accident—CVA)

943

Q *A woman in our church was paralyzed right after the birth of her last child. They said it was a stroke. How could that happen to someone so young?*

A Stroke is the name given to the damage done to the brain when a blood vessel ruptures and bleeds into it, or a blood clot blocks blood flow into or out of a localized area of the brain. Cerebrovascular accidents (CVA), despite being rare in young people, still account for about 10 percent of maternal deaths. They occur most often in the third trimester and in the weeks shortly after delivery.[80] There are many different types and causes of stroke.

Pregnancy is a hypercoagulable state, meaning that blood clots form more easily. (See this section: DVT) Cerebral embolism is the most common cause of stroke in pregnant women. It occurs more frequently in the third trimester and in the month following delivery. The most common underlying cause is an embolic clot from a damaged heart valve in someone who had rheumatic heart disease as a child. Care is supportive, and often involves the use of anticoagulants such as heparin to prevent further events.

Hemorrhagic stroke is most often associated with bleeding into the brain tissue itself as a complication of severe preeclampsia. Bleeding onto the surface of the brain, known as subarachnoid hemorrhage, is usually due to rupture of a congenitally weak vessel called an aneurysm, or rupture of an abnormal connection between the arteries and veins called an arteriovenous malformation (AVM). This type of stroke occurs about one in ten-thousand cases and thus is the second most common form of stroke associated with pregnancy.[81]

SKIN DISEASES

(See also Section 2: Skin)

944

Q *I'm thirty-six weeks pregnant and broke out in a rash last week that started on my abdomen and now has spread to my thighs. It's itching like crazy. Is there anything I can do?*

A PUPP (pruritic urticarial papules and plaques of pregnancy) is the most common rash unique to pregnancy. Raised, red patches spread from the abdomen and may spare only the face. It may be intensely itchy. Treatment includes oral antihistamines and when these fail, as they usually do, either topical or oral steroids such as prednisone or medrol are required. (See Section 5: Anti-inflammatories) The rash resolves quickly after delivery, and will almost never recur in future pregnancies.

945

Q *My friend had a rash and her doctor said it was herpes. Can you really get herpes all over like that?*

A No, and your friend didn't have herpes all over. Herpes gestationis (HG) is a skin disease peculiar to pregnancy, and it is incredibly rare (one in fifty-thousand). In fact, you are ten times more likely to die in pregnancy than to get herpes gestationis. It occurs in late pregnancy and the eruption blisters and itches intensely. These blisters may be tiny, widespread, and on a reddened raised patch, or large, tense, raised areas called vesicles, or bullae. It is the blistering tendency that earns the rash its name, even though it has nothing to do with a herpetic viral infection. Unlike PUPP, this skin disease always recurs in future pregnancies.

Treatment always requires oral steroids such as prednisone. It is possible that HG is associated with an increased incidence of preterm labor, but that is controversial.[82]

Another rare pregnancy rash is Impetigo herpetiformis, which may actually be related to psoriasis. The lesions are reddened patches with multiple, small, sterile pustules (blisters with pus in them); these begin in the crease of the elbow, behind the knee, and in the groin, and then spread, often to the mucous membranes of the mouth and vagina. Systemic symptoms include nausea, vomiting, diarrhea, chills, and fever. This process may continue until weeks after delivery.

OBESITY

(See also Section 2: Dietary Guidelines and Weight Gain)

946

Q *What sort of problems can I expect starting pregnancy at 250 pounds and only 5'3" tall?*

A Obesity is an increase in the percentage of body fat, while overweight means an increase in body weight over an arbitrary standard. The body mass index (BMI) is the weight in kilograms divided by the height in meters squared (kg/m^2). (See Appendix B) Obesity has been defined as higher than the 85th percentile on the BMI chart. That would be a BMI of 27.3 for women twenty to twenty-nine years old.

In your case, at 250 pounds and 5'3", your BMI is about 43. You then have increased risks of diabetes, hypertension, hyperlipidemia, heart disease, stroke, gout, sleep apnea, osteoarthritis, and many forms of cancer, as well as certain complications of pregnancy.

You, and all obese pregnant women, have the following increased risks:

1. Diabetes
2. Hypertension (and with it, an increased risk of congestive heart failure)
3. Post-term pregnancy
4. Need for oxytocin induction
5. Macrosomic infant (heavier than 4,500 grams, or nine pounds fourteen ounces)
6. Shoulder dystocia (shoulders stuck after the head delivers; a potentially lethal complication for the baby)
7. Cesarean section
8. Wound infection
9. Excessive blood loss

947

Q *If I start out pregnancy obese, do I really have to gain at least fifteen pounds?*

A Probably not. Work at the University of California at San Francisco revealed in a review of almost seven-thousand term pregnancies that weight gain (not starting weight) had no effect on birth weight.[83] This contradicts the commonly observed finding that inadequate weight gain in underweight or normal-weight women leads to babies of significantly lower birth weight.

Still, the recommendations of the Institute of Medicine, Food, and Nutrition Board are for at least a fifteen-pound weight gain in obese women, as opposed to a weight gain of twenty-five to thirty-five pounds in women who have a normal Body Mass Index.

948

Q *Are there other problems in treating the obese pregnant woman besides the medical complications listed above?*

A Absolutely. Various tests and procedures are rendered less effective by increased abdominal wall fat. Ultrasonography, used for many reasons in pregnancy (Section 3: Ultrasound, Tests of Fetal Well-Being), may be rendered extremely ineffective by obesity. This impairment may lead to problems evaluating the fetal cord, heart, and spinal column in particular.[84]

External cephalic version may be much more difficult. Fortunato found only 37 percent success in obese women as opposed to a norm of about 70 percent.[85]

Measurements of fundal height at prenatal visits may be considerably less accurate, so that IUGR may be more likely to be overlooked.

Decreased exercise tolerance is a self-fulfilling prophecy, and the lack of exercise contributes to the risk of gestational diabetes, deep vein thrombosis, constipation, and hemorrhoids.

Operative complications at the time of cesarean section, including wound dehiscence (wound coming apart), wound infection, pelvic infection, pulmonary embolism, pulmonary edema, and deep venous thrombosis, are all increased. At the time of surgery, 60 percent of pregnant women over three-hundred pounds require cesarean deliveries, and there is an increased risk of prolonged and difficult surgery for them. Additionally, they have increased blood loss and often need repeated attempts at epidural placement. One fourth of morbidly obese women are placed on intravenous heparin to try and avoid DVT and pulmonary embolus.[86]

949

Q *Is there an increased danger for my baby if I'm obese?*

A The biggest problem for the fetus stems from the fact that obese mothers give birth to larger babies. This in turn gives the baby an increased risk of asphyxia (decreased oxygen), shoulder dystocia, birth trauma, and hypoglycemia (low sugars shortly after birth, which can lead to seizures). In fact, perinatal mortality is doubled in the macrosomic infant weighing more than 4,500 grams.[87]

COLLAGEN VASCULAR DISEASES (CONNECTIVE TISSUE DISEASES)

Systemic Lupus Erythematosis

950

Q *I have lupus and want to get pregnant. What do I need to know?*

A Systemic Lupus Erythematosis (SLE) is a disease that is characterized by the destruction of tissues throughout the body, but especially the kidneys, heart, joints, skin, and brain, due to the deposition of immune complexes formed by autoantibodies. In other words, the immune system of the person with SLE attacks his or her own tissues, leading to chronic disease. It is a disease almost exclusively of women, and often in their reproductive age. There is good evidence that lupus does not worsen simply due to pregnancy, as was previously thought, as long as you stay on your medicines.[88]

If your kidney function is essentially normal, then there is about an 80 percent chance that it will stay normal, a 10 percent chance it will worsen but you will recover, and about a 10 percent chance that it will worsen and stay worse than before your pregnancy.

Your steroids and/or azothiprine should not be stopped in pregnancy; in fact, some doctors recommend that the doses be increased in labor and continued at higher levels for eight to ten weeks after delivery.

Your fetus is at risk due to your lupus, but it seems to correlate with the severity of your kidney disease. With large amounts of proteinuria and/or significantly reduced creatinine clearance (See Section 2: Urinary Tract) almost one-fourth of pregnancies end in stillbirth; one-third deliver prematurely, and another one-third have IUGR. With normal creatinine clearance and serum creatinine lower than 1.5 milligrams per deciliter, as well a

clinical remission for more than six months before conception, outcomes were much improved.[89]

951

Q *How would I know if I might have lupus before I try to get pregnant?*

A SLE is diagnosed with a positive antinuclear antibody test (ANA), as well as a 70 percent incidence of a positive anti-DNA antibody. The antibody Anti-Sm is specific for lupus, but present only 30 percent of the time.

If any four of the following eleven conditions are present, the diagnosis is felt to be assured: Malar (butterfly) rash, discoid rash, photosensitivity, painless oral ulcers, arthritis in two or more joints, serositis with inflammation of lung lining (pleurisy) or sac around heart (pericarditis), kidney disease with proteinuria, presence of seizures or psychosis, hematologic disorder with either hemolytic anemia, low white cells (leukopenia), or low platelets (thrombocytopenia), immunologic disorder with positive anti-DNA, anti-Sm, or false positive syphilis test, or a positive ANA.

Fibromyalgia

952

Q *What will happen to my fibromyalgia when I get pregnant?*

A Fibromyalgia is a diffuse pain syndrome which seems to involve nerve endings throughout the body, but especially at certain "trigger points." Eighteen such points have been identified, and pain in response to pressure in at least eleven of these must be documented to entertain the diagnosis. It is a disorder of young women primarily, with onset at about twenty-nine to thirty-seven years old. It is frequently associated with a previous trauma such as a motor vehicle accident. Common accompanying symptoms include chronic headache about half the time, irritable bowel syndrome about one-third to one-half of the time, and Raynaud's Phenomenon (peripheral blood vessel constriction) about one-third of the time.

Pregnancy usually causes a near-complete remission as is often the case with other autoimmune processes, although specific antibodies have not been identified with this syndrome. The diagnosis itself as a legitimate entity is only recently gaining acceptance among mainstream medicine. (See Resources at the end of this section.)

CANCER

953

Q *Are cancers common enough to be a problem in pregnant women?*

A Unfortunately, about 15 percent of all female cancers occur during the reproductive years. In women fifteen to twenty-four years old, Hodgkin's lymphoma, thyroid cancer, and melanoma are the most common. For women twenty-five to forty-four years old, breast and cervical cancers are more frequent than melanoma.

Concerns include issues before, during, and after pregnancy. When cancer is found, should pregnancy be allowed afterward? If cancer is diagnosed in early pregnancy, should the pregnancy be terminated or allowed to continue? What effects could the cancer therapy have on the fetus if treatment progresses during pregnancy? Will I be able to get pregnant again after radiation or chemotherapy?

954

Q *Won't cancer chemotherapy treatments harm the fetus?*

A Almost all the antineoplastic (anticancer) drugs are classified in Category D, meaning they have been shown to cause birth defects in humans. However, these adverse effects are essentially confined to the period from five weeks to ten completed weeks of gestation. (See Section 5: Introduction) After the first trimester, there are surprisingly few adverse fetal effects from cancer chemotherapy.[90]

955

Q *I realize that diagnostic X-rays are usually at a dose so low that they don't pose a problem, but surely radiation therapy is harmful to the fetus?*

A Radiation therapy certainly may pose dangers to the fetus. The National Council on Radiation Protection and Measurements concluded that radiation exposure at levels of less than 5 rads do not pose a risk of birth defects or later problems.[91] However, even scatter radiation from therapeutic fields used for breast cancer can add up to 100 rads if the uterus has grown large enough. Radiation therapy directly to the pelvis is always contraindicated in pregnancy unless abortion has been chosen.

Breast Cancer

956

Q *My sister was diagnosed with breast cancer at twenty-two weeks of gestation. Does the fact that she's pregnant worsen her prognosis?*

A About one in three-thousand pregnancies will be complicated by breast cancer. Since the 1940s, study after study has shown that pregnancy does not influence the course of breast cancer.[92]

The problem is that women don't do their self-examinations, and even when they find a lump, they tend to dismiss it as a pregnancy change. Then they breast-feed for a year and discover an invasive cancer, which they have ignored for eighteen to twenty-four months. Naturally, these cancers tend to be at a more advanced stage than normally encountered in a nonpregnant woman of the same age.

Keep doing your self-examination, and don't minimize anything you find that concerns you, even a little. Any breast lump in pregnancy should be brought to the attention of your doctor, and if the cause is not clear-cut, the diagnosis should be aggressively pursued with fine-needle biopsy, core-needle biopsy, or open-surgical biopsy.

957

Q *How should my sister with breast cancer be treated at twenty-two weeks?*

A After biopsy confirmation, surgical excision, whether lumpectomy or modified radical mastectomy, combined with lymph node dissection, should not be delayed. Furthermore, chemotherapy either for node-positive disease or preventively for node-negative disease, should be given any time after twelve weeks of gestation without waiting for delivery.[93]

958

Q *I had breast cancer four years ago at age thirty and now I want to have a baby. Will pregnancy increase my chance of a recurrence?*

A The overwhelming majority of evidence would seem to suggest that the answer is "no." [94] Most medical oncologists today, however, recommend waiting at least two to three years before attempting conception after treatment for breast cancer.

Cervical Cancer

959

Q *How often does cervical cancer occur in pregnancy?*

A Cervical cancer occurs in only about one in 2200 pregnancies, but carcinoma in situ is the most advanced form of precancerous cervical intraepithelial neoplasia (CIN III) (severe dysplasia) and occurs in as many as two to five in one-thousand pregnancies.[95] Pregnancy itself does not appear to worsen the prognosis for cervical cancer.[96]

960

Q *What causes cervical cancer?*

A Human papilloma virus (HPV) is now felt to be the causative agent of about 90 to 95 percent of cervical cancers. This sexually transmitted virus has over sixty different subtypes, not all of which can progress to cancer, but most of which can cause vulvar or cervical venereal warts. (See this section: Infections) Once the virus infects your cervix, it may take only a few years to show up as an abnormal Papanicolaou (Pap) smear and then progress to cancer. Or it could take many years for this to happen. Since you have no way of knowing, you should get Pap smears yearly.

961

Q *What do we do if my Pap smear at my first pregnancy visit is abnormal?*

A If the Pap smear suggests dysplasia, colposcopy (looking at the cervix with special lenses) is performed. Suspicious areas may then be biopsied in the office with little discomfort or risk. Cone biopsy or LEEP excision in the office is usually avoided in pregnancy if possible, but may be done if needed to differentiate between severe dysplasia and invasive cervical cancer.

962

Q *How is cervical cancer treated if I'm already pregnant?*

A Severe dysplasia or carcinoma in situ is both diagnosed and treated with LEEP excision. If LEEP reveals microinvasive cervical cancer, definitive treatment may be delayed until after vaginal delivery at term. Only with frankly invasive cervical cancer (greater than a three-millimeter invasion into the tissue) is consideration given to terminating a pregnancy of less than twenty weeks by performing a radical hysterectomy (more tissue out to either side of the uterus is removed than with a simple hysterectomy) and lymph node dissection (sampling), with termination of the fetus still in the uterus. After twenty weeks, definitive surgical therapy is delayed until term delivery when a radical hysterectomy may be performed at time of cesarean, or after a six-week delay.[97]

Radiation therapy has a much higher complication rate peripartum and the surgical approach is uniformly preferred today.

Hodgkin's Lymphoma

963

Q *What happens if I get Hodgkin's disease while pregnant?*

A Hodgkin's disease is the most common type of lymphoma to affect young women of childbearing age and occurs in about one in six-thousand pregnancies. Symptoms include enlarged, nontender lymph nodes, especially in the neck and under the arms. Systemic symptoms include generalized itching night sweats, fever, and fatigue, and sometimes weight loss. Neither the incidence nor the prognosis is changed by pregnancy.

MRI is used to evaluate the extent of disease in pregnancy. Usually local radiation would be used to treat isolated nodal involvement without evidence of disease elsewhere, but not necessarily in pregnancy. Local irradiation to head and neck appears safe with shielding, but not safe when dosing the mid-chest region.[98]

With widespread disease, chemotherapy should be started at diagnosis, or delayed until ten completed weeks of gestation.

Fertility returns about half the time after chemotherapy. Women with Hodgkin's are also at considerable risk (about 20 percent) for recurrence of other types of cancer, especially leukemia.

SKELETAL PROBLEMS

964

Q *I've had scoliosis since I was a teenager. I had Harrington rods placed and now I'm pregnant. Will I have trouble with labor and delivery and can I have an epidural?*

A Scoliosis is a curvature of the lower spine, which, when severe enough, is often treated with the placement of metal rods. There is no reason to believe you will have any increased difficulty with labor or delivery. While the rods do not actually cover the access to the epidural space, they do limit your ability to bend forward and open the spaces between the vertebral bodies, making epidural placement sometimes impossible. Harrington rods do not prohibit the placement of spinal anesthetic for delivery or cesarean.

965

Q *I've had a lumbar discectomy for a herniated lumbar disc in the past. Can I have an epidural?*

A Previous herniated disc surgery is a relatively common complication of labor and delivery, especially as the American childbearing age has increased to include many women over thirty-five. Anesthesiologists and obstetricians who might place your epidural catheter are worried about several potential problems.

If there is scarring in the epidural space, the catheter may not thread, the medicine may not distribute equally, or the needle or catheter might have an increased risk of puncturing a vein or entering the spinal fluid space, resulting in the possibility of a dangerously high block, or a postpartum spinal headache.[99] This does not necessarily mean that you may not have an epidural, and each case must be individualized.

966

Q *I was in a car accident when I was sixteen and fractured my pelvis in several places. Will I be able to deliver vaginally?*

A Pelvic fracture is a fairly frequent occurrence, particularly in automobile accidents. Most women with previous multiple pelvic fractures can deliver vaginally, at least barring other nonrelated reasons for requiring a cesarean. Your doctor may wish to review your X-rays taken at the time of injury, but I have never had to refuse a trial of labor on the basis of a previous fracture.

TRAUMA IN PREGNANCY

Motor Vehicle Accidents/Seat Belts/Falls

967

Q *I was in a car accident and I'm twenty-eight weeks pregnant. I feel a little bruised and the baby's moving. Do I need to go the hospital? Another pregnant friend fell on the ice, is her baby at risk?*

A Motor vehicle accidents are by far the greatest cause of traumatic injury to both mother and fetus. If you were wearing your seat belt and shoulder harness, in all probability your fetus is fine, since the amniotic fluid provides an excellent cushion for the baby. However, car accidents at high speeds cause rapid deceleration, which can shear off vessels in your brain, chest, and abdomen. Obviously this can prove fatal to you and the baby, but deceleration can also shear vessels in the placenta and lead to placental abruption. (See Section 8: Placental Abruption)

Your doctor may wish to monitor your contractions and the fetus's heart rate for a couple of hours. He or she may also wish to do a blood test called a Kleihauer Betke test to determine if any of the fetus's blood has mixed with your bloodstream, possibly indicating a hidden abruption. If your blood type is Rh-negative, your doctor may also wish to administer a shot of 300 micrograms of Rhogam to prevent sensitization. (See Section 8: Rh Disease)

If, after two to four hours of observation on a fetal monitor, you have no worrisome fetal heart rate changes, less than five contractions per hour, a nontender uterus, and no vaginal bleeding or leaking fluid, you can safely be discharged.[100]

Patients fall frequently in pregnancy due to altered center of gravity. Almost any fall from ground level under 25 weeks is rarely a concern for the fetus, no matter which part of your anatomy contacts the ground! The baby is incredibly well protected. After 25 weeks it is possible to rupture your membranes or stimulate pre-term contractions, but even late in pregnancy falls almost never cause a problem directly the pregnancy. After 25 weeks you should describe the fall to your doctor's office and they will let you know if you need any monitoring at all.

968

Q *I heard that if there is an accident, the shoulder harness can compress the uterus and hurt the baby. Besides, it's uncomfortable, and I don't wear it, especially since we have air bags. Is that protection enough?*

A Shoulder harness seat belt restraints in all probability save more babies each year than all the obstetricians and midwives combined. Every year about 50,000 people are killed in automobile accidents in the United States alone, with another 150,000 permanently impaired. Seat belts, automatic seat belt restraints, and air bags all save lives and reduce serious injury, and yet 50 percent of Americans refuse to wear them.[101] Incredibly, seat belt use goes down during pregnancy, despite the fact that pregnant women are now responsible for another life inside them.

Automobile accidents certainly can direct force to the abdomen, but seat belts, properly worn, do not increase the risk of injury to the fetus.[102] Being ejected from the vehicle when unrestrained accounts for 25 percent of all motor vehicle accident deaths.

Air bags alone are not adequate protection for your baby. They may help little with crashes which occur from the side, and the explosive force of the air bag could potentially be a problem late in pregnancy in the same way it has been for small children in front-or rear-facing car seats. Pregnant women should move their seats as far away from the air bag as possible. Never hold a baby in your lap! In a head-on collision with both vehicles only going twenty-five mph, a 7 1/2 pound newborn would feel instantly like 150 pounds and would not be possible to hold on to!

969

Q *How should I wear my seat belt when my belly's so huge?*

A The seat belt lap restraint should be worn across the upper thighs and under the pregnant abdomen and as snug as possible. The shoulder restraint should go over the shoulder and between the breasts.

Blunt Abdominal Trauma (Battery)

970

Q *My boyfriend beat me up and hit me in the stomach. I'm twenty-three weeks pregnant and worried about my baby because he hasn't been moving ever since that happened. Could he be hurt?*

A With no symptoms other than bruising, your fetus probably has not been seriously injured. Fetuses do not move consistently, daily, often until after twenty-five weeks. Nevertheless, you should see your obstetrician immediately, since very occasionally there could be hidden problems.

As many as one in twelve women in the inner city are assaulted and battered during pregnancy.[103] Placental abruption can occur with relatively minor trauma to the abdomen.[104]

If placental abruption were occurring in you, frequent symptoms would be vaginal bleeding, uterine tenderness and contractions, and fetal heart rate abnormalities such as tachycardia and late decelerations. Even if you have little pain and no bleeding, you should be evaluated by your obstetrician after any blow to the abdomen. However, it remains extremely likely that your fetus is fine. If your blood type is Rh negative, your doctor may consider giving you Rhogam to prevent sensitization. (See Section 8: Rh Disease)

If, after two to four hours of observation on a fetal monitor, you have no worrisome fetal heart rate changes, less than five contractions per hour, a non-tender uterus, and no vaginal bleeding or leaking fluid, then you can safely be discharged.[105]

You need to ditch your current boyfriend. If that means moving out, do it today. If you're scared, call your County Health Department and ask them to help you contact a woman's shelter. Your local hospital, as well as the local police force, can give you those references also. The most important thing to remember is if your "boyfriend" or husband could do this even once, next time he could kill you or your baby.

SUGGESTED RESOURCES

American Cancer Society
1-800-227-2345

American College of Obstetricians and Gynecologists
ACOG Web site: http://www.acog.com
Main Switchboard: 800-673-8444, (206) 658-5577
Order Desk: 800-762-2264

American Diabetes Association
Website: http://www.diabetes.org/
1660 Duke Street
Alexandria, VA 22314
1-800-DIABETES

American Heart Association
Website: http://www.amhrt.org/
7320 Greenville
Dallas, TX 75231
1-214-373-6300

For more information on Pregnancy and Seat Belts or Infant Restraints:

American Academy of Pediatrics, Office of Public Education, Evanston, IL

American College of Obstetricians and Gynecologists
ACOG Website: http://www.acog.com
Main Switchboard: 800-673-8444, (206) 638-5577
Order Desk: 800-762-2264 Ask for: Car safety for you and your baby.
ACOG Patient Education Pamphlet AP018, 1988

WEBSITES

Asthma and Pregnancy
http://www.emedicinehealth.com/asthma_in_pregnancy/article_em.htm
http://www.nlm.nih.gov/medlineplus/asthma.html

AIDS and Pregnancy
http://www.nlm.nih.gov/medlineplus/aidsandpregnancy.html

Bell's Palsey
http://www.nlm.nih.gov/medlineplus/bellspalsy.html

Breast Cancer and Pregnancy

http://www.meb.uni-bonn.de/Cancernet/105380.html

Carpal Tunnel Syndrome

http://www.ninds.nih.gov/disorders/carpal_tunnel/ detail_carpal_tunnel.htm

Cervical Cancer and HPV

http://www.nlm.nih.gov/medlineplus/hpv.html

http://www.nlm.nih.gov/medlineplus/cervicalcancer.html

Congenital Heart Disease

http://www.nlm.nih.gov/medlineplus/congenitalheartdisease.html

Diabetes and Pregnancy

http://www.nlm.nih.gov/medlineplus/diabetesandpregnancy.html

Gastrointestinal Disease and Pregnancy

http://www.nlm.nih.gov/medlineplus/crohnsdisease.html

http://www.nlm.nih.gov/medlineplus/ulcerativecolitis.html

Headache

www.americanpregnancy.org/pregnancyhealth/headaches.html

Heart Disease and Pregnancy

http://www.americanheart.org/presenter.jhtml?identifier=4688

http://www.nlm.nih.gov/medlineplus/heartdiseaseinwomen.html

Hypertension and Pregnancy

http://www.nlm.nih.gov/medlineplus/highbloodpressureinpregnancy.html

Infections in Pregnancy

http://www.nlm.nih.gov/medlineplus/infectionsandpregnancy.html

Lupus and Pregnancy

http://www.nlm.nih.gov/medlineplus/lupus.html

http://www.betterhealth.vic.gov.au/bhcv2/bhcarticles.nsf/
pages/ Lupus_and_pregnancy?OpenDocument

Mammograms in Pregnancy

http://www.pregnancy.org/article.php?sid=1388

Mitral Valve Prolapse

http://www.nlm.nih.gov/medlineplus/mitralvalveprolapse.html

Neurologic/Seizure Disorders

http://www.nlm.nih.gov/medlineplus/epilepsy.html

http://www.emedicine.com/med/topic3433.htm

Section Ten

After the Delivery

(See Also Section 6: Bonding)

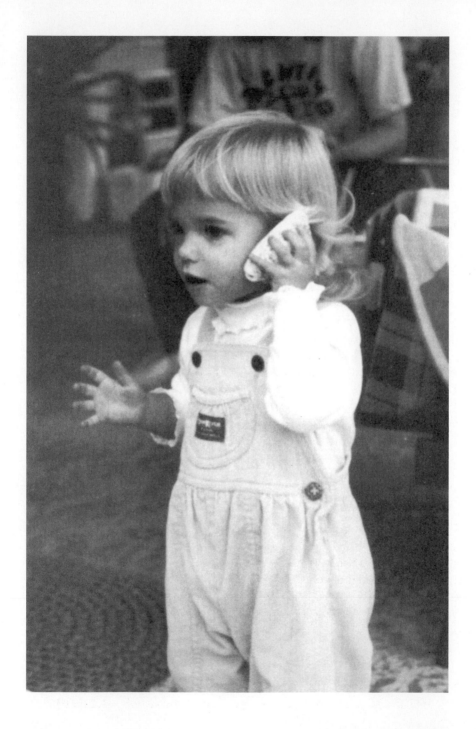

971

Q *How long will I stay in the hospital, and what will go on while I am there?*

A A hospital stay for a vaginal delivery is usually about twenty-four to forty-eight hours; for a cesarean the stay is about seventy-two to ninety-six hours. The time you need will vary with your particular delivery. American insurers, as of January, 1998, are mandated by Congress to provide maternity benefits, which include coverage for a minimum of forty-eight hours for vaginal and ninety-six hours for cesarean delivery.

So, when you contact your insurer, be sure to ask how many nights they will pay for your circumstance, not how long you can stay. They will only tell you that they can't make medical decisions, and you can stay as long as your doctor recommends.

For the first twenty-four hours, you will be observed closely for any sign of fever, excessive bleeding, or incision problems. Your temperature, pulse, and blood pressure will be taken frequently, and the nurses will also be firmly massaging your uterus to make sure that it is adequately contracted to minimize bleeding. If you had an episiotomy, or simply swelling from pushing for a long time, an ice bag will be placed on the perineum. After twelve hours, this will be replaced by sitz bathing (your bottom is in hot water), often followed by the soothing warmth of a "perilamp" positioned between your legs for twenty minutes, two to three times a day. Once you're at home, since you probably don't own a perilamp, a handheld hair dryer directed on your episiotomy after sitz bathing will do just as well.

If you and the baby are both healthy, almost all institutions will allow you to keep the baby with you after his/her initial evaluation and check-in. (See Section 6: Bonding; Section 7: Admissions Nursery) However, fewer women than you might expect choose to have twenty-hour rooming-in. Labor is often an exhausting process, and all your friends and relatives will be inadvertently expecting you to be the "hostess with the mostess" when they drop by. If you breast-feed, the baby will be brought to you when he or she cries (on demand), or at least at about midnight and four A.M. You'll need every moment of sleep that you can get.

972

Q *I don't have any idea how to take care of a baby. How do I learn what to do?*

A There is no question that God provided for this! After about a week, you will know what every cry, twitch, and gurgle means better than anyone else in the world. (Even better than your mother-in-law!) Keeping a baby warm, fed, and changed are just about all you need to know early on. All hospitals will have baby care classes to help you with diaper changes, first bath, and feeding, whether by breast or bottle. Encourage your husband to join the class at least for the diaper part.

Your pediatrician will need to see the baby again at about two weeks of life and can tell you how you're doing at that time. Remember, telephones work twenty-four hours a day after you leave the hospital, and no question is too stupid to ask.

Postpartum Instructions

973

Q *How do I take care of my body after a vaginal delivery?*

A Postpartum instructions are pretty simple. Your doctor will want to see you six weeks after delivery, or earlier if necessary. You will usually be given a narcotic painkiller to take home with you, and you may need it for several days. You may drive a car after seven to ten days when your bottom doesn't hurt and you're not taking narcotics.

Do not let yourself get constipated. Drink a lot of water, and if you haven't had a bowel movement by forty-eight to seventy-two hours after delivery, consider using milk of magnesia or Dulcolax suppositories (unless you've had a fourth-degree tear or an episiotomy into the rectum). Colace may be taken as a stool softener once or twice per day, beginning the day after delivery.

Exercise may include walking right away, and swimming whenever your bleeding stops. Bleeding may continue for up to six weeks, but don't use tampons.

Restrictions include no tampons and no parts of other people's anatomy in your body. In other words, no messing around until you have returned for your checkup in four to six weeks.

974

Q *Is there anything different to watch out for after a cesarean?*

A Usually a cesarean incision will be closed with stainless-steel staples, which are removed on the second or third day; removal is almost painless. Sometimes your incision will be closed with subcuticular stitches with sutures that reabsorb and don't need removal. Newer skin adhesives that work like clear glue may replace both of these methods soon.

Remember that a cesarean is closed in seven layers. The fascia, strong connective tissue that holds your insides in, is put together with a very strong semipermanent suture. Your skin incision is more for decoration than support. You should let your doctor know if any redness or swelling above your incision gets larger rather than smaller after your discharge from the hospital. Call if you have any yellowish fluid leaking from the wound. A small amount of bloody spotting from the staple holes is not worrisome.

Avoid heavy lifting, meaning anything heavier than a newborn baby, for the first four weeks. You may walk for exercise as soon as you are able. In general, let pain be your guide and follow the same restrictions as indicated above for vaginal delivery.

Postpartum Discomforts

975

Q *I know why my bottom hurts after a vaginal delivery, but why does my stomach cramp so much?*

A After-birth pains are uterine contractions that get progressively more intense after each pregnancy. They are especially noticeable when you breast-feed, since stimulation of the nipple releases oxytocin, the hormone involved in initiating labor. (See Section 7: Normal Labor and Delivery) Sometimes you can relieve the pain by changing position, lying with a pillow under your abdomen, keeping your bladder empty, and taking your pain pills about thirty minutes *before* breast-feeding. The narcotic in your milk will not have any significant effect on the baby

976

Q *I delivered three days ago, and my breasts hurt and feel extremely full. Am I doing something wrong?*

A You're not doing anything wrong. Your milk takes about forty-eight to seventy-two hours to come in. Prior to that only colostrum is present, which may start leaking only after delivery, or it may have been present in small amounts in one or both breasts since as early as twenty weeks of pregnancy. Wear a good support bra and continue to breast-feed. Your breasts will adjust to the baby's demand very quickly.

If you're not going to breast-feed, you may be advised to bind your breasts with an elastic bandage in place of wearing a support bra, apply plastic bags of crushed ice to ease the pain and swelling, or take a medicine to suppress lactation. Even if your milk comes in and you get engorged, the pain and hardness will only last about twenty-four to seventy-two hours.

Although Parlodel lost FDA approval for lactation suppression in 1995, a newer medicine, carbegoline (Dostinex) became available in 1997. The FDA has not approved it for lactation suppression, but your doctor may choose to use it anyway because it is given as a one-time dosage instead of the Parlodel dosage of twice per day for two weeks.

977

Q *My hemorrhoids got worse with delivery, which I wouldn't have thought possible. Is there anything I can do?*

A Witch hazel compresses such as Tuck's pads can help. Commercial creams such as Preparation H, Anusol HC, and Tronolane may provide some relief. Substituting medicated wipes such as Rantex or flushable baby wipes for plain toilet paper is an extremely good idea.

RETURN TO NORMAL

978

Q *How long will it take for my body to get back to normal?*

A Your body will go through just as many changes now that you are not pregnant as when you became pregnant and you shouldn't expect it to happen overnight. Your cervix stays open more than normal for several weeks after a vaginal delivery. No matter how you delivered, your uterus will be easily felt at about the level of your navel for several days after delivery. It feels like a firm lump about the size of a large cantaloupe. At this point, it weighs about two and a half to three pounds, but by six to eight weeks it will weigh only six ounces.

Your abdominal skin and muscles were stretched to accommodate your enlarged uterus, and the same type of exercises suggested for early pregnancy will help to gradually tone these muscles over several months.

You will have a vaginal discharge made up of blood and the shedding lining of your uterus for weeks after delivery. The discharge is referred to as lochia, and will change from bright red after three to four days to pinkish brown to yellowish by ten to fourteen days. You may have intermittent bleeding for six weeks. If you have had several babies before, you may even pass some clots from time to time, especially about seven to ten days after delivery. The discharge and bleeding usually stop in about six weeks.

Your hair may come out in larger amounts than usual when you brush it or shower. This is a common hormonal phenomenon and resolves by itself. By six months, your hair growth will usually be back to normal. (See Section 2: Hair)

979

Q *I had a scheduled cesarean and wasn't swelling at all before I had the baby, but now that's changed. When will the swelling go away?*

A When you have a C-section, and to a lesser extent, when you deliver vaginally, a considerable amount of Lactated Ringer's Solution is placed in your IV. Basically, this is salt water and after your surgery you've had the equivalent of about twenty pizzas without benefit of the cheese. Overhydration, done on purpose, lets you bleed diluted blood and you actually lose fewer red blood cells and relatively more serum made from water. You have been given a huge salt load, which takes several days to a week for your kidneys to excrete. This intravenous hydration, or volume load, also helps prevent episodes of low blood pressure while you are under the regional anesthesia of an epidural or a spinal.

So if you feel like a dirigible after a C-section, be reassured that you'll lose at least several pounds in edema fluid over the next week or so.

980

Q *When will I have my first period?*

A Your first menses postpartum is usually about seven to ten weeks after delivery. If you are breast-feeding full time, you may have no return of periods at all, or they may be unpredictable. Remember, you can become pregnant again (oh, there's a pleasant thought), even before your six-week postpartum visit, if you're not careful. Breast-feeding decreases the frequency of ovulation to about one-third of normal, but you ovulate when you least expect it with no periods or irregular ones.

981

Q *What will we do about birth control after the baby is born?*

A If you are breast-feeding, an all-progestin minipill called Micronor may be taken each day, without stopping to have menstrual periods. It should be started at least two weeks before you make love. Micronor fails only about to 3 percent of the time in the breast-feeding woman, as opposed to a 10 to

15 percent failure rate for diaphragm or condoms. Other minipills, called Nor-QD and Ovrette, are commercially available as well. Once you have weaned to two or fewer feedings per day, you should switch to a regular estrogen-progestin birth-control pill. It is perfectly safe to wean while you are taking the regular pill. In fact, many doctors may recommend use of the regular pill even while you are breast-feeding. The only concern is the potential for decreased milk supply in the first few weeks.

If you are bottle-feeding, the combined estrogen-progestin pill may be started several weeks after delivery to avoid the slight increased risk of blood-clotting problems in the peripartum period.

IUDs may be placed at the postpartum visit, although traditionally waiting until ten weeks for the uterus to return to normal size has been recommended. IUDs should be in place for one cycle before depending on them for birth control.

DepoProvera may be used as early as several days after delivery so that protection is effective by your postpartum visit. Likewise, Norplant may be inserted subcutaneously at any time after delivery.

As of 1996, the spermicidal Today sponge is no longer commercially available in the United States.

Don't be surprised if sexual intercourse hurts. Sex won't feel like it once did until up to six months after you give birth, but by four to six weeks after delivery, someone in your family is going to be very interested in sex! While it may not be you, intercourse can be much more comfortable if you use an excellent sexual lubricant such as Astroglide. Especially when you are breast-feeding, the vagina does not respond to sexual excitation with the normal engorgement, lengthening, and lubrication. Patience, gentleness, and external lubrication are the best approach. Use position to your advantage. Side-to-side or woman astride allows you more control of penetration and may be less painful to the episiotomy site. Sex after a cesarean will also hurt in the vaginal area unless you use external lubrication, especially if you are breast-feeding.

982

Q *I haven't delivered yet, but my husband and I want me to get a tubal ligation after the baby is born. How is that done?*

A Postpartum tubal ligation is a poor term for a procedure in which the tubes are actually transected and a piece of each tube sent to the pathologist. Shortly after delivery, usually about thirty minutes, you may be taken to an operating room, where a small incision is made in the lower part of your navel for surgical sterilization. This can be done under local anesthetic, epidural or general. The tubes are grasped with an instrument and brought up through the two-centimeter incision. Then the tubes are ligated, or tied, in two places about an inch apart and the intervening portions excised. If you had a cesarean, no additional incision has to be made.

983

Q *I know my husband has my postpartum visit circled in red on his calendar, but I just don't feel like making love at all. He's been wonderful, but somehow I'm almost repulsed by his touch. What am I going to do?*

A Relax. You've been in demand not only from your baby, but from every relative and friend you've ever had over the last six weeks. It's natural to be exhausted. Often, you need your personal space more than ever before. A decreased desire for sex (decreased libido) may not just be limited to the couple of months postpartum either. Your attention is focused on your newborn, and rightly so. Although you may love your husband just as much as ever, it's almost impossible to avoid his playing second fiddle to your baby. After all, your newborn really is helpless and totally dependent on you for food, protection, and mobility. Your husband, as much as he may act like it, is not totally helpless.

Be sure to discuss these issues with your husband. He will feel less rejected if he understands your decreased libido in terms of focus and a need for personal space. Most women who had a satisfying sexual relationship before the baby will have one again, even if there are a few changes. Overcome your aversion to sexual relations at least intermittently, even if it takes a conscious effort in the beginning. Get a baby-sitter and have a romantic evening out together as soon as possible after you feel comfortable leaving the baby briefly. Time alone with your husband outside of bed will be critical to arousing your interest in sex once again.

Most of all, don't panic. Everything takes time. Even if you fear intercourse, remember that other forms of sexual play can be just as satisfying to your partner when there has been no sexual contact for many weeks or months.

984

Q *I'm about five weeks postpartum and I want to jump my husband every night when he comes home. The problem is, for the first time ever, he just doesn't seem interested. Could I be that unappealing now?*

A In all probability, you're not unappealing, just scary. Many men who were intensely fearful of hurting the fetus with sex during pregnancy are still wary after delivery. Now they're afraid of hurting you, afraid you won't like it anymore, or afraid sex may not feel the same. Some men are even turned off by the milk letdown that accompanies sexual stimulation.

In the first weeks and sometimes months postpartum, it's not your sex appeal that's the problem, it's usually a mismatch and/or miscommunication about what you both fear or want, physically, from each other. Discuss this together, even if it's embarrassing. If you experience hurt feelings, remind yourself that your husband's fear of hurting you or his initial distaste for some of your physical changes is temporary and is not a sign that he has stopped thinking of you as attractive. Remember, love is patient and it really does conquer all.

SIGNS OF PROBLEMS

985

Q *What kinds of problems warrant a call to my doctor's office?*

A Postpartum warning signs include painful urination (symptom of bladder infection common after catheterization in labor), bleeding heavier than a period (symptom of subinvolution of the uterus or weak contracting), a hot, reddened tender area in the breast (symptom of mastitis, a breast infection that spreads out from the nipple), worsening pain around your episiotomy (symptom of infection or hematoma), swelling and pain in your leg, or coughing with chest pain with or without coughing up blood (symptom of thromboembolism), nausea and vomiting after a cesarean, or a fever of over 100.4 degrees Fahrenheit.

You may have problems that are psychological rather than physical in nature. Usually these mood changes are self-limited, but occasionally you will need special help. (See this section: Postpartum Depression)

BREAST-FEEDING

986

Q *What considerations will help me decide whether I should breast-feed?*

A Breastfeeding is of course what God had in mind, but it may not be for everyone. One thing you can stop worrying about is where you can breast-feed. The United States Congress passed a bill in 1997 that makes it legal to breast-feed everywhere. This supersedes older laws in those states and municipalities that forbid nursing in public. A little decorum, however, in the form of a baby blanket or cloth diaper draped over the nursing infant's head and your breast, is probably wise.

It is thought that breast milk provides the perfect source of nutrition for your growing baby. Most women also find breast-feeding more convenient than having to lug around bottles and formula. But some women find it difficult to breast-feed full time once they return to work, and they may either be unable to or lack the desire to pump their breasts in order to store milk.

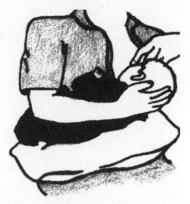

Some women cannot breast-feed because of previous surgery, most often a breast reduction in which the nipple has been transplanted. Even in this circumstance, most women can breast-feed because the milk ducts have been left intact on purpose. Breast augmentations usually pose no problem whatsoever in breast-feeding.

The decision, if you are physically able to breast-feed, has to do with time, comfort, convenience, work, and attitude. If you decide to breast-feed, try it for

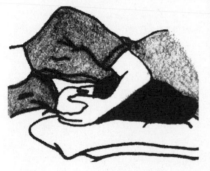

a minimum of at least six weeks. Once breast-feeding is well established, your nipples no longer hurt, your milk supply exactly meets your baby's needs, and you may find that you enjoy the experience immensely. Many women feed for a year or more comfortably, adding solids to their baby's diet as tolerated.

Hundreds of studies on the topic have demonstrated that breast-feeding is somewhat protective against gastroenteritis (diarrhea), and to a lesser extent, upper respiratory infections, in the first year or so of life. This can be demonstrated with as little as two months of breast feeding.[1]

However, unlike many other mammals, breast-feeding is certainly not essential for passage of immune capability in humans. The majority of a newborn's immune protection is in the form of IgG antibodies, which are passed to him or her across the placenta. These antibodies help protect the newborn against systemic infection until the baby's body can start manufacturing antibodies on its own.

Breast milk contains secretory IgA antibodies, which appear to be useful for protecting the gut and possibly upper airways to a statistically significant extent over bottle-fed infants. Additionally, lactoferrin is a breast-milk protein that helps prevent diarrhea.[2]

However, babies born with a congenital absence of IgA do not have significantly increased morbidity, while babies born without the ability to make IgG have an almost invariably fatal outcome.

987

Q *When can I start breast-feeding and is it true that breast-fed babies have fewer problems with allergies later in life?*

A You may put the baby to breast moments after delivery if your baby is healthy and the circumstances allow. You will have only colostrum present until three to five days after delivery. The baby may suckle right away, or show virtually no interest at all. Either of these is normal and is no cause for worry.

Atopy is a term used to describe those allergic reactions, with a tendency to be hereditary, caused by pollens, foods, animal dander, insect venom, and other irritants. There is some evidence that breast-feeding for as little as 70 days reduces the risk of atopy in later infancy but that longer breast-feeding does not impart additional benefit.[3]

988

Q *I've heard that I should only let the baby feed on each breast for five to ten minutes until my nipples get tougher. Is that correct?*

A Opinions have changed about several different aspects of breast-feeding in recent years. Prevailing opinion in 1997 seems to be that you should feed from one breast for as long as the baby will take the breast. When the baby is satisfied, stop. When he or she either demands feeding again by fussing, or it is time to feed again on a schedule, offer the other breast. (A safety pin on your gown or nursing bra will help you remember which breast you used last, although once your milk is fully in, it should be obvious.) Once your milk is fully in you may divide your feedings evenly between both breasts.

Different "experts" will give you different opinions about demand feeding versus scheduled feeding. Although some pediatricians feel that scheduled feeding ensures adequate intake, others feel that this only applies for bottle-feeding. Demand feeding triggers exactly the correct volume of milk for your baby under usual circumstances. Each time the baby sucks on the nipple, it triggers the release of hormones that regulate the amount of milk required. Breastfeeding probably should be on demand, but at least every one and a half to three hours for the first six weeks. Most babies will need to breast-feed about ten to twelve times over twenty-four hours. Babies may later tolerate feedings as infrequent as every four hours, but early on, this may lead to inadequate milk supply.

989

Q *How do I know that my breasts are providing enough milk?*

A If your baby is satisfied for one and a half to three hours, your supply is probably doing the job. Pay attention to your baby's diapers for a day or two. In the first six weeks, your baby should wet five or six disposable diapers and have two bowel movements every twenty-four hours. If this is the case, you may be assured that your baby is receiving adequate nutrition and hydration.

990

Q *What's the controversy about bottles and pacifiers?*

A Nipple confusion is the term given to the phenomenon in which a breastfeeding baby is fed intermittently from a bottle and then subsequently prefers the easy flow from the bottle. This could then lead to decreased milk supply and, as a consequence, to bottle-feeding as necessary for adequate nutrition.

In addition to recommending that you avoid the bottle for water or formula in the early days to weeks of breast-feeding, some lactation nurses recommend avoiding pacifiers as well. The leap from condemning the use of a bottle to condemning the use of a pacifier is a large one indeed. The rationale for avoiding the bottle when trying to bring the mother's milk in is a logical one. The condemnation of pacifiers is not quite so clearly founded.

Sucking is a universally pleasurable and appreciated human activity. Witness everything from lollipops to cigarettes to human sexual response. A baby gets no nutritional value from a pacifier and will remain just as hungry before and after its use. Yet it may be comforting to him or her when the breast is not available.

In any event, the only opinion that really matters in your case is yours (and your husband's) and your baby's.

991

Q *My daughter is five days old, but my breasts are hard as rock and the nipples are really sore. Will the soreness continue? What should I do?*

A Breast engorgement occurs naturally as your milk comes in with a vengeance about three to five days after delivery. Use hot compresses or a hot shower with massage of the areola to soften the nipple before each feeding. Between feedings, try putting plastic bags with crushed ice on the breasts, and use a good support bra to hold the ice bags in place. This engorgement lasts only a day or two while your brain figures out exactly how much milk your baby needs.

Sore nipples are a very frequent occurrence. There are a few ways to minimize the pain. It is important to keep the nipples dry. You can use your handheld hair drier to dry the nipple and areola right after feeding. Be sure you use your hand to support the breast while feeding, and check to make sure the baby has both chin and nose touching the breast simultaneously. Try to get as much of the areola in the baby's mouth as possible, not just the nipple. Be sure to use your finger to break the suction before pulling the baby off the nipple. If the baby falls asleep at the breast, remove it from his or her mouth and air-dry the nipple.

When nursing is painful, use the same breathing you used to handle contractions in labor, and start with the least sore nipple first. Many experts recommend avoiding the breast pumps shaped like a bugle as well as avoiding plastic breast shields, which used to be recommended.

Be alert to the possibility of mastitis, the symptoms of which are a fever, chills, and a hot, sore red patch extending out from the nipple area. Mastitis is an infection of the breast due to bacteria that live in the back of your baby's throat. Usually staph or strep bugs, they enter through the nipple itself or through cracks in the nipple. Mastitis may usually be treated conservatively with oral antibiotics from your doctor, hot compresses, and continued breast-feeding from the affected side. While continued breast-feeding may be extremely painful, it will hasten the resolution of the infection and keep your breast from drying up. You must keep emptying the breast.

992

Q *I've been breast-feeding for ten days and my milk still doesn't come out for a long time after the baby starts. Is there anything I can do?*

A You can try expressing your milk manually right before nursing, which might take time. A commercial preparation that helps with slow milk "let-down," a nasal spray called Syntocin, can be used thirty minutes before intended nursing. Syntocin is simply oxytocin, which was also responsible for allowing labor to begin. Most lactation experts would resort to this only as a last-ditch effort to keep you breast-feeding, since your immediate letdown mechanism may not be fine-tuned for a month or so. After a month, your "letdown" may be more immediate than you'd like— you'll probably discover this the first time a stranger's baby cries while you're standing in line at the grocery store!

993

Q *What exactly is a colicky baby?*

A If your baby has been home for at least a couple of weeks but continues to be inconsolable, with long periods of crying broken only by occasional sleep, he or she may be "colicky."

Pediatricians have different opinions about how to respond, but most agree that the mother should discontinue any dairy products from her diet for about a week. If this fails to help, try discontinuing iron supplements for a week and, finally, try eliminating caffeine for a week.

994

Q *If I want to take my husband at his word and let him help with some middle-of-the-night feedings, how do I go about it?*

A You may pump your breasts at anytime and store the milk in a plastic bottle in the refrigerator if you plan to use it within three days. Breast milk may be stored in the freezer portion of a refrigerator for up to three months.

At feeding time, your husband should defrost the milk by holding the bottle with the frozen milk first under tap water, then lukewarm water. He should not refreeze the remainder after a feeding, but discard it instead.

995

Q *My baby is only three weeks old, but he seems irritated all the time. Am I doing something wrong?*

A Babies can be awfully cute, but they can be awfully grumpy as well. They have mood changes and get fussy for reasons they just can't always share with us. You may think your milk is inadequate, but remember the wet-diaper and two-bowel-movement rule. By a couple of weeks of age, your baby can get annoyed by lots of things besides hunger.

If the baby is grumpy but won't nurse, then try changing rooms, walking, rocking and/or playing with him or her. Screw up your face into different expressions, grin and coo a lot, pump the baby's legs like a bicycle, blow on feet and tummy, help the baby use his or her hands to touch your eyes, lips, nose, and hair. Let the baby grasp your fingers, then gently extend his or her arms out in front, over the head, and down to the sides.

If your child would rather fuss than play, bring him or her with you in a carrier while you get something done. The baby's natural curiosity may not provide adequate distraction, in which case, you can try an old-fashioned rocker, an infant swing, or a pacifier. After three weeks, breast-feeding will be well established and few would argue that "nipple confusion" is a legitimate issue any longer.

The baby who was so "serene" at the hospital may seem to sleep less and keep you awake more. What's going on is that your baby sleeps for roughly twenty of the first twenty-four hours of life, and only gradually wakes up and starts to interact with the world.

In the first few hours after birth, babies are in the quiet alert state, in which their bodies are at rest, but their eyes are looking all around. The active alert state is one in which the baby is still curious, but now moves all the extremities and is easily distracted. After this activity, he or she may get sleepy, or really feisty. The crying state may follow this phase. Marshall Klaus in *The Amazing Newborn* states that you may head off the crying state by using a front pack or a sling. Rocking chairs and automated infant swings help some annoyed babies. And yes, some babies do very well with pacifiers, which pose no risk to breast-feeding if it is already well established.

The baby may become drowsy as a result of rocking or rhythmic motion. When sleep finally comes, it will alternate between quiet sleep and active sleep every thirty minutes or so.[4]

996

Q *I have inverted nipples and it's really hard to get the baby to latch on. What can I do?*

A Inverted nipples (turned-in nipples) may make it more difficult to breast-feed, but not impossible. Inverted nipples retract rather than protrude in response to sexual excitation, cold, or sucking. The baby grasps the entire areola, not just the nipple. While the nipple may help stimulate the suck reflex by touching the roof of the mouth, it is compression of the areola that helps eject the milk. A special plastic nipple shield may be worn in the bra during the daytime to help evert the nipple. If you cannot get the baby to suckle successfully no matter what you try, talk to your doctor about formula feeding instead. Don't let anyone shame you into feeling inadequate if you decide to bottle-feed. Your baby can sense when you are upset, tense, and overtired, and it's wrong to torture yourself because you think you must breastfeed.

997

Q *I'm going back to work in about ten days and I want to breast-feed as much as possible. At least several feedings will be at the day-care center. How do I go about pumping?*

A Breast pumps come in many different forms, from the inexpensive plastic bugle-or bicycle-horn-shaped models operated by hand suction or batteries to the glass cylinder types on electric pumps. Bugle-or bicycle-horn-shaped pumps are considered fairly traumatic to the nipple. Battery-operated models often require that you break the suction intermittently by altering the vacuum manually to roughly simulate the suck-release cycle of the newborn.

With a rented electric pump such as the Medela Pump, both breasts may be emptied simultaneously, and intermittent suction helps protect the nipples from damage.

Manual expression is still probably the safest way to empty your breasts, although it requires some effort and a little more time. Massage your breast with both hands in a circular motion, moving gradually from the chest wall out toward the nipple. Place your thumb and index finger on the areola about one to one and a half inches back from the nipple and press gently inward toward the chest wall while you roll the thumb and finger forward, almost in a wide pinching motion. Keep repeating at different angles around the areola until all of the ducts have been emptied. This same massage may help with letdown shortly before pumping.[5]

Your milk may be frozen up to three months in your refrigerator's freezer compartment, but once the milk is thawed, it should not be refrozen. To thaw it, run the container under warm water, but never use a microwave or stove to heat breast milk. If the milk is to be used in the next three days, it can be kept in the refrigerator.

998

Q *I've chosen not to breast-feed. What can I do to keep my milk from coming in?*

A Simply avoiding stimulation to the breast, wearing a good support bra, or binding your breasts with an elastic bandage may keep your milk from coming in. Then again, it may not. When your milk comes in after five days or so and your breasts blow up like balloons but feel like rocks, resist the temptation to empty them with manual massage if you want to suppress lactation. The same applies while weaning. Use crushed ice in plastic bags and narcotic pain relievers if you must. Remember that your temperature may go up to well over 100 degrees Fahrenheit when your milk is coming in. This does not imply infection. The discomfort will usually last only twenty-four to seventy-two hours.

Lactation suppression was pharmacologically done years ago with injection of estrogens, but this lead to an increased risk of thromboembolism. For about fifteen years, bromocryptine (Parlodel) was used routinely, but recent evidence suggesting an increased risk of problems with blood pressure and stroke led to its withdrawal by the FDA for this indication. Milk also came in after the two weeks on Parlodel about 60 to 70 percent of the time anyway.

Carbegoline (Dostinex) was released in 1997, and while it also has no FDA indication for lactation suppression, there is no reason to think that the onetime oral dose of one milligram of Dostinex is dangerous.

EMOTIONS

Baby "Blues"

999

Q *My baby's only four days old. She's perfect, my husband has been a doll, and I can't stop crying. What's wrong with me?*

A The baby "blues" are real. If your mood defies logic, you really don't have anything to be unhappy about, and your easy crying or sad episodes are fleeting, even if frequent, probably nothing is wrong. You are simply having mood swings in response to hormonal changes. When the placenta separated, your estrogen levels fell about fifteen-hundred-fold and your progesterone levels fell about four-hundred-fold over the course of a day. Shucks, we blame mood changes in menopause on estrogen drops of only one fold and that is over many months!

Many factors other than hormones come into play also. You may have a sudden realization that everything is different, and will never be the same. Your mind may be whirring with "what ifs." What if I don't ever look the same? What if my husband, who's gaga over the baby won't ever be gaga like that over me again? What if I can't do my job anymore? What if my husband and I can't do anything alone together anymore? Because the results of any change are unknown, even a change that you expect to bring you happiness can feel frightening.

You may feel as if your labor and delivery didn't live up to your expectations. In fact, you may feel like your part in the process was somehow inadequate, or even a failure.

You *will* be exhausted. Not only is labor and delivery (vaginal or cesarean) an exhausting experience, but nobody seems to want to let you sleep afterward. You have to be the hostess with the big smile and perfect makeup for your husband's college roommate's cousin's best friend who just dropped by to say congratulations at the hospital at six A.M. on his way to work. You have to feed the screaming, little, red, wrinkled (but beautiful) bundle of humanity you've created. The nurses, aides, housekeeping staff, food service personnel, and doctors drop by about twenty times in the first day.

And hey, soon you get to go home to face laundry, dishes, the pets, your other children, and all those things that dad isn't so good at! Also when you get home, you'll have nothing to wear except for baggy maternity clothes or a bathrobe. That's probably all that will fit. Given the circumstances, baby "blues" are an entirely appropriate reaction.

1000

Q *How long do the "blues" usually last?*

A Luckily, the answer to that one is only about two to three days, although emotional swings that include easy crying can certainly go on for several weeks postpartum.

1001

Q *Is there anything I can do to help with the baby "blues"?*

A The most important thing is to tell your husband, closest friends, and parents about the "blues" ahead of time. Everyone's first reaction is likely to be to try cheering you up. They want to be around you and assure you that you're fine.

Let people cheer you up by doing rather than counseling. Ask someone to bring you casseroles. Let them take your other children, clean your house, write thank-you notes and announcements, do the dishes, and so on.

Don't be afraid to say, "I really love you. Now leave me alone for an hour, please." All the furor and excitement around delivery can leave you with a deep yearning to be alone. Your husband needs to understand that this time alone may even mean without him present, or if present, just quietly reading and being available should you need something.

After a few days at home, try and get some time alone with your husband to have a romantic dinner either out or at home. Have it sent in if you choose to be at home. Let your husband know that he's still your guy, even though there's a little one around now.

Go and hide when you need to breast-feed. If people think it's modesty, great! Only you need to know that it's really a chance to put your feet up, close your eyes, and float for a while.

Postpartum Depression

1002

Q *How do I tell if the "blues" is really postpartum depression?*

Postpartum depression is a completely separate entity from the baby "blues." Although it is thought to occur with less than 0.5 percent of births, some doctors feel that it may be overlooked too often. Contrary to the transient nature of the "blues," postpartum depression may have begun as early as a few days after delivery, and it never seems to lift. If you still feel sad, but also have feelings of worthlessness, hopelessness, and frustration at more than a month postpartum, you need to call your doctor and ask his or her advice. Contemplation of suicide, sleeplessness unrelated to the baby's needs, and even feelings of a violent nature toward your newborn are all serious warning signs.

1003

Q *I had postpartum depression so severely last time that I was almost hospitalized. Now I'm thirty-four weeks pregnant and terrified that it might happen again. What can I do?*

A While postpartum depression does have a recurrence rate, it is more likely that it won't occur than that it will. Nevertheless, the fear of the loss of control that accompanies true postpartum depression may be significant enough that it alters your abilities as a parent, wife, and homemaker during the rest of this pregnancy. Certainly where your doctor and possibly a therapist agree that your risk is significant and already affecting you in this pregnancy, you may be safely started on the serotonin reuptake inhibitors, such as Prozac, Zoloft, and Paxil (See Section 5: Antidepressants) in the second and third trimesters of pregnancy.

Your Husband

1004

Q *Can my husband get the baby "blues" too?*

A Although your husband won't have the same hormonal drop that you can have, he certainly is subject to feelings resulting from the tremendous change he has just experienced.

Just like you, he'll be excited and a little scared about a new baby. Just like you, he may have feelings of inadequacy about supporting you during the pregnancy, labor, delivery, or immediate postpartum period. He wants to help, but doesn't want to get in the way either.

He can feel like a fifth wheel, especially if your mother and his have decided to pay extended visits and relive their own memories through their grandchild's birth. He can also feel left out when it comes to breast-feeding, bathing, and clothing the baby.

1005

Q *What can I do to keep my husband from feeling left out?*

A Although your husband can't breast-feed, he certainly can help with any supplementary feeding. Bottle-feeding breast milk in the middle of the night can give him some time alone with the baby as well as giving you a little of the sleep you so desperately need. You have many opportunities to be alone with your new little one and he may have very few. Time alone with the baby will reinforce the fact that the baby is his to, and allow him the time he needs to "bond" separately from you.

Don't let your husband sleep through the night if you're not. You may think you're being sweet by not waking him, since he's got to go to work in the morning, but remember, so do you. Fathers like to be up in the middle of the night with you as you learn about the new baby. Wake your husband and ask him to help with whatever needs doing. (We dads actually cannot hear the baby crying at night—honest!)

Finally, keep reassuring him that you love him. Reassure him that despite never seeming to have a moment alone together, you want that as much as he does. Contrary to public perception, we guys can benefit from snuggling without sex. Sure, some spontaneity in your lives is gone, from movies to making love. When you were dating, there was no spontaneity either. You had to arrange a time to be together, and those times weren't so bad, were they? So, arrange time together again. It takes a little effort, but it brings back some of that excitement that went along with dating.

Raising your child together as your capacity for love and understanding broadens and deepens can be the most satisfying date you'll ever have.

SUGGESTED RESOURCES AND READING

American College of Obstetricians and Gynecologists. *Breast Feeding Your Baby; You and Your Baby; Prenatal Care, Labor and Delivery; Postpartum Care.* ACOG Website: http://www.acog.com
Main Switchboard: 800-673-8444, (206) 638-5577
Order Desk: 800-762-2264

Amis, Debby, and Jeanne Green. *Prepared Childbirth the Family Way.* The Family Way Publications: Plano, TX 75093.
To Order: (972) 403-0297

Brott, Armin. 1995. *The Expectant Father, Facts, Tips and Advice for Dads to Be.* Abbeville Press.

Caplan, Frank. 1993. *The First Twelve Months of Life.*

Misri, Shaila. 1995. *Shouldn't I Be Happy?*

WEBSITES

Post Partum Depression

http://www.nlm.nih.gov/medlineplus/postpartumdepression.html

Breast Feeding

http://www.breastfeeding.com/

http://www.nlm.nih.gov/medlineplus/breastfeeding.html

APPENDIX A

*Recommended Daily Dietary Allowances for Women
Before and During Pregnancy, and Lactation*

NUTRIENT	NON-PREGNANT	PREGNANT	LACTATING
Kilocalories	2200	2500	2600
Protein (g)	55	60	65
Fat-soluble vitamins			
A (mg)	800	800	1300
D (mg)	10	10	12
E (mg)	8	10	12
K (mg)	55	65	65
Water-soluble vitamins			
C (mg)	60	70	95
Folate (mg)	180	400	280
Niacin (mg)	15	17	20
Riboflavin (mg)	1.3	1.6	1.8
Thiamin (mg)	1.1	1.5	1.6
B6 (mg)	1.6	2.2	2.6
B12 (mg)	2.0	2.2	2.6
Minerals			
Calcium (mg)	1200	1200	1200
Phosphorus (mg)	1200	1200	1200
Iodine (mg)	150	175	200
Iron (mg)	15	30	15
Magnesium (mg)	280	320	355
Zinc (mg)	12	15	19

From the Food and Nutrition Board of the National Academy of Sciences/National Research Council.

APPENDIX B

Optimum Body Weight = BMI 21-22

WEIGHT (LB.)	HEIGHT (FT. IN.)								
	4'10"	5'0"	5'2"	5'4"	5'6"	5'8"	5'10"	6'0"	6'2"
125	26	24	23	22	20	19	18	17	16
130	27	25	24	22	21	20	19	18	17
135	28	26	25	23	22	21	19	18	17
140	29	27	26	24	23	21	20	18	18
145	30	28	27	25	23	22	21	19	19
150	31	29	27	26	24	23	22	20	19
155	32	30	28	27	25	24	22	20	20
160	34	31	29	28	26	24	23	21	21
165	35	32	30	28	27	25	24	22	21
170	36	33	31	29	28	26	24	22	22
175	37	34	32	30	28	27	25	23	23
180	38	35	33	31	29	27	26	24	23
185	39	36	34	32	30	28	27	25	24
190	40	37	35	33	31	29	27	25	24
195	41	38	36	34	32	30	28	26	25
200	42	39	37	34	32	30	29	27	26
205	43	40	38	35	33	31	29	27	26
210	44	41	38	36	34	32	30	28	27
215	45	42	39	37	35	33	31	29	28
220	46	43	40	38	36	34	32	29	28
225	47	44	41	39	36	34	32	30	29
230	48	45	42	40	37	35	33	31	30

©1996 Wyeth-Ayerst Laboratories 604 86–00. Printed in USA May, 1995

APPENDIX C

American College of Obstetricians and Gynecologists
INDICATIONS FOR ULTRASOUND IN PREGNANCY★

1. Estimation of gestational age
   For patients with uncertain clinical dates
   For verification of dates in those patients about to undergo scheduled cesarean
   For scheduled induction
   For elective termination of pregnancy
2. Evaluation of fetal growth
3. Vaginal bleeding of undetermined etiology
4. Determination of fetal presentation
5. Suspected multiple gestation
6. Adjunct to performance of amniocentesis
7. Uterine size dates/discrepancy
8. Pelvic mass
9. Suspicion of molar pregnancy
10. Adjunct to cerclage placcmcnt
11. Suspected ectopic pregnancy
12. Adjunct to special procedures (such as Dilatation and Evacuation—D&E; cordocentesis)★★
13. Suspected fetal death
14. Suspected uterine anomaly
15. IUD localization
16. Biophysical Profile for evaluation of fetal well-being
17. Observation of intrapartum events
18. Suspected polyhydramnios or oligohydramnios
19. Suspected abruption placenta
20. Adjunct to external version for breech
21. Estimation of fetal weight and/or presentation in PROM and/or preterm labor
22. Abnormal alpha fetoprotein value
23. Follow-up observation of fetal anomaly (such as choroid plexus cyst)★★
24. Follow-up evaluation of placental localization for identified placenta previa
25. History of previous congenital anomaly
26. Serial evaluation of fetal growth in multiple gestation
27. Evaluation of fetal condition in late registrants for prenatal care

★ *From ACOG. Ultrasonography in Pregnancy, ACOG Technical Bulletin, Number 187, Dec. 1993*
★★ *Author's comments in parenthesis*

ABOUT THE AUTHOR

Doctor Thurston is a Board Certified obstetrician and gynecologist in the private practice of medicine at Presbyterian Hospital in Dallas, Texas, with Walnut Hill Ob/Gyn Associates. He currently serves as an Associate Clinical Professor of Ob/Gyn at University of Texas Southwestern Medical School and is actively involved in teaching medical students and residents.

Doctor Thurston is a cum laude graduate of Rice University and a magna cum laude graduate of Baylor College of Medicine in Houston. He is past President of the Beta Texas Chapter of the Alpha Omega Alpha Honor Medical Society (AOA). His postgraduate training was at the University of California, San Francisco, where he served his internship and residency, and then served as the Administrative Chief Resident in 1985. Thus far, he has attended the delivery of more than 7,000 babies.

Doctor Thurston lives in Dallas with his wife Pat and their four children. He is also the author of *Death of Compassion* (WRS Publ., Waco, TX, 1996) and *Disrobe Completely* (Brown Books, Plano, TX 2006), in which he discusses the detrimental effects of managed care on the doctor-patient relationship.

Doctor Thurston is currently pursuing his Master of Biblical Studies at Dallas Theological Seminary and worships at Bent Tree Bible Fellowship in Carrollton. His hobbies include reading, shooting, hunting, and he is an avid sailor having recently earned his Merchant Marine Captain's License from the U.S. Coast Guard rated at 100 Ton Master. Doctor Thurston sails a Catalina 350 on Lake Texoma.

Find more about his practice at http://www.walnuthillobgyn.com/home

REFERENCES

SECTION TWO.

1   Erick, M. *Nausea & Vomiting in Pregnancy.* ACOG Clinical Review. Vol. 2. Issue 3. May/June 1997.
2   Eric, M. et al. IBID.
3   Depue, RH et al. AmericanJ Obstetric Gynecology 156:1137 1987.
4   Stein, Z. et al. *Nutrition and Mental Performance.* Science 178:708.1972 and Smith, CA. *Effects of Maternal Undernutrition in Holland.* AJOG 30:229. 1947.
5   *Nutrition During Pregnancy.* ACOG Technical Bulletin #179 April 1993. 4.
6   Teratogens. ACOG Educational Bulletin. No.236. April, 1997.
7   Cunningham et al., Williams Obstetrics 19th Ed. Appleton & Lange. 1993 257-259.
8   Cunningham, G. et al. Williams Obstetrics. 19th Ed. Appleton & Lange. 1993 258.
9   Committee on Maternal Nutrition of the National Research Council. 1989.
10 Sorensen, et al. *Fetal heart function in response to short term maternal exercise.* British Journal of Obstetric Gynecology. 93:310. 1986.
11 Clapp, et al. *Fetal heart rate response to running in mid and late pregnancy.* American Journal of Obstetric Gynecology 153:251. 1985. Lotgering et al. The *Interactions of Exercise and Pregnancy: A Review.* American Journal of Obstetric Gynecology 149:560. 1984 Huch. et al. *Pregnancy and Exercise—Exercise and Pregnancy: A short Review.* British Journal Obstetric Gynecology. 97:208. 1990.
12 Adapted with additions from: *ACOG Guide to Planning for Pregnancy. Birth and Beyond.* ACOG. Washington, DC 1990.
13 *Air Travel During Pregnancy.* ACOG Committee Opinion Num 443 Oct 2009.
14 Voitk et al. *Carpal Tunnel Syndrome in Pregnancy.* Can Med Assoc Jrnl: 129:277 1983.
15 Ekman-Oredeberg. et al. *Carpal tunnel syndrome in pregnancy: a prospective study.* Acta Obstetric Gynecology Scand. 66:233. 1987
16 McGregor et al. Bell's *Palsy in Late Pregnancy etc.* Obstetric Gynecology: 69:435. 1987
17 Ueland & Metcalf. *Circulatory Changes in Pregnancy.* Clinical Obstetric Gynecology. 18:41. 1975.
18 Diczfalusy et al. *Influence of Oophorectomy on steroid excretion in early pregnancy.* Journal Clinical Endocrinol. 21:1119. 1961.

SECTION THREE.

1   ACOG Opinion #241, Sept 2000.
2   Briggs et al. Drugs in *Pregnancy and Lactation.* Fourth Ed. 1994. 864.
3   ACR Practice Guidelines, ACR, 2007, pg.1025-1033.
4   ACOG Opinion #223, Oct. 1999.
5   Philip, J et al., Obstetrics and Gynecology, 103, No. 6, June 2004, p. 1164.
6   Report of the Third International Workshop-Conference on Gestational Diabetes. Held in Chicago. 1990.

SECTION FOUR.

1   Bromley,B. et al. *Choroid Plexus Cysts and risk of Chromosomal Abnormality. Ultrasound* Obstetric Gynecology October 8, 1996. (4) :232.
2   Dagan, R. et al. *Relationship of breast feeding vs. bottle feeding with ER visits and hospitalizations for infectious disease.* European Journal of Pediatricians. November, 1982. 139(3): 192-4.
3   Fallot, ME., et al. *Breast feeding: Reduction in incidence of hospital admissions for infection in infants.* Pediatricians. January, 1980. 65(6): 1121-4.

SECTION FIVE.

1   Teratology. ACOG Educational Bulletin. No.236. April, 1997.
2   Teratology. ACOG Educational Bulletin. No.236. April, 1997.
3   Briggs, GG. et al. Drugs in Pregnancy and Lactation. 4th Ed. 1994 . 308/d.
4   Erick, M. *Nausea & Vomiting in Pregnancy.* 3. May/June 1997.
5   Briggs, et al. *Drugs in Pregnancy and Lactation.* 4th Ed. 1994. 64/a.
6   Stone, D. et al. *Aspirin and Congenital Malformations. Lancet* 1976. 1:1373-5.
7   Committee on Drugs. APA. *The transfer of drugs and other chemicals into human milk.* Pediatrics. 1994.93:137.
8   Briggs, et al. *Drugs in Pregnancy and Lactation.* 4th Ed. 1994. 2/a-6/a.
9   Ibid. Briggs.
10 Heinonen, OP, et al. Birth *Defects and Drugs in Pregnancy.* Littleton, MA:Publishing Sciences Group. 1977.
11 Cordero, JF. Is *Bendectin a teratogen?* JAMA. 1981:245:2307.
12 Rayburn, WE et al. *Uterine and fetal doppler flow changes from a single dose of long acting nasal decongestant.* Obstetric Gynecology 1990. 76: 180-2.
13 Rosenberg L. et al. *Selected birth defects in relation to caffeine containing beverages.* JAMA 1982. 247:1429-32.
14 Narod, et al. *Coffee during pregnancy: A reproductive hazard?* American Journal Obstetric Gynecology 164:1109. 1991.
15 Committee on Drugs. APA. *The transfer of drugs and other chemicals into human milk.* Pediatrics. 1994.93:137-50.
16 Briggs, G.G., et al. Drugs in *Pregnancy and Lactation.* 4th Ed. 1994 177/c.
17 Splete, Heidi, *PPIs might raise risk of cardiac birth defects* OB.Gyn.News, Vol 45 No. 14, Dec 2010
18 Linn, S. et al. *The Association of Marijuana Use with Outcome in Pregnancy.* AmericanJ Public Health 73:1161. 1983 &' Greenland, S. et al. *The effects of marijuana use during pregnancy.* Drug Alcohol Depend 11:359. 1983.
19 Heinon, et al. Birth *Defects and Drugs in Pregnancy.* Littleton, MA Publishing Sciences Group. 1977.
20 ACOG. *Cocaine Abuse: Implications for Pregnancy.* ACOG Committee Opinion. No 81. 3/90.
21 Ostrea, EM. et al. *Perinatal problems in maternal drug addiction.* Journal Pediatr 1979.94:292-5.
22 Naeye, RL. et al. *Fetal complications of maternal heroin addiction.* Journal Pediatr 1973.83:1055-61.
23 Briggs, GG. *Drugs in Pregnancy and Lactation.* 4th Ed. Williams & Wilkins. 510/1.
24 Mattson, MP. et al. *Degenerative and axon out growth altering effects of PCP in human fetal cerebral cortical cells.* Neuropharm. 1992. 31:279-91.
25 ACOG Technical Bulletin. No 195. July, 1994.
26 Cunningham et al. Williams Obstetrics.19th Ed. 1993. 264.
27 *Teratogens.* ACOG Educational Bulletin. No.236. April, 1997.
28 Barlow, S. et al. *Reproductive Hazards of Industrial Chemicals.* New York. Academic Press. 1982.
29 Taskinen, et al. *Effects of Ultrasound. Shortwaves, and physical exertion on pregnancy outcome.* Journal Epedimiol Community Health 44:196. 1990.
30 Brent R.L. The *effect of embryonic and fetal exposure to X-ray, microwaves and ultra-sound.* Semin Oncol 1989. 16:347-368.
31 Miller, RW. *Epidemiologic conclusions from radiation toxicity studies.* Fry RJM, et al. *Late Effects of Radiation.* London. Taylor & Francis. 1970.

32 July, 1997 NEJM.

33 Tynes, T. et al. *Electromagnetic fields and cancer in children residing near Norwegian high voltage power lines.* AmericanJ Epidemiology February 1997. 145(3): 219-26. Robert, E. Teratology Update: EM fields. Teratology December 1996. 54(6):305-13.

34 Rosermass, E. et al. *Protection against UV-B by UV-A induced tan.* Arch Dermatol 1982. Jul:118(7): 483. Dergren, M.S., et al. *Tanning, protection against sunburn and Vii D formation with UV-A "sun-bee* Br Journal Dermatol 1982 Sep 107(3): 275. Fairchild, et al. *Safety information provided to customers of NYC suntan salons.* AmericanJ Prey Med 1992 Nov-Dec. 8(6) : 381.

35 ACOG Committee Opinion No 438, August 2009.

36 Snider, DE. et al. *Treatment of Tuberculosis During Pregnancy.* Amer Rev Respir Dis. 1980. 122:65.

37 Briggs, GG. et al. *Drugs in Pregnancy and Lactation.* 4th Ed. Williams & Wilkins. 1994. 13a.

38 Scott, LL. et al. *Acyclovir suppression to prevent Cesarean Section delivery after 1st episode genital herpes.(HSV).*

39 Cunningham, G. et al. Williams *Obstetrics.* 19th Ed. Appleton & Lange 1993. 964.

40 Rosa, FW et al. *Pregnancy outcomes after 1st trimester vaginitis drug therapy.* Obstetric Gynecology. 69:751. 1987a.

41 Briggs, GG. et al. *Drugs in Pregnancy and Lactation.* 4th Ed. W&W. 1994.18a.

42 NIH. Executive Summary: *Management of Asthma During Pregnancy.* Publication 93-3279A March, 1993. 5.

43 Briggs, GG. et al. *Drugs in Pregnancy and Lactation.* 4th Ed. W&W. 1994. 714/p.

44 Collaborative Group on Antenatal Steroid Therapy. J. Pediatric 1984. 104:259-267.

45 Briggs, Ob.Gyn. News, April 15, 2005, pg. 17.

46 Briggs, ObGyn News, April 15, 2005, pg. 71.

47 Briggs, GG. et al. *Drugs in Pregnancy and Lactation.* 4th Ed. 1994. 80/a.

48 Briggs. Ibid. 242c.

49 Heinonen, OP. et al. Birth *Defects and Drugs in Pregnancy.* Littleton, MA Publishing Science Group. 1977:336.

50 Rubin, PC., et al. *Atenelol in the treatment of chronic hypertension in pregnancy.* Br Journal Clinical Pharmacy. 1982. 14:279. Butters, L et al. *Atenelol in essential hypertension in pregnancy.* Br. Med. Journal. 1990. 301:587.

51 ACOG Opinion #211, Nov. 1998.

52 Hall, JG. et al. *Maternal and Fetal Sequelae of anticoagulation in pregnancy*, American Journal of Medicine 1980.68:122-40.

53 ACOG Technical Bulletin #219, Jan. 1996

54 Safra, MJ. et al. *Valium: An Oral cleft teratogen?* Cleft Palate Journal 1976: 13:198-200.

55 *Use of psychiatric medicines during pregnancy and lactation.* ACOG Practice Bulletin Number 92 April 2008.

56 Milkovich, L et al. *Effects of prenatal meprobamate and chlordiazepoxide on human embryonic and fetal development.* NEJM.1974:291:1268-71.

57 Kohen at al., Ob/Gyn News, 9/15/04

58 Hallberg et al. 2005

59 Ibid, Briggs. 39/1. 259/d. 636/n

60 Weinstein, MR. et al. Recent Advances in Current Clinical Psychopharmacology. Lithium Carbonate. Hosp Form. 1977.12:759.

61 Ibid. Briggs. 723/p.

62 Briggs, GG. et al. *Drugs in Pregnancy and Lactation.* 4th Ed. Littleton. 1994. 166/c.

63   Briggs, GG. et al. *Drugs in Pregnancy and Lactation.* 4th Ed. Littleton. 1994. 777/s.
64   Friedman, W. et al. *Potential human teratogenicity of commonly prescribed drugs.* Obstetric Gynecology 1990.75594-9.
65   Wilson, JG. et al. *Are female sex hormones teratogenic?* American Journal of Obstetric Gynecology 1981. 141: 567-80.
66   Cunningham, et al. Williams Obstetric. 19th Ed. Appleton 1993. 970.
67   Van Waes, A et al *Safety evaluation of haloperidol in the treatment of hyperemesis.* Journal Clinical Pharmacy 1969. 9:224-7.
68   Slone, D. et al. *Antenatal exposure to the Phenothiazines.* American Journal of Obstetric Gynecology 1977.128:486-8.

SECTION SIX.

1   Caldwell, WE., Moloy, HC. *Anatomical variations in the female pelvis.* American Journal of Obstetric Gynecology 28:482. 1934.
2   Amis, D. *Prepared Childbirth.* The Family Way. 5th Ed. Family Way Publications. 1996. 24.
3   IBID.
4   IBID.
5   IBID.
6   IBID.
7   ACOG Committee Opinion No. 441 September, 2009.
8   Leveno, K. *Prospective comparison of selective and universal electronic fetal monitoring in 34,995 pregnancies.* NEJM 315:615. 1986.
9   *Intrapartum Fetal Heart Rate Monitoring.* ACOG Practice Bulletin Num 106 July 2009.
10   Taddio, et al. *Efficacy and Safety of Lidocaine-Prilocaine Cream for circumcision. N.* England Journal of Medicine 1997 . 24. 336 (17): 1197-201.

SECTION SEVEN.

1   Crane, J. et al. *The effectiveness of sweeping membranes at term: a prospective trial.* Obstetric Gynecology 1997. April, 1989. (4): 586-90.
2   Thorp, JA et al. *The effect of intrapartum epidural analgesia on nulliparous labor.* American Journal of Obstetric Gynecology. 169:851. 1993. Chestnut DH et al. *Does early administration of epidural analgesia affect Obstetric outcome in nullips receiving intravenous oxytocin?* Anesthesiology. 80:11931200. 1994. Chestnut et al. *Does early administration of epidural analgesia affect Obstetric outcome of nullips in spontaneous labor?* Anesthesiology 80:1201-1208 Morton, SC, et al. *Effect of epidural analgesia for labor on Cesarean delivery rate.* Obstetric Gynecology 83:1045-1052. 1994.
3   Seidman, DS. et al. *Long term effects of vacuum and forceps.* Lancet 337:1583. 1991.

SECTION EIGHT.

1   Miller, et al. *Classification and staging of gestational trophoblastic tumors.* Obstetric Gynecology Clinical. NorthAmerican. 15:477. 1988.
2   Wexler, P. et al. *Early diagnosis of placenta previa.* Obstetric Gynecology. 54:231. 1979.
3   Cotton, et al. *The conservative aggressive management of previa.* American Journal Obstetric Gynecology. 137:687, 1980.
4   Creasey, R. et al. *Maternal Fetal Medicine.* 3rd Ed. WB Saunders. 1994. 610.
5   Cunningham, et al. *Obstetrical Hemorrhage in Willimas Obstetric.* 19th Ed. Appleton & Lange. 1993. . 829.
6   Pritchard, et al. *Genesis of severe placental abruption.* American Journal of Obstetric Gynecology 0108:22. 1970.

7   Walsh, SW. *Preeclampsia: An imbalance in placental prostacyclin and thromboxane pro-duction.* American Journal of Obstetric Gynecology. 152:335. 1985.

8   Sibai et al. *Reassessment of IV MgSO₄ therapy in preeclampsia.* Obstetric Gynecology. 57:199. 1981.

9   Spitz, et al. *Low dose aspirin.* American Journal of Obstetric Gynecology. 159: 1035. 1988.

10   Imperiale, et al. *A meta-analysis of low dose aspirin for the prevention of PIH.* JAMA 266:260. 1991.

11   CLASP *Collaborative Group: A randomized trial of low dose aspirin in 9364 women.* Lancet 343:619-29. 1994. Sibai, BM. et al. Prevention *of preeclampsia with low dose AM in healthy nulliparous pregnant women.* N Engl Journal Medicine 329:1213-8. 1993.

12   Cunningham, et al. Williams Obstetrics. 19th Ed. Norwalk. CT. Appleton & Lange. 1993. 878.

13   *Fetal Lung Maturity.* ACOG Practice Bulletin Num 97 Sept 2008.

14   ACOG Committee Opinion No. 404, April, 2008.

15   Kochanek. et al. *Advance report of final mortality statistics.* 1992. Monthly Vital Stats Report. Vol. 43. No.6. suppl. Hyattsville. Maryland: National Ctr for Health Statistics. 1995.

16   Ventura. et al. *Advance report of final natality statistics.* 1993. Monthly Vital Stats Report. Vol.44. No.3. suppl. Hyattsville. Maryland: National Ctr for Health Statistics. 1995.March of Dimes Birth Defects Foundation. *March of Dimes Statbook: statistics for healthier mothers and babies.* White Plains. New York: MODBDF. 1993.

17   Colton. T. et al. *A metaanalysis of home uterine activity monitoring.* American Journal of Obstetric Gynecology 1995.173: 1499-1505.

18   Home Uterine Activity Monitoring. ACOG Committee Opinion. Number 172. May 1996.

19   Cox. et al. *Randomized investigation of MgSO₄ for prevention of preterm birth.* American Journal Obstetric Gynecology 163:767. 1990.

20   Besinger. RE. Niebyl. J. et al. *Randomized comparative trial of indomethacin and rito-drine.* American Journal Obstetric Gynecology 164:981. 1991.

21   Murray. C. et al. *Nifedipine for treatment of preterm labor: a historic prospective study.* American Journal Obstetric Gynecology 167:52. 1992.

22   Duscay et al. *Effects of calcium entry blockers.* American Journal Obstetric Gynecology 157:1482. 1987.

23   ACOG Committee Opinion, No. 419, October, 2008.

24   Macones. GA et al. *Efficacy of oral beta agonist maintenance therapy in preterm labor: a meta-analysis.* Obstetric Gynecology 1995.85:313-17.

25   Effect of *corticosteroids for fetal maturation on perinatal outcomes.* NIH Consensus Development Panel. JAMA 1995.273:413-418.

26   ACOG Committee Opinion No. 402, March 2008

27   Cox. S. et al. *The Natural history of preterm rupture of membranes.* Obstetric Gyne-cology 71:558. 1988.

28   Lonky. et al. *A Proposed mechanism for premature rupture.* Obstetric Gynecology Sury 43(0:22. 1988.

29   Minkoff et al. *Risk factors for prematurity and PROM.* American Journal Obstetric Gynecology 150:965. 1984.

30   ACOG Committee Opinion No. 402, March, 2008

31   Garite. et al. *A Randomized trial of ritodrine vs expectant mgt in pts with pre-term PROM.* American Journal Obstetric Gynecology 157:388. 1987.

32   Duff. et al. *Mgt of PROM and unfavorable cervix in term pregnancy.* Obstetric Gynecology 63:697. 1984.

33   Ray. et al. *Prostaglandin E2 for induction of labor in patients with PROM at term.* American Journal Obstetric Gynecology 166:836. 1992.

34   Leveno. et al. *Prolonged pregnancy: Observations.* American Journal Obstetric Gynecology 150:465. 1984. Phelan. J. et al. *The role of ultrasound assessment of amniotic fluid volume in the mgt of postdates pregnancy.* American Journal Obstetric Gynecology 151:304. 1985.

35   Barss. et al. *Stillbirth after nonstress testing.* Obstetric Gynecology 65:541.1985. Devoe. JD et al. Post dates pregnancy: Assessment of fetal risk. Journal Reprod Med 28:576. 1983.

36   *Management of Stillbirth.* ACOG Practice Bulletin Num 102 March 2009.

37   Goldberg, et al., The Infectious Origins of Stillbirth. AJOG 189(3):861-73.

38   ACOG Technical Bulletin. Induction of Labor. #217

39   *Fetal Lung Maturity.* ACOG Practice Bulletin Num 97 Sept 2008.

40   McColgin. et al. *Stripping membranes at term.* Obstetric Gynecology 76:678.1990 El-Torkey. et al *Sweeping of the membranes is an effective method of induction.* Br Journal Obstetric Gynecology 1992:99:455-458.

41   Crane. J. et al. *The effectiveness of sweeping membranes at term: a prospective trial.* Obstetric Gynecology 1997. Apr 89 (4): 586-90.

42   Rayburn. et al. *Prostaglandin E2 gel for cervical ripening.* American Journal Obstetric Gynecology 1989. 160:529-534.

43   *Induction of Labor.* ACOG Practice Bulletin Num 107 August 2009.

44   Bakos. et al. *Induction of labor. a prospective randomized study into amniotomy.* Ada Obstetric Gynecology Scand 1987.66:537-541.

45   Eastman. NJ. *The role of Frontier America in the development of cesarean section.* American Journal Obstetric Gynecology 24:919. 1932.

46   Frigoletto. et al. *Maternal Mortality Rate associated with cesarean section.* American Journal

47   Katz, Vern L., *Maternal Mortality, the Correct Assessment is Everything.* Obstetrics and Gynecology, Vol. 106, No. 4, October 2005.

48   Rosen. et al. *Consensus Task Force on Cesarean Childbirth.* NIH Publication No. 82-2067. 1981.

49   Stafford. et al. *Alternative strategies for wrangling rising C-section rates.* JAMA 263:683. 1990.

50   Silbar et al. *Factors relating to the increasing cesarean section rate.* American Journal Obstetric Gynecology 154:1095. 1986.

51   Clarke. et al. *State Variations in Rates of Cesarean and VBAC.* Statistical Bulletin Metropol Ins. Co. 1996 Jan-Mar 77(1):28-36.

52   Thorp. JA. et al *The effect of intrapartum epidural analgesia on nulliparous labor.* American Journal Obstetric Gynecology 169:851. 1993. Chestnut. DH et al. *Does early administration of epidural analgesia affect Obstetric outcome in nullips receiving intravenous oxytocin.* Anesthesiology 80:11931200. 1994 Chestnut et al. *Does early administration of epidural analgesia affect Obstetric outcome of nullips in spontaneous labor?* Anesthesiology 80:1201-1208 Morton, SC. et al. *Effect of epidural analgesia for labor on Cesarean delivery rate.* Obstetric Gynecology 83:1045-1052. 1994. See also Hoult et al. *Lumbar epidural analgesia in labour* Br Med Jrnl 1:14. 1977 Cox et al. Epidural anesthesia during labor. Tex Med 83:45. 1987.

53   Wong, Cynthia, et al., *The Risk of Cesarean Delivery with Neuraxial Analgesia Given Early versus Late in Labor,* NEJM, February 17, 2005, 352:655-665.

54   Leveno. K. *Prospective comparison of selective and universal electronic fetal monitoring in 34,995 pregnancies.* NEJM 315:615. 1986.

55   Haverkamp et al. *A controlled trial of the differential effects of intrapartum fetal monitoring.* American Journal Obstetric Gynecology 134:399. 1979.

56   *Fetal Lung Maturity.* ACOG Practice Bulletin Num 97 Sept 2008.

57   Nelson,K.B.,et al., *Can We Prevent CP?* NEJM, Oct 2003, 349(18):1765-9.

58 Clarke. et al. *State Variations in Rates of Cesarean and VBAC.* Statistical Bulletin Metropol Ins. Co. 1996 Jan-Mar 77(0:28-36.

59 Flamm. BL. et al. *Elective repeat cesarean vs trial of labor: a prospective multicenter study* Obstetric Gynecology 1994. 83:927-932.

60 Flamm. BL et al. *Elective repeat Cesarean vs trial of labor: a prospective multicenter study.* Obstetric Gynecology 1994. 83:927-932. Cowan. RK. et al. *Trial of labor following cesarean delivery.* Obstetric Gynecology 1994.83:933-936.

61 Hoskins. et al. *Correlation between maximum cervical dilation at Cesarean and subsequent VBAC.* Obstetric Gynecology 89(4):591-3. 1997.

62 Rosen. MG. et al. Vaginal birth after Cesarean: a meta analysis of morbidity and mortality. Obstetric Gynecology. 1991. 77: 465-70. Leung. AS. et al. *Risk factors associated with uterine rupture during trial of labor after Cesarean delivery: a case control study.* American Journal Obstetric Gynecology 1993.168:1358-1363.

63 Blanco. JD. et al. *Prostaglandin E2 gel induction of patients with a prior low transverse cesarean section.* American Journal Perinatol 1992.9:80.

64 O'Sullivan et al. *Vaginal Delivery after Cesarean.* Clin Perinat 8:31. 1981.

65 Rosen. MG. et al. *Vaginal Birth after Cesarean: A meta-analysis of morbidity and mortality.* Obstetric Gynecology 77:475. 1991.

66 McMahon. M.J. et al. *Comparison of a trial of labor with an elective second Cesarean section.* NEJM 1996. Sep. 5. 335(10): 689-98.

67 Gardeil. F et al. *Uterine Rupture in Pregnancy Reviewed.* European Journal Obstetric Gynecology Reprod Biol 1994. Aug. 56 (2):107.

68 Pitkin. R. *Once a Cesarean?* Obstetric Gynecology 77:939. 1991 Scott JR. et al. *Mandatory trial of labor after Cesarean? An alternate viewpoint.* Obstetric Gynecology 77:811. 1991 Jones. R.O. et al. *Rupture of low transvers Cesarean scars during trial of labor.* Obstetric Gynecology 77: 815. 1991.

69 ACOG. *Vaginal delivery after a previous cesarean birth.* ACOG Committee Opinion No. 143. Washington. DC. ACOG 1994.

70 Sachs. BP et al. *Maternal Mortality in Mass Trends and prevention.* NEJM 316:667 1987.

71 Dickason. LA. et al. *Red blood cell transfusion and Cesarean section.* American Journal Obstetric and Gynecology 167:327. 1992.

72 Gilbert. WM. et al. *Angiographic embolization in the management of hemorrhagic complications of pregnancy.* American Journal Obstetric Gynecology 166:493. 1992.

73 Andres. et al. *A reappraisal of the need for autologous blood donation in the Obstetric patient.* American Journal Obstetric Gynecology 163:1551. 1990.

74 *Multiple Gestation Pregnancies.* Healthdyne Maternity Management Pamphlet. Marietta. Ga. 30067. No. PSO441-7/1995.

75 Derom. et al. *Increased monozygotic twinning rate after ovulation induction.* Lancet 1:1237. 1987.

76 MacLennan et al. *Routine hospitalization in twin pregnancies between 26 and 30 weeks.* Lancet 335:267. 1990. Andrews. et al. *Elective hospitalization in the management of twin pregnancies.* Obstetric Gynecology 77:826. 1991.

77 Ashworth. et al. *Failure to prevent preterm labour and delivery in twin pregnancy using prophylactic oral salbutamol.* Br Journal Obstetric Gynaecol 97:878. 1990.

78 *Home Uterine Activity Monitoring.* ACOG Committee Opinion Number 172. May. 1996.

79 Laros. RK. Dattel. BJ. *Management of Twin Pregnancy: The vaginal route is still safe.* American Journal Obstetric Gynecology 158:1330. 1988. Blickstein. et al. *Vaginal Delivery of the second twin in breech presentation.* Obstetric Gynecology 68:774. 1987.

80 *Later Childbearing.* ACOG Patient Education Pamphlet. NoAP060. ACOG. Sept 1992

SECTION NINE.

1   Balducci. J. et al. *Pregnancy outcome following 1st trimester varicella.* Obstetric Gynecology. 79:5. 1992.
2   DeNicola. et al. *Congenital and Neonatal Varicella.* Editorial. Journal Pediatr 94:175. 1979.
3   Briggs. et al. *Drugs in Pregnancy and Lactation.* 4th Ed. Williams & Wilkins. 12/a. 1994.
4   Weller. T.H. et al. *The cytomegaloviruses.* N Eng Jrnl Med 285:203.267. 1971.
5   Demmler. et al. *Summary of a workshop on surveillance for CMV disease.* Rev Infect Dis. 13:315. 1991.
6   Balfour. CL et al. *CMV is not an Occupational risk for Nurses.* JAMA 256:1909. 1986.
7   Humphrey et al. *Severe nonimmune hydrops secondary to parvovirus B19 infection.* Obstetric Gynecology. 78:900.1991.
8   CDC: *Risks associated with human parvoB19.* MMWR 38:81. 1989.
9   Creasey. B. et al. *Maternal Fetal Medicine.* 3rd Ed. W.B. Saunders. 1994. 691.
10 Kulhanjian. et al. Identification of women at unsuspected risk. NEJM:326:916. 1992
11 Scott. LL et al. *Acyclovir suppression to prevent Cesarean Section delivery after 1st episode genital herpes. (HSV).*
12 *Management of Herpes in Pregnancy.* ACOG Practice Bulletin Num 82 June 2007.
13 Creasey. R. et al. *Maternal Fetal Medicine.* 3rd Ed. WB Saunders. 1994. 673.
14 Ricci. et al. *Congenital Syphilis.* Obstetric Gynecology. 74:687. 1989.
15 Creasey. R. et al. Maternal Fetal Medicine. 3rd Ed. WB Saunders. 1994. 683.
16 Creasey Ibid. 684.
17 Crombleholme. W et al *Amoxicillin therapy for C trachomatis.* Obstetric Gynecology. 75:72. 1990.
18 Creasey Ibid. 681.
19 Sempirini. et al. *HIV infection mid AIDS in newborn babies of mothers positive for HIV* Prey Med 294:610. 1987.
20 Minkoff et at *Pregnancy outcomes among women infected with HIV and matched controls.* American Journal Obstetric Gynecology. 153:1598. 1990.
21 Giaquinto. et al. *Natural history of pediatric HIV infection.* 4th Intl Conference on AIDS. Stockholm. 1988 Abstract 7227.
22 Gravett. MG. et al. *Preterm Labor associated with bacterial vaginosis.* Obstetric Gynecology 67:229. 1986a.
23 Carey. JC et al. *Antepartum cultures are not useful.* American Journal Obstetric Gynecology 164:728.1991.
24 Baker. CJ et al. *Infectious Diseases of the fetus and newborn infant.* 4th Ed. Philadelphia. WB Saunders. 1995:980-1054.
25 Allen, UD. et al. *Effectiveness of intrapartum penicillin prophylaxis in preventing early onset Grp B strep infections.* Can Med Assoc Jrnl 1993.149:1659.
26 ACOG Committee Opinion. No.173. June. 1996 Also ACOG Patient Education Pamphlet AP105. August. 1994. ISSN 1074-8601.
27 Sibai. et al. *A comparison of no medication vs methyldopa or labetalol in chronic hypertension during pregnancy.* American Journal Obstetric Gynecology 162:960. 1990.
28 ACOG Committee Opinion No. 421, October 2008.
29 *Anemia in Pregnancy.* ACOG Practice Bulletin, Num 95 July 2008.
30 Cunningham. et al. Williams Obstetrics. 19th Ed. Appleton & Lange. 1994. 1184.
31 Powars. et al. *Pregnancy in Sickle Cell Disease.* Obstetric Gynecology 67:217. 1986.
32 Cunningham. et al. Williams Obstetrics. 19th Ed. Appleton & Lange. 1993. 1112.
33 ACOG: *Thromboembolism in Pregnancy.* ACOG Educational Bulletin. Number 234. March. 1997.

34 Haeger. K. *Problems of acute deep venous thrombosis.* Angiology. 1969. 20:219.

35 Ginsberg. et al. *Venous thrombosis in pregnancy: Leg and trimester of presentation.* Throemb Haemost 67:519. 1992.

36 ACOG: *Thromboembolism in Pregnancy.* ACOG Educational Bulletin. Number 234. March 1997.

37 Bell. et al. *The clinical features of submassive and massive* PE. American Journal Med. 57:355. 1977.

38 Andreoli. et al. *Cecil Essentials of Medicine.* 4th Ed. WB Saunders. 1997. 147.

39 Scott et al. *Doppler Ultrasound II: Clinical applications.* Radiology. 174:310. 1990.

40 PIOPED Investigators: Value of the V/Q Scan in acute pulmonary embolism. JAMA 263:2753. 1990.

41 NIH: *Executive Summary: Management of Asthma During* Pregnancy. Publ # 93-3279A 1993.1.

42 Greenberger. PA et al. *The outcome of pregnancy complicated by severe asthma.* Alergy Proc 1988 Sep-Oct. 9 (5): 539-43Schatz. M. et al. *Intrauterine growth is related to pulmonary function in pregnant asthmatic women.* Kaiser Permanente Asthma in Preg. Study Group. Chest 1990 Aug.98 (2): 389-92.

43 NIH *Consensus Statement on Genetic Testing for CF.* May. 1997. World Wide Web at http://consensus.nih.gov.

44 Scarbeck. Kathy. NIH *Panel Pushes for CF Test for all Pregnancies.* Ob/Gyn News. June 1 1997.

45 Medchill. et al. *Diagnosis and management of tuberculosis during pregnancy.* Obstetric and Gynecology Survey. 44:81. 1989.

46 ACOG: *Diabetes and Pregnancy.* ACOG Technical Bulletin.No.200 Dec. 1994 .

47 Lucas. MJ. et al. *Early pregnancy glycosylated hemoglobin, severity of diabetes, and malformations.* American Journal Obstetric Gynecology 161:426. 1989. Kitzmiller. JL et al. *Preconception care of diabetes: Glycemic control prevents congenital anomalies.* JAMA 265:731. 1991.

48 Diamond. et al. *Reassessment of White's Classification and Pedersen's prognostic bad signs of diabetic pregnancy in IDDM pregnancies.* American Journal Obstetric Gynecology 156:599. 1987.

49 Andreoli. et al. *Cecil Essentials of Medicine.* 4th Ed. WB Saunders. 1997. 493.

50 Hayslip. et al. *The value of serum antimicrosomal antibody testing in screening for symptomatic postpartum thyroid dysfunction.* American Journal Obstetric Gynecology 159:203. 1988.

51 Moltich. et al. *Pregnancy and the hyperprolactinemic women.* N Eng Journal Med 312: 1364. 1985.

52 Cunningham. et al. Williams Obstetrics. 19th Ed. Appleton & Lange. 1993. 1148.

53 Podolsky. et al. *Inflammatory Bowel Disease* (parts I & 2) N Engl Journal Med 325:928 & 1009. 1991.

54 Miller. JP. *Inflammatory Bowel Disease in Pregnancy: A Review.* Journal Roy Soc Med 79:221. 1986.

55 Woolfson. et al. *Crohn's Disease in Pregnancy.* Dis Colon Rectum 33:869. 1990.

56 Mazze. et al. *Appendectomy during pregnancy: A Swedish Registry Study of 778 cases.* Obstetric Gynecology 77:835. 1991.

57 Greenberger. et al *Diseases of the Gallbladder and Bile Ducts.* In *Harrison's Principles of Internal Medicine.* 12th Ed. New York. McGraw Hill. 1991. p 1358.

58 Landers. et al. *Acute Cholecystitis in Pregnancy.* Obstetric Gynecology. 69:131. 1987.

59 Cunningham. et al. Williams Obstetrics. 19th Ed. Appleton & Lange. 1993. 1153.

60 Fisk. et al. *Maternal Features of Obstetric cholestasis: 20 years experience.* Aust NZ Jrnl Obstetric Gynecology 95:1137. 1988.

61 Hirvioja. et al. *The treatment of intrahepatic cholestasis of pregnancy with dexamethasone.* Br Journal Obstetric Gynaecol 99:109. 1992.

62 Snyder. RR. Hankins. G. *Etiology and treatment of acute fatty liver of pregnancy.* Clin Perinatol 13:813. 1986.

63 Cunningham. et al. Williams Obstetrics. 19th Ed. Appleton & Lange. 1993. 1130.

64 Cunningham. et al. *Pulmonary injury complicating antepartum pyelonephritis.* American Journal of Obstetric Gynecology. 156:797. 1987.

65 Cox. S. et al. *Mechanisms of hemolysis and anemia associated with acute antepartum pyelonephritis.* American Journal of Obstetric Gynecology 164:587. 1991.

66 Hendricks. S. *An algorithm for diagnosis and therapy of mgt and complications of urolithiasis during pregnancy.* Surg Gynecology Obstetric. 172:49. 1991.

67 Grunfeld. JP et al *Acute Renal Failure in Pregnancy.* American Journal Kid Dis. 9:359. 1987.

68 Shorvon. SD. *Epidemiology, classification, natural history, and genetics of epilepsy.* Lancet 363:93. 1990.

69 Hiilesmaa. VK. et al. *Obstetric outcome in women with epilepsy.* American Journal of Obstetric Gynecology. 1985. 152:499-504.

70 Nakane. Y. et al. *Multi-institutional study on the teratogenicity and fetal toxicity of antiepileptic drugs: a collaborative study group in Japan.* Epilepsia 1980. 21:663-680.

71 Hanson. JW. et al *The fetal hydantoin syndrome.* Journal Pediatr 1975. 87:285-290 DiLiberti. JH. et al. *The fetal valproate syndrome.* American Journal Med Genet 1984. 19:473-481.

72 Jones. KL et al. *Pattern of malformations seen in the children of women treated with carbamazepine during pregnancy.* N Engl Journal Med 1989. 320:1661.

73 Firma. RH. et al *Clinical and experimental studies linking oxidative metabolism to phenytoin induced teratogenesis.* Neurology 1992. 42 (Suppl 5). 25-31.

74 ACOG: *Seizure Disorders in Pregnancy.* ACOG Educational Bulletin. Number 231. December 1996.

75 Delgado-Escueta. AV. *Consensus guidelines: preconception counseling, management, and care of the pregnant woman with epilepsy.* Neurology 1992. 42 (Suppl 5):149-160.

76 ACOG: *Seizure Disorders in Pregnancy.* ACOG Educational Bulletin. Number 231. December 1996.

77 Annegers. JF. et al. *Seizure disorders in offspring of parents with a history of seizures-maternal paternal difference?* Epilepsia 1976:17:1-9.

78 Birk, K. et al. The *clinical course of multiple sclerosis during pregnancy and the puerperium.* Arch Neurol 47:738. 1990.

79 *Committee on Obstetrics: Maternal Fetal Medicine.* ACOG Committee Opinion Number 83: Mgt of labor & delivery for patients with spinal cord injury' May. 1990.

80 Rochat et al. *Maternal Mortality in the United States: Report from the Maternal Mortality Collaborative.* Obstetric Gynecology 72:91. 1988.

81 Dias. et al. *Intracranial hemorrhage from aneurysms and AVMs during pregnancy and the puerperium.* Neurosurgery 27:855. 1990.

82 Shomick JK. *Herpes Gestationis* Journal from the American Academy of Dermatology. 17:539. 1987.

83 Abrams & Laros. *Prepregnancy weight, weight gain, and birthweight.* American Journal of Obstetric Gynecology 154503. 1986.

84 Ramin. S. et al. *Obesity in Pregnancy.* Williams Obstetrics Supplement No. 13. June/July, 1995.

85   Fortunato. SJ. et al. External *Cephalic Version with tocolysis: Factors associated with success.* Obstetric Gynecology 7259. 1988.

86   Hood. DD. et al. *Anesthetic and Obstetric Outcome in Morbidly Obese parturients.* Anesthesiology 79:1210. 1993. Konje. et al. *Pregnancy in Obese women.* Journal Obstetric Gynecology 13:413. 1993.

87   Spellacy. WN. et al. *Macrosomia-Maternal characteristics and infant complications.* Obstetric Gynecology 66:158. 1985.

88   Varner. MW. *Autoimmune disorders and pregnancy.* Semin Perinatol 15:238. 1991.

89   Niddin. JL. *SLE and pregnancy at the Royal Women's Hospital.* Brisbane 1979–1989. Aust NZ Obstetric Gynecology 31:128. 1991.

90   Doll. DC. et al. *Management of Cancer during Pregnancy.* Arch Intern Med 148:2058. 1988.

91   Brent. RL. *Ionizing Radiation.* Contemp Ob/Gyn 30:20. 1987.

92   Zemlickis et al. *Maternal and Fetal Outcome after breast cancer in pregnancy.* American Journal of Obstetric Gynecology 166:781. 1992. King. RM. et al. *Carcinoma of the breast associated with pregnancy.* SurgGynecology Obstetric 160:228. 1985.

93   Hoover. HC Jr. et al. *Breast Cancer during pregnancy and lactation.* Surg Clin N Amer 70:1151 1990.

94   Sutton. R. et al. *Pregnancy and offspring after adjuvant chemotherapy in beast cancer patients* Cancer 65:847. 1990. Donegan. WL. Cancer and Pregnancy. CA 33:194. 1983.

95   Jolles. CJ. *Gynecological Cancer associated with pregnancy.* Semin Oncol 16:417. 1989.

96   Hacker. NE et al. *Carcinoma of the cervix associated with pregnancy.* Obstetric Gynecology 59:735. 1982.

97   Greer. BE. et al. *Fetal and maternal considerations in the mgt of Stage I-B cervical cancer during pregnancy.* Gynecology Oncol 34:61. 1989.

98   Jacobs, C. et al. *Management of the Pregnant patient with Hodgkin's Disease.* Ann Intern Med 95:669. 1981.

99   Daley. MD. et al. *Epidural anesthesia for Obstetrics after spinal surgery.* Reg. Anesth 15:280. 1990.

100   Williams. JK. et al *Evaluation of blunt abdominal trauma in the third trimester of pregnancy: Maternal and fetal considerations.* Obstetric Gynecology 1990.75:33-37.

101   *Automobile Passenger Restraints for Children and Pregnant Women.* ACOG Technical Bulletin. Number 151. January. 1991.

102   Crosby et al. *Safety of lap restraint for pregnant victims of automobile collisions.* N Engl Journal Med 1971.284(12):632-636.

103   Helton. et al. *Battered and Pregnant: A prevalence study.* AmericanJ Publ Health 1987. 77:13371339.

104   Goodwin. TM. et al. *Pregnancy outcome and fetomaternal hemorrhage after nomatostrophic trauma.* American Journal of Obstetric Gynecology 1990. 162:665 Pearlman. MD. et al. *A prospective controlled study of outcome after trauma during pregnancy.* American Journal of Obstetric Gynecology 1990. 162:1502.

105   Williams. JK. et al. *Evaluation of blunt abdominal trauma in the third trimester of pregnancy: Maternal and fetal considerations.* Obstetric Gynecology. 1990. 75:33-37.

SECTION TEN.

1   Dagan, R. et al. *Relationship of breast feeding vs bottle feeding with ER visits and hospitalizations for infectious disease.* European Journal Pediatricians. November, 1982. 139(3) : 192-4.

2   Fallot, ME. et al. *Breast feeding: Reduction in incidence of hospital admissions for infection in infants.* Pediatrician. January, 1980. 65(6): 1121-4.

References

3   Savilahti, E. et al. *Prolonged exclusive breast feeding and heredity as determinants in infant atopy*. Arch Dis Child. March, 19182. 62(3). 269-73.

4   Kraus, Marshall and Phyllis. *The Amazing Newborn*.

5   Amis, Debby and Jeane Green. *Prepared Childbirth the Family Way*. Family Way Publications Inc. Plano. Tx 1996. 56.

INDEX

Note: Numbers are question numbers, not page numbers